DERMATOLOGICAL FORMULATIONS

DRUGS AND THE PHARMACEUTICAL SCIENCES

A Series of Textbooks and Monographs

Edited by

James Swarbrick
School of Pharmacy
University of North Carolina
Chapel Hill, North Carolina

Other Volumes in Preparation

DERMATOLOGICAL FORMULATIONS

Percutaneous Absorption

BRIAN W. BARRY

University of Bradford,
Bradford, West Yorkshire
England

MARCEL DEKKER, INC.   New York and Basel

Library of Congress Cataloging in Publication Data

Barry, Brian W. , [date]
    Dermatological formulations.

    (Drugs and the pharmaceutical sciences ; v. 18)
    Includes bibliographical references and indexes.
    1. Dermatologic agents. 2. Skin absorption.
I. Title. II. Series [DNLM: 1. Skin absorption.
2. Dermatologic agents--Metabolism. 3. Biological
availability. W1 DR893B v. 18 / QV 60 B279d]
RM303.B37 1983   615'.778   83-5154
ISBN 0-8247-1729-5

MARCEL DEKKER, INC.
270 Madison Avenue, New York, New York 10016

Current printing (last digit):
10 9 8 7 6 5 4 3 2 1

PRINTED IN THE UNITED STATES OF AMERICA

To Betty and Simon

PREFACE

The theme of this book is how the physicochemical properties of a drug combined into a dosage form affect the percutaneous absorption of the drug after we apply the combination to the skin of a man or an animal. In this context it is necessary to appreciate that for topical therapy, as for other routes of administration, the dosage form of the drug acts as a delivery system. As a consequence any change in the system (either through formulation alterations or through interactions with the organism or the environment) may alter the delivery rate of the drug to the receptor site, together with the total amount of medicament transported to the locus of its action. In dermatological therapy we may refer to the bioavailability of a topical drug as the relative absorption efficiency for the agent. This bioavailability is determined by the release of the drug from the formulation (ointment, cream, lotion, etc.) followed by its penetration through the dead stratum corneum into the viable epidermis and dermis, where the molecule usually produces its characteristic pharmacological response. The ultimate aim in dermatological biopharmaceutics is to design active drug molecules (or prodrugs) with selective permeability, to be incorporated into vehicles which ensure that the medicament arrives at the active site in the biophase at a controlled rate. At the receptor, the drug should maintain a sufficient concentration for the required time.

This book developed from the author's interest in dermatological formulations, and the approach used is a discussion of the fundamental principles of percutaneous absorption rather than specific examples. Many papers in the scientific literature on percutaneous absorption represent a complex blend of physicochemical theory and physiological practicalities. The reader must integrate in his or her mind these two main streams so as to assess the worth of the conclusions. Before this amalgamation can be produced, the reader needs to appreciate the subtleties of the biological and the physicochemical approaches; this book will provide the groundwork for this endeavor.

Chapter 1 introduces the reader to the structure, function, and diseases of human skin and the text provides a brief condensed review of common topical medicaments. A discussion of the basic principles of diffusion through membranes leads on to considerations of skin transport, the routes by which drugs penetrate through the skin, and the role of the epidermal reservoir. Chapter 4 deals with the whole complex of factors that influence percutaneous absorption, classified on the basis of biological or physicochemical considerations. A review of the methods by which we determine the permeation of drugs through skin precedes a discussion on the formulation of dermatological vehicles. The final chapter is rather specialized, as it deals with the flow properties of topical bases; the information presented is directed mainly toward quality control and research and development scientists in the pharmaceutical and cosmetic industries.

The text does not consider specifically the pharmacokinetics of topical therapy or the pharmacodynamics of drug interactions at receptor sites. Pharmacological textbooks and monographs, including Volume 1 and Volume 7 (Chapter 3) in this series, "Drugs and the Pharmaceutical Sciences," present information on these important topics.

The modern trend for scientific books is for an expert to write each chapter so as to provide comprehensive, authoritative treatments. As for other extensive areas of science, it is impossible for any one person to possess a detailed knowledge of all aspects of topical therapy. In contrast, this book is a single-authored text and I trust that the continuity of treatment obtained through an individual aim will compensate for a lack of expertise in specific detail and an inevitable concentration on areas of personal interest.

It is hoped that the book will be useful to pharmacy students and to pharmacists, whether employed in hospital, industry, or community practice, with regulatory authorities, or in teaching and research institutions. Much of the information is also relevant to cosmetic and veterinary scientists and to investigative dermatologists. In particular, the text aims to present a general introduction to the complex subject of percutaneous absorption for those scientists involved in developing topical formulations.

I would like to express my appreciation to Mrs. Marion Firth for her excellent typing, her assistance with the proofreading, and her profound patience in dealing with the many changes made during the preparation of the manuscript. My thanks are also due to Mr. Christopher Bowers and the staff of the Graphic Unit for drawing the diagrams and Mr. J. Merrick and his staff in the Photographic and Film Unit at Bradford University for their help.

Brian W. Barry

CONTENTS

DERMATOLOGICAL FORMULATIONS

— 1 —

STRUCTURE, FUNCTION, DISEASES, AND TOPICAL TREATMENT OF HUMAN SKIN

I. INTRODUCTION

The skin, the heaviest single organ of the body, combines with the mucosal linings of the respiratory, digestive, and urogenital tracts to form a capsule which separates the internal body structures from the external environment. This flexible, self-repairing shell defends the stable internal milieu of living tissues, bathed in their body fluids, from a hostile external world of varying temperature, humidity, radiation, and pollution. The integument not only physically protects the internal organs and limits the passage of substances into and out of the body but also stabilizes temperature and blood pressure with its circulation and evaporation systems. The skin mediates the sensations of touch, pain, heat, and cold; it expresses the redness of anger and embarrassment, the sweating of anxiety, and the pallor of fear; and the integument identifies individuals through the characteristics of the hair, odor, texture, and color shades particular to man.

We may combine these many roles into two purposes: communication between the inside and the outside environments, and control of the former. Now the study of communication and control forms the science of cybernetics (Weiner, 1948), which is therefore an appropriate technology for examining the skin. Mier and Cotton (1976) have reviewed cybernetic concepts in dermatology with particular emphasis on the biochemistry of skin cells.

In the light of the many requirements which the skin must fulfill, it is not surprising that anatomists find that the integument is a very unhomogeneous organ. For an average 70-kg human with a skin surface area of 1.8 m², a typical square centimeter covers 10 hair follicles, 12 nerves, 15 sebaceous glands, 100 sweat glands, 3 blood vessels with 92 cm total length, 360 cm of nerves and 3×10^6 cells (Lubowe, 1963; Wells and Lubowe, 1964).

Because the skin is the most accessible tissue of the body, we easily damage it, mechanically, chemically, biologically, and by radiation. Thus, we cut, bruise, and burn it. We often expose the tissue to organic solvents, detergents, chemical residues, and pollutants and to contact allergens produced by bacteria, yeasts, molds, fungi, and plants. Insects and animals sting and bite it. Toiletries, cosmetics, topical and systemic drugs, together with a myriad of skin diseases, may all harm the skin.

In order that we may appreciate and may control the biopharmaceutics of dermatological formulations, and so that we can answer questions regarding the therapeutic and cosmetic properties of the many topical preparations available in the market or on prescription, we need first to understand the skin. We require at least a knowledge of the basic principles of skin anatomy, physiological function, and chemical composition. We also want to know how common diseases and damage alter the skin's properties, in particular its selective barrier function. In general, it is not essential for the formulator to appreciate all the biochemical and molecular subtleties of skin derangements. This chapter presents a simple introduction to the skin, together with a scheme by which we may approach the science of topical formulation, with a simple listing of those topical agents which we commonly employ in dermatology.

II. ANATOMY AND PHYSIOLOGY

The human skin comprises two distinct but mutually dependent tissues, the stratified, avascular, cellular epidermis and an underlying dermis of connective tissue. At the bottom of the dermis lies the fatty, subcutaneous layer (Fig. 1.1). In transverse section, the dermoepidermal junction undulates because a series of thickened epidermal ridges (the rete ridges) project downwards into the dermis. The ridges inscribe characteristic patterns in different regions of the body (Szabo, 1967), which we see best in split skin preparations (Montagna and Parakkal, 1974).

Human skin displays two main types. Hairy skin encloses hair follicles and sebaceous glands, but there are no encapsulated sense organs. Glabrous skin of the palms and the soles constructs a thick epidermis with a compact stratum corneum, but the integument lacks hair follicles and sebaceous glands and the dermis supports encapsulated sense organs. Ridges groove hairless skin into individually unique configurations termed dermatoglyphics. Besides providing identification, for example, fingerprints, dermatoglyphics may aid diagnosis or they may indicate that a patient has an increased tendency to develop certain diseases, for example, alopecia areata or psoriasis (Cummins and Midlo, 1961; Cummins, 1964; Holt, 1968; Verbov, 1968, 1970).

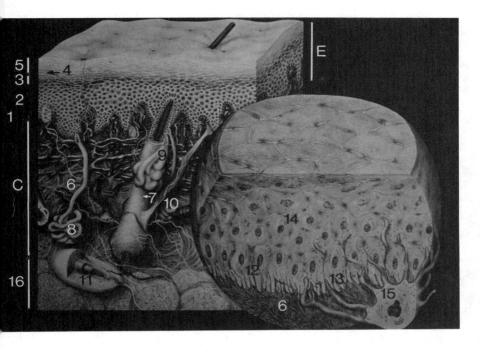

FIG. 1.1 The complex nature of human skin. The inset sphere shows in greater detail the differentiation, development, and keratinization of cells. Key: (E) Epidermis—(1) stratum basale; (2) stratum spongiosum; (3) strtum granulosum; (4) stratum lucidum; (5) stratum corneum. (C) Corium—(6) collagen fibers; (7) hair roots; (8) sweat glands; (9) sebaceous glands; (10) apocrine glands; (11) Pacini corpuscles; (12) basal membrane; (13) cylindrical basal cells with rete pegs; (14) keratinocytes attached by desmosomes; (15) melanocyte exposed from basal membrane; (16) fat cells. (Reproduced with the kind permission of I.C.I. Pharmaceuticals Ltd.)

A. The Epidermis

The multilayered envelope of the epidermis varies in thickness, depending on cell size and the number of cell layers, ranging from about 0.8 mm on the palms and the soles down to 0.06 mm on the eyelids. Cells which provide epithelial tissue differ from those of all other organs in that as they ascend from the proliferative layer of basal cells they change in an ordered fashion from metabolically active and dividing cells to dense, dead, keratinized protein. We can trace this crucial process if we consider the individual layers in the order in which they form.

1. The basal layer (stratum germinativum)
and the dermoepidermal junction

The basal cells are nucleated, columnar, and about 6 μm wide, with their long axis at right angles to the dermoepidermal junction; they connect by cytoplasmic intercellular bridges.

Mitosis of the basal cells constantly renews the epidermis and this proliferation in healthy skin balances the loss of dead horny cells from the skin surface. The epidermis thus remains constant in thickness. Although there are difficulties in calculating epidermal turnover times (Halprin, 1972), workers use tritiated thymadine to selectively label nuclear DNA and thereby they estimate that a cell from the basal layer takes at least 14 days to reach the stratum corneum. In the rapidly proliferating epidermis of psoriasis, the transit time is only 2 days (Epstein and Maibach, 1965; Weinstein and Van Scott, 1965). Radioactive glycine studies indicate that the normal turnover time in the stratum corneum is some 13 or 14 days, with the residence time in psoriatic stratum corneum shortening to 2 days (Rothberg et al., 1961). Therefore, the total turnover times, from the basal layer to shedding, average 28 days in healthy skin and only 4 days in psoriatic skin. The mitotic rate also increases within 24 to 36 hr of injuries such as radiation damage or removal of the stratum corneum by adhesive tape stripping, scrapings, and incisions (Pinkus, 1951, 1952; Weinstein and Frost, 1971). Jarrett (1973) has reviewed epidermal kinetics, and Potten (1975) has estimated the minimal transit time for four regions of the epidermis in mice.

The basal cell layer also includes melanocytes, which produce and distribute melanin granules to the keratinocytes in a complex interaction. The skin requires melanin for pigmentation, a protective measure against radiation (see Sec. III.B.3). Melanocytes lose their activity in vitiligo and hyperactive melanocytes produce tanning, chloasma, freckles, moles, and malignant melanomas (Riley, 1974). Although the melanocyte is the best studied of mammalian cells after the erythrocyte (Fitzpatrick, 1965), for our purposes we need not consider it further here.

Below the basal cell layer lies the complex dermoepidermal junction, which constitutes an anatomic functional unit (Briggaman and Wheeler, 1975). In electron micrographs, the junction spans four components: (1) the basal cell plasma membrane with its specialized attachment devices, the hemidesmosomes; (2) the lamina lucida; (3) the basal lamina; and (4) the fibrous components below the basal lamina, which include anchoring fibrils, dermal microfibril bundles, and collagen fibrils. The "basement membrane" revealed by light microscopy corresponds to the fibrous zone below the basal lamina.

The junction serves the three functions of dermal-epidermal adherence, mechanical support for the epidermis, and control of the passage of cells and some large molecules across the junction. Thus, diseases which operate at this level can markedly reduce the adhesion of the epidermis to the dermis (Briggaman and Wheeler, 1973; Pearson et al., 1974), as can some experimental techniques (Kahl and Pearson, 1967; Briggaman et al., 1971; Jensen and Moffet, 1970). Investigators who use suction to produce blisters in the lamina lucida conclude that the major stabilizing force at the dermo-epidermal junction is a highly viscous bond (Küstala and Mustakallio, 1967; Lowe and Van der Leun, 1968; Peachy, 1971a,b; Hunter et al., 1974; Van der Leun et al., 1974).

We can best consider the barrier function of the junction in terms of three species—small molecules, large molecules, and cells. There is no evidence that the junction significantly inhibits the passage of water, electrolytes, and other low-molecular-weight materials. To do so would, of course, lead to serious consequences with respect to the supply of nutritional materials to the epidermis via the dermal blood vessels. Large molecules also cross the junction [e.g., horseradish peroxidase, a water-soluble protein of molecular weight 40,000 (Schreiner and Wolff, 1969; Squier, 1973) and ruthenium red (Hashimoto and Lever, 1970)]. However, an even larger substance such as thorotrast mainly stays beneath the basal lamina (Wolff and Honigsmann, 1971). It is well established that dermal cellular elements traverse the junction in normal skin and that passage is pronounced in some pathological conditions (Wolff, 1973). The sequence of events is that an area of basal lamina disintegrates, a gap forms in the junction between adjacent cells, and the invading cell penetrates. Finally, basal cells on either side close the gap.

2. The prickle cell layer: the keratinocytes
(stratum germinativum)

As the cells produced by the basal layer move outward, they alter morphologically and histochemically. The cells flatten and their nuclei shrink. We call these polygonal cells prickle cells because they interconnect by fine prickles. Each prickle encloses an extension of the cytoplasm, and the opposing tips of the prickles of adjacent cells adhere to form intercellular bridges—the desmosomes. These links maintain the integrity of the epidermis. Between the desmosomes, a capillary space full of tissue fluid separates neighboring cells and the void permits nutrients and oxygen to pass outward. The desmosomes can break and reform to allow migrating melanocytes and leukocytes to pass (De Vargos Lindres and Burgos, 1964).

In spongiosis of early eczema, the intercellular spaces swell with tissue fluid (intercellular edema) but the desmosomes mainly remain intact. With increasing severity of the disease, the desmosomes disrupt and larger spaces (vesicles) form in the epidermis; the process often involves the death and autolysis or premature keratinization of cells. Acantholysis is the separation of individual cells by fracture of desmosomal linkages; this cleavage is a feature of the pemphigus group of blistering diseases.

3. The granular layer (stratum granulosum)

As the keratinocytes approach the surface, they manufacture basic-staining particles, the keratohyalin granules. It was suggested that these granules represent an early form of keratin (Brody, 1960; Matoltsy and Matoltsy, 1962; Odland, 1964; Reaven and Cox, 1965), but they may be cell organelles partially destroyed by hydrolytic enzymes (Jarrett and Spearman, 1964, 1967; Jarrett, 1967, 1968, 1973). This keratogenous or transitional zone is a region of intense biochemical activity and morphological change. The dynamic operation manufactures the keratin to form the horny layer by an active rather than by a degenerative process (Winkelmann, 1969). The term "transitional zone" is convenient in that we can define a region between living cells and dead keratin, even when no granules form. This is the condition in psoriasis when the epidermis produces a parakeratotic tissue. Polypeptide building blocks of keratin, formed in the prickle cell layer, aggregate in the transitional zone to form insoluble, fibrous keratin molecules.

4. The stratum lucidum

In the palm of the hand and the sole of the foot, an anatomically distinct, poorly staining hyalin zone forms a thin, translucent layer immediately above the granular layer. This region is the stratum lucidum.

5. The horny layer (stratum corneum)

As the final stage of differentiation, epidermal cells construct the most superficial layer of the epidermis, the stratum corneum. Man owes his ability to survive in a nonaqueous environment to the almost impermeable nature of this refractory horny layer (Blank and Scheuplein, 1964). On general body areas the membrane provides 10-15 layers of much flattened, keratinized dead cells, stacking them in highly organized units of vertical columns (MacKenzie, 1972; Christophers, 1971; Menton and Eisen, 1971). The horny layer may be only 10 μm thick when dry (less than half the thickness of an average piece of paper), but it swells in water to several times this thickness. When dry, it is a very dense tissue, about 1.5 g cm^{-3}. Each thin, polygonal cell measures approximately 0.5 to 1.5 μm thick, with a diameter ranging from 34 μm on the forehead to 46 μm on the thigh axilla (Plewig and Marples, 1970). The cells lie tangential to the skin surface and interdigitate their lateral edges with adjacent cells so as to form cohesive laminae. Besides containing keratin, the cells are the final repository of the end products of epidermal metabolism. They enclose sebaceous and sweat gland secretions, all accommodated in a highly organized structure.

We can distinguish two types of horny layer by anatomic site, function, and structure. The horny pads of the palms and soles adapt for weight bearing and friction, and the membranous stratum corneum over the remainder of the body is flexible but impermeable. The horny pads are at least 40 times thicker than the membranous horny layer, and the cells stack vertically in a much less regular fashion. The cells of the pads contain less water-soluble substances, they are very brittle when dry, and they are more permeable to water and to chemicals. Certain compounds, and mechanical trauma, dissociate callus cells more easily and their membranes dissolve more readily in alkali. The protection provided by the pads is very much a function of their thickness. Much of the older published data on the physicochemical properties of stratum corneum have been derived from studies on callus, which is more readily available and more easily handled. We should modify such data when we apply them to the more prevalent membranous horny layer.

We constantly shed the outermost layers of the stratum corneum as lipid-soaked, horny flakes with an average daily loss from the whole body surface of 0.5 to 1 g (Kligman, 1964; Goldschmidt and Kligman, 1964). Even in generalized exfoliative diseases, daily losses are only of the order of 9 to 17 g (Freedberg and Baden, 1962). Thus the skin functions economically, demanding insignificant amounts of body nitrogen.

The stratum corneum plays a crucial role in controlling the percutaneous absorption of drug molecules. The selective permeability of its elegant structure provides a central theme in many aspects of the study of the biopharmaceutics of topical products.

6. Other cells of the epidermis

Langerhans' cells are dendritic cells with a lobular nucleus, a clear cytoplasm containing characteristic Langerhans' cell granules, and well-developed endoplasmic reticulum, Golgi complex, and lysosomes. Langerhans' cells may be concerned with the organization and function of the squamous epidermis. In recent years, much evidence has been presented that these cells are also involved in the immune response in the skin; thus they bind antigens, probably modify them, and transport them to the lymph nodes for lymphocyte activation (Ebling, 1979b; Parish, 1979). Merkel's corpuscles attach to adjacent epidermal cells by numerous desmosomes; they are associated with the sensation of touch (Ebling, 1979b; Cunliffe, 1979a).

B. The Dermis

The dermis (or corium), at 3 to 5 mm thick, is much wider than the overlying epidermis which it supports, and the corium thus makes up the bulk of the skin. The dermis consists essentially of a matrix of connective tissue woven from fibrous proteins (approximate composition: collagen, 75%; elastin, 4%; and reticulin, 0.4%) which embed in an amorphous ground substance of mucopolysaccharide providing about 20% of the mass (Wilkes et al., 1973). Blood vessels, nerves, and lymphatics cross this matrix and skin appendages (eccrine sweat glands, apocrine glands, and pilosebaceous units) penetrate it. In man, the dermis divides into a superficial, thin, papillary layer (composed of narrow fibers) which forms a negative image of the ridged lower surface of the epidermis, and a thick underlying reticular layer made of wide collagen fibers. In regions of the body such as the penis, scrotum, nipple, and perineum, the reticular layer contains smooth muscle fibers which, when contracted, produce wrinkling.

1. Dermal components

a. Collagen Fibroblasts secrete collagen into the surrounding tissue in the form of a precursor, soluble tropocollagen. This is a rod-shaped molecule in the form of a triple polypeptide helix, with a molecular weight of 300,000 to 360,000, a length of about 280 nm, and a width of only 1.5 nm (Lewis and Piez, 1963; Piez, 1967; Schmitt, 1955; Wood, 1964). In living skin, tropocollagen molecules aggregate to form, in sequence, filaments (composed of three to five molecules), microfibrils, and fibrils. Bundles of these fibrils assemble into the collagen fibers, which we see in light microscopy as colorless, branching, wavy bands with faint longitudinal striations.

Collagen is the generic name for a family of proteins which accounts for a third of total human protein. It is the main fibrous constituent of skin, bone, cartilage, tendon, and ligament; collagens from different connective tissues differ only slightly in their amino acid composition. Collagen lacks cystine, but it is rich in the amino acids glycine, proline, and hydroxyproline (Fleischmajer and Fishman, 1965).

b. Elastin In humans, the dermis abounds with elastic fibers which stretch relatively easily and which revert to their original shape when the stress subsides. The elastic fibers form a framework in the dermis, so that the mechanical properties of connective tissues depend on the presence of both the collagen and the elastic fibers.

Elastic fibers incorporate two components—an inner amorphous medulla composed of the protein elastin (derived from a precursor, tropoelastin) and an outer cortex consisting of nonelastin protein microfibrils. These two portions differ markedly in amino acid composition, and neither resembles collagen (Ross and Bornstein, 1969). Elastin possesses the unique amino acids desmosine and isodesmosine (Thomas et al., 1963), which probably form a special kind of cross-link within the molecule; the resulting product is insoluble and very stable. Adult animals retain their elastin for life.

Theories concerning the nature of elastin structure have been summarized with the aid of various molecular models (Partridge, 1970b; Sandberg et al., 1971; Hall, 1971).

c. Ground substance The amorphous ground substance, in which the cells and fibers lie, contains a variety of lipid, protein, and carbohydrate materials. The most important are the mucopolysaccharides hyaluronic acid and dermatan sulfate (chondroitin sulfate B), together with a small amount of chondroitin-6-sulfate. The molecular weight of the hyaluronic acid depends on the tissue source and the method of preparation; it may be several millions. Dermatan sulfate has a molecular weight of not more than 40,000. Both compounds are single-chain, linear polymers (Ebling, 1979a).

d. Cells Fibroblasts are the most numerous cells inhabiting loose connective tissue (Branwood, 1963; Jarrett, 1974; Porter, 1964). Mast cells and histiocytes also occur (Wilkes et al., 1973; Woodburne, 1965).

2. The vascular supply

The dermis needs a rich blood supply which regulates temperature and pressure, delivers nutrients to the skin and removes waste products, mobilizes defense forces, and contributes to skin color. Branches from the artery network (the arterial plexus) convey blood to the hair follicles, the sweat glands, the subcutaneous fat, and the dermis itself (Woodburne, 1965).

The blood supply reaches to within 0.2 mm of the skin surface, so that it readily absorbs and systemically dilutes most chemicals which penetrate past the stratum corneum and the viable epidermis. The vascular surface available for the exchange of materials between local tissues and the blood is about 1-2 cm^2 per cm^2 of skin surface, with a blood flow rate of about 0.05 ml min^{-1} per cm^3 of skin (Scheuplein and Blank, 1971; Rothman, 1954).

Of particular relevance to biopharmaceutical studies is the fact that this generous blood volume usually functions as a "sink" with respect to the diffusing molecules which reach it during the process of percutaneous absorption. This sink condition ensures that the penetrant concentration in the dermis remains near zero and therefore the concentration gradient across the epidermis is maximal. As the concentration gradient provides the driving force for diffusion, an abundant blood supply assists percutaneous absorption. However, vasoconstrictors such as topical steroids may restrict the local circulation and vasodilators such as the nicotinic acid esters may widen the capillaries to increase further the blood flow (see Chap. 4, Sec. II. E).

The lymphatic system forms a vascular network with the primary function of removing plasma proteins from the extravascular spaces, together with particulate and other matter (Foldi, 1969; Kinmonth, 1972; Yoffey and Courtice, 1970; Champion, 1979a).

3. The neural supply

A liberal nerve supply serves the skin, with great variations from region to region. The face and the extremities are richly innervated, whereas the bank of the trunk carries a sparse network. Cutaneous nerves, nerve endings, and capillaries modulate the sensations of pain, pruritus (itching), touch, and temperature (Cunliffe, 1979a). A point made by Winkelman (1961) is that the skin is a physiological paradox, as it serves two mutually exclusive functions—protection from the environment (which requires minimal sensory perception), and recording of the surroundings (needing sensitive nervous responses).

C. The Subcutaneous Tissue

The subcutaneous fat (hypoderm, subcutis) spreads all over the body as a fibrofatty layer, with the exception of the eyelids and the male genital region. The sheet of fat lies between the relatively flexible skin and the unyielding, deep fascia, and its thickness varies with the age, sex, endocrine, and nutritional status of the individual. The cells manufacture and store lipids in large quantities and bundles of collagen fibers weave between aggregates of fat cells to provide flexible linkages between the underlying structures and the superficial skin layers. The subcutis provides a thermal barrier and a mechanical cushion; it is a site of synthesis and a depot of readily available high-energy chemicals (Jeanrenaud, 1963; Renold and Cahill, 1965; Cunliffe and Bleehen, 1979).

D. The Skin Appendages

The highly vascularized dermis and the epidermis support several appendages: the eccrine, apocrine, and sebaceous glands, the hair follicles, and the nails.

1. Eccrine sweat glands

Eccrine sweat glands develop over the skin surface but not over mucous membranes. Their anatomy and physiology have been reviewed by Grice and Verbov (1977), Kuno (1956), Montagna and Parakkal (1974), Rothman (1954), Sato (1977), and Champion (1979b). The gland density varies greatly with skin site; for example, the thighs possess about 120 glands per cm^2 and the soles of the feet have about 620 per cm^2 (Szabo, 1967). The average fractional surface area which these glands occupy is only of the order of 10^{-5} or less (Scheuplein, 1967). Total body numbers lie between 2 and 5 million.

The gland arises as a secretory coil in the lower dermis and subcutaneous tissue, forms a duct leading through the dermis to the intraepidermal sweat duct unit, and exits on the skin surface as a pore invisible to the naked eye. The coil manufactures a watery solution from plasma, which the duct subsequently modifies. The sodium pump in the gland can generate a pressure equivalent to 500 mmHg (Dobson and Sato, 1970). The composition and the quantity of the sweat varies greatly with subject, time, environmental conditions, exertion, and skin site (Gordon and Cage, 1966; Robinson and Robinson, 1954; Rothman, 1954). The liquid is a dilute, hypotonic solution (containing 99% or more of water), the most important constituents being Na, Cl, K, urea, and lactate, at a pH of 4.0 to 6.8. The gland may also occasionally secrete a variety of other substances, such as drugs (Comaish and Shelley, 1965; Thayson and Schwartz, 1953) and various proteins, antibodies, and antigens (Berrens and Young, 1964; Page and Rimington, 1967; Sultzberger, 1952; Champion, 1979b).

The output of sweat may fall as low as 1 liter per day, but under maximal stimulation the body can produce up to 12 liters in 24 hr or, for short periods, 3 liters hr^{-1}; this rate exceeds the ability of man to drink (Schmidt-Nielsen, 1964). Sweat production accounts for about 80% of the water lost through the skin, with the transepidermal flux contributing the remainder (Ebling, 1963). If the sweat glands block, prickly heat (miliaria) and heat stroke may intervene.

The principal function of the gland is to assist in heat control, as high external temperatures and vigorous exercise stimulate secretion. However, because the autonomic nervous system innervates the glands, emotional stress can also provoke sweating, that is, the clammy palm syndrome.

2. Apocrine sweat glands

Apocrine sweat glands are epidermal appendages which develop throughout the skin of the embryo as part of the pilosebaceous follicle. Most of the glands subsequently disappear so that the characteristic adult distribution is in the axilla (armpit), the perianal region, and the areola of the breasts (Biempica and Montes, 1965; Hurley and Shelley, 1960; Montagna, 1964; Woodburne, 1965; Montagna and Parakkal, 1974; Champion, 1979b). The glands develop poorly in childhood but enlarge with the onset of puberty. Apocrine glands are about 10 times bigger than the eccrine sweat glands and extend well into the subcutaneous tissue. Each structure consists of a tubule and a duct; most ducts open into the neck of a hair follicle above the sebaceous gland, but a few exit onto the surface of the skin.

The apocrine gland secretes a small quantity of a milky or oily fluid which may be colored. The secretion contains lipids, proteins, lipoproteins, and saccharides. Surface bacteria rapidly metabolize this odorless liquid to produce the characteristic body smell (Kligman and Shehadek, 1964). The glands play no part in thermoregulation, and we can consider them to be vestigial secondary sex organs which now have no apparent function in man.

The epithelium of the secretory coil varies its rate of secretion under hormonal control, e.g., in menstruation and in pregnancy. We may expel apocrine sweat continuously, or emotional stimuli may provoke discharge.

3. Hair

Although hair serves no vital purpose in humans, its psychological functions are all important. Genetically disposed men accept, somewhat reluctantly, scalp baldness, but the loss of hair from the head distresses women as much as the growth of facial or body hair in amounts greater than the individual culture accepts (Ebling and Rook, 1979a).

Hair grows from follicles, invaginations of the superficial epidermis which enclose at their base a stud of dermis, the dermal papilla. The follicles slant into the dermis, with the longer ones extending into the subcutaneous fat. The arrector pili, an oblique muscle, attaches the follicle wall to the dermoepidermal junction. When the fibers contract, the hair stands upright to produce the "goose pimple" effect on skin. One or more sebaceous glands, and in some body regions also an apocrine gland, open into the follicle above the smooth muscle (Ebling, 1976; Hamilton, 1950; Lubowe, 1959; Lyne and Short, 1965; Montagna and Ellis, 1958; Montagna and Dobson, 1969).

Hair follicles develop over the entire skin surface except the palms, the soles, the red portion of the lips, and parts of the sex organs. The average fractional surface area of the openings is about 0.1% (Scheuplein, 1967; Szabo, 1962). As man grows toward adulthood, the body surface increases and the actual density of follicles falls. It is generally accepted that adult skin cannot develop new follicles. The total number of pilosebaceous units in humans is about 5 million, of which a fifth lie in the head with perhaps 100,000 in the scalp. The follicle number shows no significant racial or sexual differences (Szabo, 1968, 1967; Muller, 1971). We lose some of our hair follicles with advancing age, and there are fewer follicles in baldness (Giacometti, 1965).

The hair shaft comprises three concentric rings of tightly fused horny cells. The bulk of any hair is a thick cortex of elongated, keratinized cells cemented together; in pigmented hair these cells contain granules of melanin. Nonpigmented cells overlap in 5 to 10 layers to form a cuticle which surrounds the cortex, and a continuous or discontinuous core or medulla may exist (Bullough and Lawrence, 1958).

Hair contains "hard" keratin, which differs from the "soft" keratin of desquamating tissues in its high sulfur content (Mercer, 1958, 1961; Rudall, 1964).

The growth rate of hair varies from species to species, within one species from region to region, and with sex and age. The average rate of growth in one study ranged from 0.21 mm per 24 hr on the female thigh to 0.38 mm per 24 hr on the chin of a young male. Scalp hair grows faster in women than in men, but before puberty the tempo is greater in boys than in girls. The average rate over the whole body is quicker in men than in women. Irrespective of sex, the rate reaches a maximum between 50 and 70 years. Shaving has no effect, but endocrine factors influence hair growth. Ebling and Rook (1979a) provide references to the rate of growth of hair.

Different kinds of follicle may produce distinct types of hair, although the sort of hair which a particular follicle bears may also change with age or with hormonal variations. In humans, a prenatal coat of soft, fine hair (lanugo) is normally shed in utero. Postnatal hair is of two main types: vellus, which is occasionally pigmented, soft, and seldom more than 2 cm long; and terminal hair, a longer, coarser, and often pigmented filament. However, there is a broad range of intermediate types (Rook, 1965).

Ebling and Rook (1979a) discuss racial and individual variations in hair and its change with age, the cyclic activity of the follicle, hormonal influences, and the metabolism of hair follicles.

4. Sebaceous glands

Sebaceous glands are largest and most numerous on the forehead, face, anogenital surfaces, in the ear, and on the midline of the back. The palms and the soles are usually free of them, and glands are sparse on the dorsal surfaces of the hand and the foot. For example, the chin, cheek, forehead, and scalp support between 400 and 900 glands per cm^2; elsewhere there are less than 100 glands per cm^2 (Montagna, 1963; Ebling and Rook, 1979b).

The flasklike sebaceous glands form ducts which usually open into the neck of the hair follicle. In the so-called sebaceous follicles in which acne develops, the flask is particularly large and multilobular and it looks like a miniature cauliflower (Plewig and Kligman, 1975). Some glands open directly to the surface, for example, in the eyelids, the prepuce, the muco-cutaneous surfaces of the female genitalia, the areolae of the nipples, the tongue, and the cervix uteri (Hyman and Guiducci, 1963; Montagna, 1963).

The sebaceous gland is holocrine in that it forms its secretion, sebum, by the complete disintegration of the glandular cells. Sebum is a complex mixture of lipids which varies widely from species to species (Downing and Strauss, 1974; Nikkari, 1974). Its principal components are glycerides, free fatty acids, wax esters, squalene, cholesterol, and cholesterol esters. Several functions have been ascribed to sebum, such as controlling water loss and protecting the skin from fungal and bacterial infection. However, Kligman (1963) considers it useless in man. Section II.A of Chap. 3 provides further details of sebum composition and its claimed value to man.

In the human, during the prepubertal period, the glands are tiny, but they grow greatly at puberty when the hormonal activity rises. For example, the sebum output in men increases more than fivefold, eunuchs produce half as much sebum as normal males, and adult women manufacture a little less than average men.

We can identify four main classes of abnormal sebaceous activity: (1) excessive production of sebum (seborrhea); (2) sebaceous gland hyperplasia without clinic seborrhea; (3) obstructive disorders of the sebaceous duct and the pilosebaceous canal (acne and comedones—whiteheads or blackheads); and (4) other types of sebaceous gland dysfunction—the dyssebaceas (Ebling and Rook, 1979b).

5. Nails

The embryonic epidermis at the end of each finger and toe invaginates to fabricate the nail, and its plate is almost completely formed by the twentieth week of fetal life (Zaias, 1963; Samman, 1979). The nail plate, like hair, consists of "hard" keratin, with a relatively high sulfur content, mainly in the form of the amino acid cysteine, which constitutes 9.4% by weight of the nail (Forslind, 1970; Forslind and Thyresson, 1975). Nails grow continuously throughout life, unlike hairs, and we do not normally shed them. If we do lose one through trauma, the digit replaces the nail at about the same rate as normal plate growth, which for fingernails is between 0.5 and 1.2 mm per week. Growth is greatest in childhood and decreases slowly with aging (Bean, 1974). With respect to its permeability to n-alkanols, the nail functions as a hydrophilic matrix (K. A. Walters and G. L. Flynn, personal communication, 1979).

III. FUNCTIONS OF THE SKIN

The skin performs many varied functions, and Table 1.1 presents a brief digest of its biological role. However, insofar as we are mainly concerned here with the biopharmaceutics of topical formulations, we need only examine in more detail some aspects of the containment function and the protective role of the integument. Relevant references include Wilkes et al. (1973),

TABLE 1.1 The Main Functions of Skin

1. To contain body fluids and tissues—the mechanical function.

2. To protect from potentially harmful external stimuli—the protective or barrier function: (a) microorganisms; (b) chemicals; (c) radiation; (d) heat; (e) electrical barrier; or (f) mechanical shock.

3. To receive external stimuli, i.e., to mediate sensation: (a) tactile (pressure); (b) pain; or (c) heat.

4. To regulate body temperature.

5. To synthesize and to metabolize compounds (see Chap. 4, Sec. II.D).

6. To dispose of chemical wastes (glandular secretions).

7. To provide identification by skin variations.

8. To attract the opposite sex (apocrine secretions are evolutionarily defunct in this role).

9. To regulate blood pressure.

Source: Wilkes et al. (1973); Rushmer et al. (1966); Flynn (1979).

Rushmer et al. (1966), Tregear (1966), Rothman (1954), Thiele et al. (1974), and Flynn (1979). The interested reader may also find further information relevant to the remaining functions listed in Table 1.1 in any good text on dermatology, such as the classic Textbook of Dermatology, in two volumes, edited by Rook et al. (1979).

A. The Mechanical Function

The mechanical properties of skin, which are responsible for confining the underlying tissues and for restraining their movements, depend mainly on the dermis although the epidermis plays its part. Our skin is elastic and, for a few second, it can stretch reversibly from 1.1 to 1.5 times its unstrained dimension. As deformation takes up the slack, the skin first extends readily but then the extensibility decreases. The network of elastic fibers in the dermis probably maintains the tonus of the skin, and it is likely that the fibers also provide the small elastic forces which restore the extensibility of slack skin and which allow normal body movements. In such skin the collagen fibers probably remain bent and so play no part in maintaining the tension.

Once the skin has taken up its initial slack, it extends further with some difficulty. The integument breaks under extreme stress, but it will gradually slip if we maintain it taut for a protracted period, for example, when a boil stretches the skin. The most probable mechanism is that either individual collagen fibrils align and slip relative to each other or whole fibrils move within the related ground substance. A hypothesis which explains the resistance to slip is that movement is interfibrillar, the fibers are very long, and the ground substance is highly viscous because of its content of dermatan sulfate. In hyperelastic skin, such as in Ehlers-Danlos syndrome, the collagen mechanism breaks down. The striae distensae of adolescence, pregnancy, and Cushing's syndrome involve a disruption of fibril overlap (Ebling, 1979b; Cunliffe, 1979b).

We can compress the skin. If we press a blunt point into the cutis it forms a depression which remains for some time after we remove the instrument. The skin molds around the object so as to reduce the pressure at any one point, primarily through the flow of ground substance between the collagen fibers in the dermis.

With age, the dermal structural fibers change their nature and their organization so that their solubility decreases and various physical properties alter (Elden, 1968; Jackson, 1965; Verzar, 1964). The skin becomes more rigid, the tensile strength increases, and the integument wrinkles. One theoretical scheme proposes that during aging progressive transesterification causes the intrastrand linkages in the collagen to change first into interstrand links and then to alter into intermolecular links, without any supplementation to the total number of ester bonds (Gallop, 1964; Ebling, 1979a).

The epidermis is relatively strong and its ability to withstand rupture depends primarily on the nature of the stratum corneum. The horny layer, if we judge it on a quantity normalized basis, is actually stronger than the dermal fabric. Healthy stratum corneum depends for its pliability on a correct balance of lipids, hygroscopic water-soluble substances, and (most importantly) water. Water is the principal softening agent or plasticizer within the horny layer, and the tissue requires some 10 to 20% moisture to maintain its suppleness. The water, and possibly other substances, render the horny layer soft and flexible by reducing molecular interaction between the keratin strands. The tissue becomes less "crystalline" as the water occupies space or creates gaps between the protein molecules. Without an adequate moisture supply, the integument chaps, cracks, and splits under stress (Flynn, 1979). The importance of the correct water content to the stratum corneum and the part played by the "natural moisturizing factor" are considered further in Chap. 4, Secs. III.B and III.C.1.

The dermoepidermal junction in human skin is relatively weak, and many blistering agents appear to work on the superficial collagen in the papillary layer. When investigators prepare skin membranes for in vitro diffusion experiments by heat treatment, success depends on the skin splitting at this level.

B.   The Protective Function

1.   The microbiological barrier

In its healthy state, the skin constructs a relatively dry, dense, mechanical barrier and only molecules penetrate this bastion of the horny layer to reach the water-rich viable layers of the cutis. The stratum corneum is therefore a bulwark against microorganisms, and the sloughing mechanism, which constantly sheds squames with their adherent harmless and pathogenic microorganisms, further aids the protective function. However, microbes can penetrate into the superficial cracks and fissures of the horny layer, and mechanical or disease-induced damage to the stratum corneum can provide access to the lower tissues, with the consequent risk of infection.

Sebaceous and eccrine secretions lay down an acid mantle on the skin surface, with a pH between 4.2 and 5.6 (Katz and Poulsen, 1971). For many years dermatologists thought that this acid pH provided an important defense mechanism against bacteria (Burtenshaw, 1945). However, Noble and Somerville (1974) have rejected this theory, claiming that the degree of dessication accounts for the difference in the rate at which implanted bacteria disappear from an acid and from an alkaline region; the latter site is moister. Topical infections are more prevalent in macerated skin and during the warm humid months of a tropical year, observations which emphasize the importance of a moist skin for promoting colonization.

The skin glands also secrete the short-chain fatty acids propionic, butyric, caproic, and caprylic, which are bacteriostatic and fungistatic (Peck and Russ, 1947). Lacey (1968, 1969) found that if he extracted the fatty acids from skin then the integument's resistance to colonization by staphylococci diminished, and also that neomycin can bind to some extent to fatty acids and thereby neutralize them.

The opening to the inner duct of the eccrine gland is so tiny that bacteria are unlikely to enter. However, the hair follicle and the apocrine gland are much wider, and these appendages can become infected.

Bacterial interference provides a possible defense mechanism at the surface of the skin. For example, if a strain of an organism colonizes a site, its presence can interfere with a subsequent invasion by a different strain. More than a fifth of normal subjects support some skin bacteria which secrete "antibiotics" capable of inhibiting other microorganisms; on 10% of normal human skins these antibiotic-producers predominate. However, the role of antibiotic-producing strains of bacteria in the microbial ecology of the skin is still controversial, although workers have demonstrated the potential therapeutic value of such antibiotics (Selwyn, 1975; Selwyn et al., 1976; Gerber and Nowak, 1976).

2. The chemical barrier

The most important single function of human skin is to act as a barricade in two directions, controlling the loss of water, electrolytes, and other body constituents while barring the entry of harmful or unwanted molecules from the external environment. The stratum corneum differs from other body membranes in that it is much less permeable to chemicals, often some 10,000-fold so. The horny layer usually contributes the rate-limiting step in the sequence of percutaneous absorption, although the aqueous viable tissues can hinder the penetration of very hydrophobic drugs. Chemicals can also reach the living tissues more easily via the shunt route of the appendages. We can generalize the situation and conclude that the intact skin sets up a very effective barrier to chemical permeation because the diffusional resistance of the stratum corneum is large for virtually all molecular species except gases and because the shunt route of the appendages presents only a very small fractional area (of the order of 0.1%).

We will not pursue here in any more detail the nature of the chemical barrier of the skin, as the study of this aspect of the membrane provides the biological nucleus of this book. Chapters 3 and 4, in particular, provide further specific details.

3. The radiation barrier

The component of sunlight which potentially can damage biological tissue and which the atmosphere does not filter out is the ultraviolet (UV) part of the spectrum, in particular wavelengths from 290 to 400 nm. In

photodermatology, workers generally subdivide the terrestrial UV spectrum
into two parts: (1) the section 290 to 320 nm, often called UVB, sunburn,
or erythrogenic radiation because it induces delayed erythema in normal
skin; and (2) the less damaging long-wave UVA from 320 to 400 nm.

Normal skin reacts to exposure to the sun's rays in several ways.
Some responses, such as "sunburn," a delayed erythema, develop within
a few hours while others need multiple exposures over extended time, as
in skin "aging." Sunlight (actinic radiation) may change skin in an acute or
a chronic fashion (Ramsay, 1979).

We can recognize three main acute reactions to irradiation: erythema,
pigmentation, and thickening of the epidermis. Surprisingly, the actual
cause of sunburn is unknown, although workers advocate two separate theories: the first is that the UV radiation acts directly on the dermal vessels,
while the second suggests that the light energy releases vasodilating compounds in the epidermis which diffuse to the dermis (Ramsay, 1979; Lewis,
1927). Whatever the mechanism of sunburn, the skin attempts to prevent
or to minimize further damage, mainly by pigmenting. UVA and visible
light produce immediate pigmentation soon after exposure. This browning
develops from the restoration of color in the partially bleached melanin
already deposited in the skin. The "tanning" lasts for only a few hours and
presumably does little to protect the skin from further radiation. However,
delayed pigmentation does protect the tissue against subsequent exposures.
Both UVA and UVB, but particularly the latter, stimulate the melanocytes
to produce melanin and to deposit it in the epidermis, thus developing the
tanning which certain nationalities seek as eagerly as others avoid it.
Melanin is effective in protecting the skin against further actinic radiation,
although the defense is not absolute (Kligman, 1974). For example, in a
severe photosensitive disease such as xeroderma pigmentosum the sunlight
may induce changes even in blacks, that is, subjects with intense racial
pigmentation who are therefore markedly less susceptible to sunburn. The
final protective process, an increase in epidermal thickness, follows some
days after exposure.

The chronic reactions to actinic radiation include "aging," premalig-
nancy, and malignancy. Prolonged exposure to UV stress deteriorates the
tissue (Kligman, 1969; Lund and Sommerville, 1957; Smith and Finlayson,
1965). The epidermis and the blood vessels change in an irregular and
complex fashion, and in the dermis the soluble and insoluble collagens alter
and the elastic tissue and the acid mucopolysacchardes increase.

Sun-damaged skin may develop small hyperkeratotic lesions known as
solar or actinic keratoses, which may progress to a squamous cell carcinoma. Bowen's disease, malignant melanomata, and basal cell carcinoma
may also evolve (Sanderson and Mackie, 1979). Chronic exposure to sunlight, as, for example, in Australia, almost certainly leads to many cutaneous disorders. In animals, the UVB radiation is probably responsible,
although we do not know the exact region for damage in humans; controlled
experiments would, of course, be unethical.

Ionizing radiation is destructive to tissues; therapeutic treatments employ x-rays and gamma and beta rays, but alpha rays and fast neutron beams seem to have little dermatological potential. Those pioneering scientists who investigated radioactive materials and x-rays and the victims of flash burns from atomic explosions, sustained extensive and bizarre lesions.

The damaging effects of laser burns on the skin vary with the wavelength of the laser, its power, the direction of the beam, the skin color, and the duration of the impact. Hemoglobin and melanin absorb the laser energy and lessen the effect on viable tissue. The therapeutic application of a laser produces the equivalent of a chemical burn.

4. The heat barrier and temperature regulation

The stratum corneum, although it is an excellent diffusional barrier, is so thin over most of the body that it does not effectively protect the underlying viable tissues from extremes of heat and cold. The horny layer is not an efficient heat insulator.

The skin, however, is the organ primarily responsible for maintaining the body as an isothermal system at 37°C. When man needs to conserve heat (when the external temperature drops), the skin pales as the peripheral circulation shuts down to minimize the heat loss via the blood flow at the body surface. Theoretically, if this should happen during percutaneous absorption, molecules should penetrate more slowly as the falling temperature reduces the value of the diffusion coefficient and the lowered blood volume militates against sink conditions (see Chap. 4, Secs. III.C.2 and II.E). Furry animals can contract their follicular muscles to raise their pelts and thus increase the thickness of the stagnant layer of air entrapped within the fur. This mechanism for reducing diffusive heat loss is denied man, whose vestigial response produces only "goose pimples." Shivering (involuntary rhythmic contractions of the muscles) generates energy when chilling is severe.

To lose heat in a warm environment or during vigorous exercise, the blood vessels dilate to maximize diffusive thermal loss and the skin reddens. The increased temperature of the skin and the raised blood flow could theoretically affect percutaneous absorption in a way opposite to that discussed in the previous paragraph. The eccrine sweat glands pour out their dilute saline secretion over the entire body surface, but especially on the trunk and the face (Kuno, 1956); the water evaporates and the removal of the heat of vaporization cools the body. Occlusive films retard heat loss, but more significantly they minimize evaporation and thus hydrate the skin. Both effects promote percutaneous absorption (Chap. 4, Secs. III.B.1 and III.C.1).

Extreme cold, even for a few seconds in the presence of strong winds and at high altitudes, or on contact with very cold metal, can cause frostbite—freezing of the tissues.

Only limited work has been reported which quantitatively defines the effect of burning on the permeability of skin. A recent paper which discusses the immediate influences of 60°C scalding on hairless mouse skin, and which provides a reference list, is that by Behl et al. (1980).

5. The electrical barrier

The conduction of electricity through the skin depends on the movement of endogenous ions through the most resistive layer, the stratum corneum. In dry skin, the resistance to direct current and the impedance to alternating current are much higher than in other biological tissues (Rushmer et al., 1966; Tregear, 1966). We can measure the in vivo impedance of the skin as a means of assessing the integrity of the stratum corneum barrier, as treatments which lower the impedance also generally increase the skin permeability to chemicals.

Because of the high skin impedance, electrical burns are often critical. Severe charring follows contact with 5,000 V and above; with weaker voltages the damage is delayed and is not as extensive. However, in all cases there may be more destruction at a deeper tissue level than appears likely from the superficial appearance of the lesion. Lightning burns imprint mottled, aborescent, charred lesions and burns from defective cardiac defibrillators have progressed through skin necrosis to ulcers (Sevitt, 1957; Wilkinson, 1979a).

6. Mechanical shock

We have already discussed some aspects of the response of the skin to an imposed deformation in Sec. III.A. However, investigators have not studied, to any great extent, the reaction of the tissue to a mechanical trauma which is insufficient to cause immediate, obvious injury. An acute, violent blow brings on hemorrhage (bruising) and blisters. Frictional forces initiate an adaptive response which thickens the epidermis, possibly by a chalone feedback mechanism. Repeated friction increases the cell number in the horny and granular layers and raises the epidermal turnover rate until it reaches a new steady state (MacKenzie, 1974; Schellander and Marks, 1973; Bullough, 1972). Repeated, intermittent friction of low intensity induces hyperkeratosis (hypertrophy of the horny layer) and acanthosis (increase in depth of the prickle cell layer). The hyperkeratosis develops from an increased cohesion in the cells of the stratum corneum and a reduced shedding rate (Rubin, 1949). The clinical lesions which follow are callosities and corns and, with less localized trauma in predisposed subjects, lichen simplex.

If we suddenly apply intense friction to the epidermis, blisters form. An intraepidermal bulla develops by degeneration and necrosis of the prickle cells. Fluid from the dermis floods into the splits in the epidermis to raise macroscopic blisters (Comaish, 1973; Schellander and Marks, 1973).

Accidental, minor trauma to the skin of patients on corticosteroid therapy may severely damage their skin. Even patients on a relatively low dose of these drugs over a long time can sustain hematomas and extensive lacerations which require surgery.

Wilkinson (1979a) has supplied further details of the effect of mechanical trauma, including unusual responses to injury, the presence of foreign bodies and injected material, pressure sores, and the process of wound healing in skin.

IV. COMMON DISEASES, DISORDERS, AND ABNORMALITIES OF HUMAN SKIN

In this book, we are essentially concerned with the biopharmaceutics of topical preparations, and in particular with the basic science of how to formulate effective dermatologicals so that the active therapeutic agent releases readily from its vehicle and penetrates the skin to reach its site of action. We are not concerned directly with the pharmacological mode of action of each compound, nor with the detailed biochemistry, anatomy, and pathophysiology of the diseased state. However, in order to design safe and effective formulations to treat skin maladies, we need to start with some framework which introduces scientists who are not physicians to the main types of skin disorders. To this end, Table 1.2 presents a brief outline of common dermatological disorders and other prevalent conditions; for its information and arrangement it draws extensively on the excellent treatments of Katz and Poulsen (1971) and Flynn (1979). We can note that although Table 1.2 allocates the various examples of skin disease and disorder to specific sites in the skin, the derangements will usually spread in time to involve the entire tissue. Often the disease will perturb several strata before the affliction is clinically apparent. When a formulator develops a topical for a specific disease condition, he should note in particular the state of the horny layer (absent, damaged, thickened, etc.), whether the lesion is dry or weeping, and whether the ailment has attacked the appendages. Such considerations, among many others, affect the biopharmaceutical design of the dosage form.

V. RATIONAL APPROACH TO TOPICAL FORMULATION

There are two fundamental methods by which we approach the biopharmaceutical problem of formulating a successful topical dosage form (Flynn, 1979). These two methods, as well as a third relatively recent innovation, will be considered here.

In the first process we assist or manipulate the barrier function of the skin. For example, sunscreening agents increase the power of the horny layer to protect the viable tissues from UV irradiation; topical antibiotics and antibacterials help a damaged barrier to ward off infection; and emollient

TABLE 1.2 Outline of Common Diseases, Disorders, and Abnormalities
of Human Skin

Skin disorders	Examples
1. External trauma	
A. Physical damage	
(1) Sharp and blunt instruments	Bruise, blister, cut, bite.
(2) Rubbing and scraping	Abrasion, blister, corns
(3) Pressure	Pressure sores
(4) Heat	Burns (first, second, or third degree), miliaria
(5) Cold	Chilblains, frostbite
(6) Excessive drying	Chapping, windburn
(7) UV radiation	Sunburn, pigmentation, malignancies
(8) Ionizing radiation	Pigmentation, malignancies
(9) Electricity	Burns
(10) Insects—bees, wasps, ticks, mites, lice	Bites, stings, invasion
B. Chemical damage	
(1) Immediate damage— acids, alkalis, phosphorus	Burns
(2) Solvent extraction— detergents, organic solvents	"Housewife hands"
(3) Contact dermatitis— irritant, allergic, phototoxic, photo-allergic	Redness, oozing, vesicles, itch
(4) Drug reactions	Variety of lesions
2. Abnormalities of the epidermis	
A. Stratum corneum	
(1) Decreased sloughing (thickening)	Ichthyosis
(2) Hyperkeratosis (increased division)	Corn, callus
B. Viable epidermis	
(1) General	
(a) Keratinocyte damage and inflammation	General dermatitis, eczema
(b) Fluid collection	Blister

TABLE 1.2 (continued)

Skin disorders	Examples
(c) Abnormal cell growth	Keratoses
(d) Granular layer thickening	Lichen planus
(e) Excess proliferation with incomplete keratinization	Psoriasis
(f) Malignancy	Epithelioma
(2) Melanocyte	
(a) Hyperfunction	Freckles, chloasma, tanning
(b) Hypofunction	Vitiligo (leucoderma)
(c) Congenital absence of melanin	Albinism
(d) Abnormal growth	Mole
(e) Malignancy	Melanoma

3. Abnormalities of dermoepidermal junction
   A. Lifting of the epidermis   Dermatitis herpetiformis
   B. Overgrowth of epidermis
      and elongation of dermal
      papillae   Warts (verrucae)

4. Disorders of the dermis
   A. Increased permeability of
      vasculature   Urticaria (nettle rash, hives)
   B. Fibers
     (1) Atrophy of connective
        tissue   Striae, senile atrophy
     (2) Overgrowth of collagen
        fibers   Hypertrophic scars, keloids
     (3) Disorder of collagen
        formation   Scleroderma (Lupus erythematosus)

5. Disorders of the appendages
   A. Hair follicle
     (1) Overactivity   Hirsutism
     (2) Underactivity   Alopecia, baldness
   B. Sebaceous gland
     (1) Overactivity   Seborrhea
     (2) Underactivity   Dyssebacea associated with pellagra

TABLE 1.2 (continued)

Skin disorders	Examples
(3) Blockage of sebaceous duct and pilosebaceous canal	Acne (blackheads, pimples)
C. Eccrine sweat gland	
(1) Overactivity	Hyperhidrosis
(2) Underactivity	Anhidrosis
(3) Blockage of duct	Miliaria (prickly heat)
D. Apocrine sweat gland	
(1) Blockage of duct	Fox-Fordyce disease
6. Infective conditions	
A. Bacterial	Impetigo, boils (carbuncles), folliculitis barbae
B. Fungal	Tinea (ringworm, athlete's foot), candidiasis (moniliasis, thrush)
C. Viral	Warts (verrucae), herpes zoster (shingles), herpes simplex (cold sores), chickenpox, smallpox, measles
D. Protozoal	Cutaneous amebiasis
E. Parasitic	Scabies, lice

Source: Modified from Katz and Poulsen (1971) and Flynn (1979).

ointments, creams, lotions, and baths restore the pliability of the skin after low humidity environments and detergents have dessicated the horny layer.

In the second procedure we attempt to breach the horny layer at the molecular scale so as to direct drugs to the viable epidermal and dermal tissues without using oral, systemic, or other therapies. If we do attempt systemic therapy to treat a dermatological condition, we have the problem that most drugs do not normally concentrate preferentially in the skin. We therefore usually produce drug levels in highly perfused muscles and organs which are equal to or greater than the concentration obtained within the skin. In particular, the avascular epidermis is somewhat inaccessible to systemically administered drugs. Using the systemic route we may there-fore invoke side effects because of the relatively high dosages required. In contrast, the topical route may allow a drug to diffuse to the viable cutaneous tissues in concentrations which are adequate for a therapeutic response and yet, when the medicament finally sweeps into the systemic circulation, the blood volume will so dilute it that undesirable pharmacological effects remain negligible. In addition, of course, there are many traditional, valuable dermatological medicaments which we can only apply topically, for example, tar, ichthammol, or dithranol.

The third approach is to use the skin deliberately as a portal of entry into the systemic circulation. The transdermal therapeutic system aims to provide systemic therapy for acute or chronic conditions which do not involve the skin; the transderm employs the percutaneous route instead of the more traditional oral, parenteral, pulmonary, or rectal routes. Further details are in Chap. 4, Sec. III.D.4.

We have seen, in Sec. II, that the skin develops in anatomic strata and that to a first approximation we can locate within individual layers many of the main diseases and disorders which we hope to treat (as outlined in Sec. IV). This correlation of derangements with strata is important, as it suggests that we may be able to devise a scheme which aligns our therapeutic approach with the anatomic structure of the integument. As Flynn (1979) points out, a formulation pharmacist should ask some general questions concerning any drug, preparation, or therapeutic treatment: What do we want the product to do? Where is the therapeutic target, and how accessible is it to our drug? Our general aim is the usual pharmacokinetic intention that we should try to deliver the correct pharmacological agent to the specific site in the tissue at the optimal concentration and over the most favorable time scale. However, it is worth remarking that in dermatological therapy we may not know the precise cellular or subcellular target which we must reach for maximum beneficial effect. To some extent, we often shoot blind.

At the anatomic level, we aim at five main target regions in dermatology: (1) the external objective of the skin surface; (2) the dead stratum corneum or horny layer; (3) the viable epidermis and upper dermis; (4) the skin glands; and (5) the target of the systemic circulation (Fig. 1.2). As the focus of attention moves from the skin surface toward the systemic circulation, so the receptor sites become more remote and inaccessible and pharmacological effects become more unpredictable. We will briefly survey some of the biopharmaceutical principles relevant to a therapeutic assault on these targets, so that we can lay the groundwork for the remainder of this book. The excellent review of Flynn (1979) provides a suitable framework for our commentary.

A. Surface Treatment

We can minister to the skin surface in three main ways: a simple camouflage or cosmetic application, the formation of a protective film or layer, and an assault on surface bacteria and fungi.

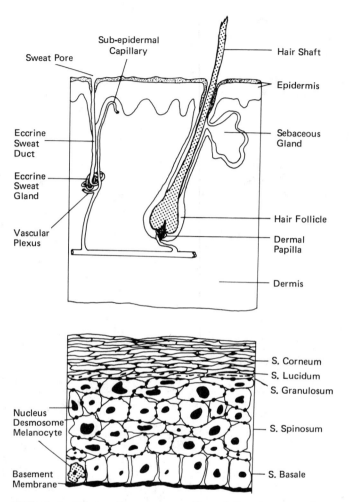

FIG. 1.2 Schematic cross-section of the skin, much simplified. The full-thickness skin is illustrated at the top, and an expansion of the epidermis is shown below. (From Dugard, 1969.)

Disfiguring lesions of the exposed skin may psychologically devastate a patient, even to the extent that an abnormality may lead to the person's social ostracism. When physicians and surgeons cannot eradicate such derangements, the patient may cover or disguise them, e.g., port wine nevi (birthmarks) and scars. Dihydroxyacetone, potassium permanganate, pickled walnut juice, or a mixture of these can disguise depigmented areas of the skin. For camouflage, the patient may blend two or more creams on the skin and then cover the area with face powder (Calnan, 1963). Of course, we may look upon simple cosmetics as forms of camouflage; such preparations enter the realms of therapy when they cause sensitization and contact dermatitis.

An example of a protective film is one which incorporates materials to absorb irritating chemicals, for example, protective pastes which absorb and neutralize the ammonia that bacteria release from infants' urine. For fair-skinned people in sunny climes, topically applied agents may protect the skin from the actinic rays in two ways: screens absorb light at specific wavelengths, and barriers ("shades"), which are opaque, reflect the radiation. Chemical screens include mexenone, para-aminobenzoic acid, quinine, salicylate esters, cinnamic acid and its compounds, and the coumarins; their protective action continues after the material diffuses into the stratum corneum. Examples of barriers include titanium dioxide or zinc oxide and red veterinary petrolatum (Alexander, 1973; MacLeod and Frain-Bell, 1971, 1975).

Another type of protective barrier hinders moisture loss from the skin and averts chapping (e.g., hydrocarbons such as petrolatum), or the application reduces friction (e.g., powder or silicone oil).

During World War II, scientists tested thousands of compounds to find the ideal insect repellent and investigated the mechanisms by which chemicals attract or repel insects (Brown, 1951; Dethin, 1947; Gilbert, 1966). We have yet to find the ideal repellent: it should remain effective for many hours and be neither an irritant nor a sensitizer. The duration of efficacy of commercially available repellents, such as dimethyl phthalate, dimethyl carbate, 2-ethyl-1,3-hexanediol, or indalone, reduces at high temperatures and in high wind velocities. Frequent applications, at intervals of not more than 3 or 4 hr, are needed.

For topical antibiotics, antiseptics, and deodorants, the surface bacteria and fungi are the therapeutic target and effective surface bioavailability is important. The formulation must release the medicament so that the antimicrobial may penetrate the surface microcracks and fissures of the skin to attack the microorganisms which lurk there. The molecules dissolve in the topical preparation (if the agent is in the form of a suspension), diffuse through the formulation matrix, and release onto the dry skin surface (or moist axillae in the case of deodorants). Only then can the bacteria and fungi take up the antimicrobial and be destroyed. Developmental studies should at least confirm that the formulation releases the active medicament and does not bind to the agent. Higuchi (1960) derived the mathematical treatment which is of most practical value for these release studies. His formal models assume that drug diffusion within the vehicle phase provides the rate controlling step in the release mechanics. Further details are presented in Chap. 4, Secs. III.D.1, 2, and 3.

B. Stratum Corneum Treatment

In the main two therapeutic activities aimed at the horny layer we try to improve emolliency and to stimulate sloughing (keratosis).

Water-impermeable films hydrate the stratum corneum and thereby increase its pliability, by inhibiting transepidermal water loss. Topical applications may also deposit "moisturizing agents" within the horny layer (see also Chap. 4, Secs. III.B.1 and III.C.1).

Salicylic acid, the classic keratolytic, seems to reduce intercellular stickiness within the stratum corneum by directly solubilizing the intercellular cement, and so causing disintegration and sloughing (Davies and Marks, 1976; Huber and Christophers, 1977). α-Hydroxy acids, propylene glycol, and sulfur are also effective.

The introduction of moisturizing agents and keratolytics into the layers of the stratum corneum involves two steps of the overall process of percutaneous absorption: (1) release of the active agent from the vehicle, and (2) penetration into the rather impermeable stratum corneum. Ideally, the medicament should not proceed further but should stop at the viable level of the skin. However, in general, only very hydrophobic drugs would not cross the viable-nonviable interface in reasonable amounts, once they had breached the horny layer.

C. Skin Appendage Treatment

We may treat hyperhidrosis of the sweat glands with antiperspirants such as aluminum salts or other metal salts, for example, aluminum chloride and aluminum hydroxychloride. Antiperspirants damage the eccrine gland reversibly, but there is little evidence that they have much effect on apocrine glands. Patients may absorb atropine-like drugs in amounts sufficient to produce a beneficial local effect without initiating systemic side effects, but the treatment is unreliable.

Acne, a condition which affects the pilsebaceous unit, is a malicious disease of adolescence. The condition may range from simple acne vulgaris, in which the patient suffers the minor irritation of the occasional blackhead and pimple, to the misery of acne conglobata, a searing, scarring disease with its horrendous variations of explosive facial acne of adult females, and tropical acne. Acne fulminans is a ferocious variety of acne with excrutiatingly tender lesions, and there are several more types which scourge the afflicted (Plewig and Kligman, 1975).

Acne patients tend to wash frequently, sometimes becoming so fanatical that they scrub themselves with soap and water as often as 8 or 10 times daily. However, there is no scientific evidence that frequent washing helps acne nor that lack of bathing worsens the condition. The most frenetic cleansing only removes surface lipids, a process which is virtually complete within half a minute. The water does not reach the deep recesses of the hair follicle where the acne organism, Propionibacterium acnes or Corynebacterium acnes, multiplies. Repeated washing with bactericidal soaps containing agents such as hexachlorophene, tricarbanilides, and chlorinated salicylanilides may reduce surface aerobic flora, but the scrubbing has no effect on the real culprit which proliferates in its follicular sanctuary.

We can use topical exfoliants in acne, such as salicylic acid, tretinoin (retinoic acid), and benzoyl peroxide. A recent introduction to the clinic is topical tetracycline in the form of Topicycline, a preparation designed to enhance the skin penetration of the antibiotic. Other topical antibiotics used to treat acne are erythromycin and clindamycin (Taplin, 1972; Wilkinson, 1979b).

Depilatories, which remove hair at the skin level, usually contain strontium or barium sulfide or thioglycollates. In addition to their cosmetic use, they are valuable in the treatment of hirsutism.

We can treat fungal diseases of the nails, together with such infections of other keratin-rich sites (stratum corneum and hair), with topical clotrimazole, miconazole, and thiabendazole.

A particular problem with skin appendage treatment is to ensure that the active ingredient penetrates to the actual site of the disease. For example, it is not easy for the treatment to achieve a high concentration of an antibiotic in a sebaceous gland when, as in acne, a horny accretion blocks the pilosebaceous follicle. Applied percutaneously, the drug may not be sufficiently hydrophobic to partition from the water-rich viable epidermis and dermis into the sebum-filled gland.

D. Viable Epidermis and Dermis Treatment

The analysis of the possible ways in which a topical drug may reach the viable epidermis and the upper dermis, and in what relative amounts, is quite complicated. In general, a molecule may penetrate to the viable tissue below the horny layer via three potential routes of entry: The medicament may pass through the pilosebacious unit or the sweat duct, or the diffusant may traverse the intact stratum corneum which lies between these appendages. Chapter 3 discusses these possible penetration pathways in more detail.

We may treat many disease states by topical application, provided that the formulation delivers drug to the site of action in sufficient amounts over a suitable time scale. However, we cannot use many potentially valuable drugs in topical therapy because they cannot cross the impermeable stratum corneum in sufficient quantities. Hence, investigators have a continuing interest in attempting to circumvent the unfavorable physicochemical properties of these drugs by developing "penetration enhancers." Such materials temporarily and reversibly diminish the barrier function of the stratum

corneum so that the weakened horny layer allows the percutaneous absorption of drugs (for further details, see Chap. 4, Sec. III. C). Another approach is for scientists to develop pro-drugs which will reach the receptor
site readily, there to release the pharmacologically active fragment of the
compound (Higuchi and Stella, 1975). The efficacy of many of the topical
steroids depends, at least in part, on the addition to the molecule of groups
which promote percutaneous absorption but which do not specifically enhance drug-receptor binding.

Examples of drug treatment at the viable tissue level include topical
steroidal and nonsteroidal agents for treating the inflamed tissues of many
dermatoses. Corticosteroids may also be used in psoriasis. Anesthetic
drugs like benzocaine reduce pain, and antipruritics and antihistamines
alleviate itch. Dermatologists may use topical 5-fluorouracil and methotrexate to selectively eradicate premalignant and some malignant skin
tumors and to treat psoriasis (Wilkinson, 1979b; Stoughton, 1974; Weinstein,
1972).

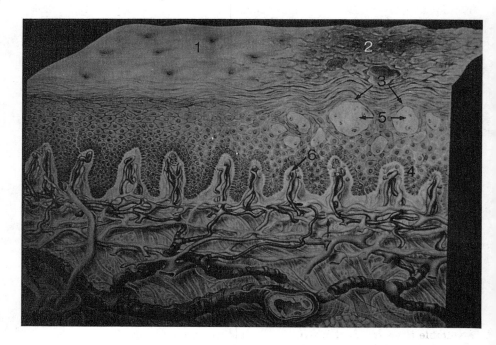

FIG. 1.3 Development of eczema vulgaris—the acute stage. Key: (1) normal
skin; (2) acute eczematous region; (3) papulovesicles; (4) interstitial serous
edema; (5) spongiosis and vesicles; (6) perivascular infiltration of lymphocytes; (7) dermal nerves. (Reproduced with the kind permission of I.C.I.
Pharmaceuticals Ltd.)

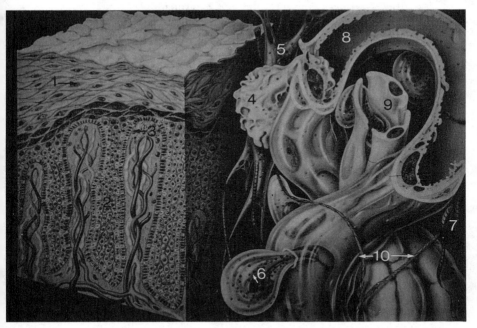

FIG. 1.4 Psoriasis—typical pathology of the disease. Key: (1) nucleated silver/gray psoriatic scales; (2) hypertrophied malpighian layer and elongated epidermal columns; (3) dilated vessels in the papilliary layer, with perivascular edema and infiltration by lymphocytes and histiocytes; (4) lymphocyte; (5) histiocyte; (6) granulocyte; (7) disintegrated collagen fibers; (8) capillary loops, which are abnormally elongated in the psoriatic plaque; (9) lymph capillary; (10) elastic fibers. (Reproduced with the kind permission of I.C.I. Pharmaceuticals Ltd.)

We may gain some concept of how two common skin complaints, eczema and psoriasis, derange the target organ by examining Figs. 1.3 and 1.4. The symptoms of acute eczema are erythema with indistinct margins, papulovesicles, vesicles, weeping, crusts, and—in the presence of secondary infection—pustules. In psoriasis, characteristic silver-gray scales overlie a hypertrophic malpighian layer and the epidermal columns are unusually long. Removal of the scales damages not only the epidermis but also the underlying capillaries, resulting in a characteristic punctate bleeding point.

E. Systemic Treatment via Percutaneous Absorption

In general, we do not use the healthy skin as a route for mounting a systemic attack on disease. Mainly, this is because the body not only absorbs
drugs slowly through the intact stratum corneum but it also assimilates
medicaments incompletely, as much of the preparation is lost by washing,
by adherence to clothes, and by shedding with stratum corneum scales. In
contrast to the 100% efficient parenteral route and the oral route, which

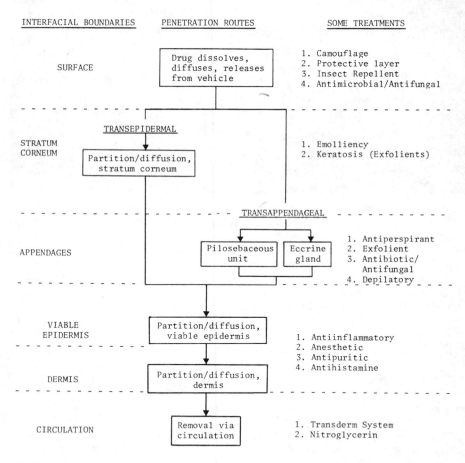

FIG. 1.5 The routes by which drugs penetrate the skin, and examples of
treatments appropriate to disorders of the various strata. Chapter 3 provides more details as to the routes of penetration, and Sec. I of Chap. 4
discusses the stages in percutaneous absorption.

may be almost as effective, the topical path may allow only a tiny fraction of a slowly diffusing drug such as a steroid to gain the systemic circulation. Other drawbacks that militate against percutaneous absorption for systemic therapy include the marked variations in the permeability of the human skin with site, age, and condition (see Chap. 4, Sec. II). Such permutations may make control difficult.

However, some investigators do use the skin route for systemic therapy, as in the treatment of motion sickness with scopolamine incorporated in the Transderm system (see Chap. 4, Sec. III.D.4). Clinicians have also controlled the pain of angina with topical applications of a 2% nitroglycerin ointment which reduced the frequency and severity of exercise-induced angina attacks and decreased the heart workload and the myocardial oxygen consumption (Parker et al., 1976; Davidov and Mroczek, 1976; Armstrong et al., 1976; Horhota and Fung, 1978, 1979; Karsh et al., 1978; Noonan and Wester, 1980).

Figure 1.5 shows diagrammatically the penetration routes available to drugs undergoing percutaneous absorption, together with examples of therapeutic treatments appropriate to disorders of the various skin strata.

VI. TOPICAL AGENTS USED IN DERMATOLOGY

Patients use a wide variety of medicaments in topical therapy, and many have been in the physician's arsenal for decades. This section is a brief, condensed review of those mainly traditional medicaments in common use. Further details on dermatological medication may be found in the texts of Brown (1970), Polano (1952), Wilkinson (1979b), Rook et al. (1979), and Wade and Reynolds (1977). Recent reviews include those of McKenzie and Wilkinson (1977c) and Ive and Comaish (1980).

A. Germicides and Antibacterial Agents

The following subsection is based on the work of Esplin (1970), Polano (1952), and Reddish (1957).

1. General

This category includes:

1. Phenols [phenol, cresol, thymol, chloroxylenol, resorcinol, pyrogallic acid, hexachlorophene—fallen into disfavor, to some extent undeservedly, because of its toxicity in babies when used in exceptional conditions; see McKenzie and Wilkinson (1977a) and Pluechahn (1973)]
2. Alcohols
3. Aldehydes (formaldehyde solution—formalin, hexamethylene tetramine—liberates formaldehyde)

4. Acids (benzoic, boric, acetic)
5. Halogens and halogenated compounds [iodine, iodoform (releases iodine, now little used), iodophors (liberates iodine), povidone-iodine (a complex between iodine and polyvinylpyrrolidone which has replaced hexachlorophene in several situations), hypochlorite, chlorhexidine (natural successor to hexachlorophene), hydroxyquinolines, i.e., chinosol, halquinol, chlorquinaldol, floraquin, diodoquin, chiniofon, clioquinol, chinoform, vioform)
6. Oxidizing agents (hydrogen peroxide, zinc peroxide, potassium permanganate)
7. Metals and their compounds (organic mercurials, lead subacetate, selenium disulfide, silver sulfadiazine, silver nitrate, zinc chloride, sulfate, and oxide)
8. Surface active agents (anionic, nonionic, amphoteric, and cationic—bactericidal; benzalkonium chloride, cetrimide, domiphen bromide, dequalinium chloride)
9. Dyes (azo, acridine, fluorescein and triphenylmethane dyes, methylene blue)
10. Miscellaneous agents [sulfur, ichthammol, chrysarobin, anthralin, polynoxylin (polyoxymethylene urea, a condensation product of formaldehyde and urea), cyclic salicylanilides)]

2. Topical antibiotics

This category includes penicillin and streptomycin (although used by surgeons, they are potent sensitizers of the skin), neomycin, framycetin, gramicidin, sodium fucidate, gentimycin sulfate, polymyxin B, and—particularly in the treatment of acne—tetracycline hydrochloride, erythromycin, and clindamycin.

3. Topical antifungals

This group includes sodium propionate, undecylenic acid and its zinc salt, tolnaftate, salicylanilide, acrisorcin, benzoic and salicylic acids, gentian violet, potassium permanganate, phenolic compounds, imidazoles (miconazole, clotrimazole, thiabendazole), nystatin, and candicidin.

4. Insect repellents and parasiticides

See Rook (1979), Dethin (1947), and Feldmann and Maibach (1970):

1. Repellents [dimethylphthalate, diethyltoluamide (deet), indalone, dimethyl carbate, 2-ethyl-1,3-hexanediol]
2. Parasiticides (benzylbenzoate, gamma benzene hexachloride, monosulfiram, crotamiton, malathion)

B. Anti-inflammatory Agents

This category comprises the topical corticosteroids (McKenzie and Wilkinson, 1977b; Munro and Wilson, 1976; Polano, 1973a; Wilson and Marks, 1976)—a wide range of compounds which may be grouped into four categories (Monthly Index of Medical Specialities, 1978):

Group I. Extremely potent (e.g., clobetasol propionate 0.05%, halcinonide 0.1%)

Group II. Potent—most fluorinated preparations (e.g., betamethasone valerate 0.1%, fluocinolone acetonide 0.025%, triamcinolone acetonide 0.025%, 1%)

Group III. Moderately potent (e.g., clobetasol butyrate 0.05%, dexamethasone 0.01%)

Group IV. Less potent (e.g., hydrocortisone alcohol or acetate, 0.1-2.5%, methyl prednisolone 0.025%)

Misuse of potent topical steroids can lead to suppression of the pituitary-adrenal function, atrophic changes, gluteal granulomas, leukoderma, and pustular psoriasis, and also to the masking of the clinical features of primary disease (Wilkinson, 1977b).

Nonsteroidal anti-inflammatories include bufexamac and benzydamine.

C. Antihistamines

The public uses topical antihistamines widely, although dermatologists condemn them because of contact sensitization. Examples include chlorcyclizine hydrochloride, diphenhydramine hydrochloride, mepyramine maleate, and phenindamine tartrate.

D. Antipuritics and Local Anesthetics

Local anesthetics of the ester type include amethocaine, benzocaine, and cocaine, with the amide type represented by cinchocaine, lignocaine, and prilocaine. Other drugs with local anesthetic activity include benzyl alcohol, chlorbutol, camphor, menthol, phenol, pramoxine hydrochloride, dimethisoquin hydrochloride, and some antihistamines.

E. Cytotoxic Agents

Physicians prescribe a number of topical cytotoxic agents to eradicate both superficial malignant conditions of the skin as well as to treat benign, proliferative conditions. Drugs include 5-fluorouracil, podophyllin, colchicine, methotrexate, nitrogen mustard, nitrosourea, and dinitrochlorobenzene. See Belisario (1964), Polano (1973b), and Zubroid (1967).

F. Antiperspirants

Aluminum chloride and aluminum hydroxychloride form the mainstay of commercial antiperspirants. Formalin (formaldehyde solution), methenamine, glutaraldehyde, and the anticholinergic agents homatropine methyl bromide and propantheline bromide have also been used. See Polano (1973c) and Shelley and Hurley (1958, 1975).

G. Astringents

Mild astringents cause the pores of the skin to close. Strong astringents in high concentrations precipitate proteins and, on mucous membranes or damaged skin, form a superficial protective layer; the body does not usually absorb them. Astringents harden the skin and check exudates and minor hemorrhages. The main agents are tannins (tannic acid) and salts of aluminum (alum, acetate, acetotartrate, subacetate, chloride, sulfate) and zinc (chloride and sulfate).

H. Keratolytics and Caustics

Agents such as benzoic acid, salicylic acid, resorcinol, and various thiols soften keratin and loosen cornified epithelium. α-Hydroxy acids (citric, glycolic, lactic, malic, pyruvic, and glucuronic), silver nitrate, and sulfur act similarly.

I.   Keratoplastic Agents

Keratoplastic agents soften and restore keratin: coal tar is used in atopic dermatitis, chronic eczema, and psoriasis; vitamin A acid (tretinoin) is employed in acne; and protagonists for urea claim that it is a moisturizer and penetration enhancer. We do not completely understand the mode of action of dithranol and its triacetate in psoriasis.

J. Rubefacients

These topical vasodilators are mainly the nicotinates (methyl, ethyl, butoxyethyl, phenethyl, and thurfyl) and the essential oils (such as mustard, turpentine, cajuput, and capsicum).

K. Pigmenting and Depigmenting Agents

The psoralens, applied topically or taken orally, are photoactive furocou-
marins which increase the production of melanin on exposure to UV light.
Dermatologists therefore use them to treat vitiligo. Trimethoxypsoralen
and 8-methoxypsoralen are also used; the latter moreover is valuable in the
treatment of psoriasis [PUVA (psoralen plus long-wave UV light) therapy]
and mycosis fungoides.

Hydroquinone and its monobenzyl ether interfere with the biosynthesis
of melanin; they are used as depigmenting agents, particularly in cosmetic
preparations.

L. Sunscreens

Sunscreens may be barriers (titanium dioxide, zinc oxide, red veterinary
petrolatum) or screens (p-aminobenzoic acid, quinine, salicylate esters,
cinnamates, anthranilates, mexenone, and naphthol sulfonic acids). See
MacLeod and Frain-Bell (1971, 1975) and Alexander (1973).

M. Epilatories and Depilatories

Epilation refers to the complete removal of the hair from the follicle
(plucking or wax treatment); depilation acts at skin level (strontium or
barium sulfide, thioglycollic acid).

N. Miscellaneous

There is a wide variety of emollients (oils, fats, hydrocarbons, waxes),
demulcents (gums, mucilages, starches), protectives, and absorbents
(dusting powders—talc, zinc oxide, zinc stearate, magnesium stearate,
starch, boric acid, insoluble bismuth salts; collodions, zinc gelatin,
dimethicone) and surfactants (anionic, cationic, nonionic, amphoteric).

VII. GLOSSARY OF DERMATOLOGICAL TERMS

This chapter concludes with a collection of brief definitions of some anatomic, physiological, and pathophysiological terms. The purpose is to
orientate readers not familiar with dermatology. For precise medical definitions, together with descriptions of the state, the body part affected, and
the etiology if known, the reader may consult standard medical dictionaries
and dermatology textbooks.

Acantholysis	Detachment of epidermal cells
Acanthosis	Increase in number of cells in the prickle-cell layer (malpighian layer)
Acne	Chronic inflammatory disease, characterized by comedones, papules, pustules, and sometimes cysts, involving the sebaceous glands and follicles
Alopecia	Lack of hair
Anhidrosis	Absence of sweat
Atopy	Marked familial tendency to allergic diseases
Atrophy	Characterized by loss of normal skin markings
Boil	Acute, painful infection of a hair follicle
Bulla	Large vesicle or blister filled with serous fluid
Callosity	Circumscribed plaques of hyperkeratosis
Carbuncle	Conglomerated mass of boils
Cheloid	Overgrowth of connective tissue
Chilblain	Itchy, red, or nodular lesion resulting from hyperactivity of the peripheral vessels in response to cold
Chloracne	Acne induced by organic chlorine compounds
Chloasma	Brownish patches on the skin
Comedo	Horny plug filling the orifice of a pilosebaceous
(pl. Comedones)	follicle (closed—whitehead; open—blackhead)
Corn	Local callosity
Crust	Dried serum and other exudates
Dermatitis	Inflammatory condition of the skin, used synonymously for eczema
Dermatitis Herpetiformis	Chronic condition characterized by grouped macules, papules, vesicles and bullae
Dermatoglyphics	Ridges in hairless skin (fingerprints)
Desmosome	Attachment plaque on cells
Dyskeratosis	Faulty keratinization with prematurely keratinized cells
Dysplasia	Congenital cellular changes in the epidermis
Eczema	Inflammatory condition of the skin (synonym: dermatitis)
Excoriation	Scratch causing bleeding
Fibroblast	Cell of loose connective tissue
Fibroma	Small, painless, well-defined nodule, usually found on the extremities in adults
Folliculitis	Infection of the hair follicles
Freckles	Yellow or brown spots
Furunculosis	Acute, usually necrotic infection of a hair follicle
Granulosis	Thickening of the granular-cell layer, as in lichen planus
Herpes Simplex	Viral infection producing grouped vesicles on red base, usually affecting lips, face, or genitalia

Herpes Zoster	Viral infection of nerves producing groups of vesicles (shingles)
Hirsutism	Abnormal, excessive hair
Hyperhidrosis	Excessive production of sweat
Hyperkeratosis	Overgrowth of the horny layer (e.g., corn)
Ichthyosis	Disease characterized by dry, rough, scaly skin (Greek: ichthus—fish)
Impetigo	Contagious superficial infection of the skin
Keloid	Overgrowth of connective tissue
Keratinocyte	Cell in the epidermis which produces keratin to construct the horny layer
Keratosis	Any horny growth
Lentigo	Small, brown, circular, or irregular macule
Leucoderma	Skin disease with light-colored (pigment-free) patches (vitiligo)
Lichenification	Acanthosis and hyperkeratosis arising from repeated rubbing of predisposed skin
Lichen Planus	Inflammatory disease with wide, shiny, flat papules
Lupus Erythematosus	Inflammation of the skin with disklike patches covered with scales or crusts
Macule	Flat, circumscribed, discolored lesion
Melanocytes	Cells which produce melanin
Miliaria	Acute inflammation of sweat glands, with pinpoint- to pinhead-sized vesicles and papules (prickly heat)
Mole	A pigmented nevus
Nevus	Circumscribed developmental defect of the skin
Nodule	Small node, solid to the touch
Papilla	Small, nipple-shaped elevation
Papule	Raised, firm circumscribed lesion
Parakeratosis	Retention of nuclei in cells of the horny layer; occurs in psoriasis and other scaly conditions
Pemphigus	Chronic disorder characterized by recurrent bullae
Pityriasis Rosea	Mild inflammatory disease characterized by macules and maculopapular lesions, which are slightly scaly
Plaque	A disk-shaped lesion
Psoriasis	Skin disease characterized by scaly red patches
Pustule	Small elevation of skin filled with pus
Rete Ridges	Thickened epidermal ridges which project into the dermis
Ringworm	Superficial infection of skin, hair, or nails by the fungus Tinea

Rosacea	Chronic inflammatory disorder of the central area of the face, usually seen with acneiform lesions and telangiectases
Scabies	Contagious disease caused by infestation by the mite Sarcoptes scabiei, characterized by intra-epidermal burrows and follicular papules, and severe itching which is worse at night
Scale	Accumulation of excess normal or abnormal keratin
Scleroderma	Disease of the skin with thickening of dermal tissue and pigmented patches
Seborrhea	Excessive activity of sebaceous glands
Sebum	Lipid secretion of the sebaceous gland
Shingles	See Herpes Zoster
Spongiosis	Intercellular edema
Striae	Atrophied strips of skin
Sweat	Secretion of the eccrine glands
Telangiectases	Literally "end vessel dilations"; permanently dilated small vessels apparent on the skin
Ulcer	More or less circumscribed loss of tissue
Urticaria	Transient weals and papules, accompanied by itching and prickling sensations (nettle rash)
Vesicle	Small sac containing fluid (blister)
Verruca	Small, solid growths arising from the surface of the skin caused by viral infection (wart)
Vitiligo	Skin disease with light-colored (pigment-free) patches (leukoderma)
Wart	See Verruca
Weal	Area of dermal edema
Wrinkle	Degeneration of elastic tissue and atrophy of the skin (particularly on the face); as a disorder of connective tissue, it is not helped by "moisturizers"

REFERENCES

Alexander, P. (1973). In Harry's Cosmeticology, J. B. Wilkinson (Ed.), 6th ed. Hill, London, p. 306.

Armstrong, P. W., Matthew, M. T., Boroomand, K., and Parker, J. O. (1976). Am. J. Cardiol. 38:474.

Bean, W. B. (1974). Arch. Intern. Med. 134:497.

Behl, C. R., Flynn, G. L., Kurihara, T., Smith, W., Gatmaitan, O., Higuchi, W. I., Ho, N. F. H., and Pierson, C. L. (1980). J. Invest. Dermatol. 75:340.

Belisario, J. C. (1964). Acta Derm. Venereol. (Stockh.) 44(Suppl. 56).

Berrens, L., and Young, E. (1964). Dermatologica 128:3.

Biempica, L., and Montes, L. F. (1965). Am. J. Anat. 117:47.

Blank, I. H., and Scheuplein, R. J. (1964). In Progress in the Biological Sciences in Relation to Dermatology, A. J. Rook and R. H. Champion (Eds.), 2nd ed. Cambridge Univ. Press, New York.

Branwood, A. W. (1963). Int. Rev. Connect. Tissue Res. 1:1.

Breathnack, A. S. (1965). Int. Rev. Cytol. 18:1.

Breathnack, A. S. (1968). Br. J. Dermatol. 80:688.

Breathnack, A. S., and Wyllie, L. M. (1967). Adv. Biol. Skin 8:97.

Briggaman, R. A., and Wheeler, C. E. (1973). J. Invest. Dermatol. 60:109.

Briggaman, R. A., and Wheeler, C. E. (1975). J. Invest. Dermatol. 65:71.

Briggaman, R. A., Dalldorf, F., and Wheeler, C. E. (1971). J. Cell Biol. 51:384.

Brody, I. (1960). J. Ultrastruct. Res. 4:264.

Brown, A. W. A. (1951). Insect Control by Chemicals. Chapman & Hall, London.

Brown, T. H. (1970). In Current Dermatologic Management, S. Madden (Ed.). Mosby, St. Louis, p. 267.

Bullough, W. S. (1972). Br. J. Dermatol. 87:187.

Bullough, W. S., and Laurence, E. B. (1958). In The Biology of Hair Growth, W. Montagna and R. A. Ellis (Eds.). Academic Press, New York, p. 171.

Burtenshaw, J. M. L. (1945). Br. Med. Bull. 3:731.

Calnan, C. D. (1963). Br. Med. J. i:437.

Champion, R. H. (1979a). In Textbook of Dermatology, A. Rook, D. S. Wilkinson, and F. J. G. Ebling (Eds.), 3rd ed., Vol. 1. Blackwell Sci. Publns., Oxford, England, p. 1103.

Champion, R. H. (1979b). In Textbook of Dermatology, A. Rook, D. S. Wilkinson, and F. J. G. Ebling (Eds.), 3rd ed., Vol. 2, Blackwell Sci. Publns., Oxford, England, p. 1675.

Christophers, E. (1971). J. Invest. Dermatol. 56:165.

Comaish, J. S. (1973). Lancet i:81.

Comaish, J. S., and Shelley, W. B. (1965). J. Invest. Dermatol. 44:279.

Cummins, H. (1964). In The Epidermis, W. Montagna and W. C. Lobitz, Jr. (Eds.). Academic Press, New York, p. 375.

Cummins, H., and Midlo, C. (1961). Finger-prints—Palms and Soles: An Introduction to Dermatoglyphics, 2nd ed. Dover, New York.

Cunliffe, W. J. (1979a). In Textbook of Dermatology, A. Rook, D. S. Wilkinson, and F. J. G. Ebling (Eds.), 3rd ed., Vol. 2. Blackwell Sci. Publns., Oxford, England, p. 1993.

Cunliffe, W. J. (1979b). In Textbook of Dermatology, A. Rook, D. S. Wilkinson, and F. J. G. Ebling (Eds.), 3rd ed., Vol. 2. Blackwell Sci. Publns., Oxford, England, p. 1611.

Cunliffe, W. J., and Bleehen, S. S. (1979). In Textbook of Dermatology, A. Rook, D. S. Wilkinson, and F. J. G. Ebling (Eds.), 3rd ed., Vol. 2. Blackwell Sci. Publns., Oxford, England, p. 1655.

Davidov, M. E., and Mroczek, W. J. (1976). Angiology 27:205.

Davies, M., and Marks, R. (1976). Br. J. Dermatol. 95:187.

Dethin, V. C. (1947). Chemical Insect Attractants and Repellents. Lewis, London.

De Vargos Lindres, C. E. R., and Burgos, M. H. (1964). Q. J. Exp. Physiol. 49:129.

Dobson, R. L., and Sato, K. (1970). Arch. Dermatol. 105:366.

Downing, D. T., and Strauss, J. S. (1974). J. Invest. Dermatol. 62:228.

Dugard, P. H. (1969). Ph.D. Thesis, Queen's University, Belfast, Northern Ireland.

Ebling, F. J. (1963). In Handbook of Cosmetic Science, H. W. Hibbott (Ed.) Pergamon Press, Elmsford, N.Y.

Ebling, F. J. (1976). J. Invest. Dermatol. 67:98.

Ebling, F. J. (1979a). In Textbook of Dermatology, A. Rook, D. S. Wilkinson, and F. J. G. Ebling (Eds.), 3rd ed., Vol. 2. Blackwell Sci. Publns Oxford, England, p. 1595.

Ebling, F. J. (1979b). In Textbook of Dermatology, A. Rook, D. S. Wilkinson, and F. J. G. Ebling (Eds.), 3rd ed., Vol. 1. Blackwell Sci. Publns Oxford, England, p. 5.

Ebling, F. J., and Rook, A. (1979a). In Textbook of Dermatology, A. Rook, D. S. Wilkinson, and F. J. G. Ebling (Eds.), 3rd ed., Vol. 1. Blackwell Sci. Publns., Oxford, England, p. 1733.

Ebling, F. J., and Rook, A. (1979b). In Textbook of Dermatology, A. Rook, D. S. Wilkinson, and F. J. G. Ebling (Eds.), 3rd ed., Vol. 2. Blackwell Sci. Publns., Oxford, England, p. 1691.

Elden, H. R. (1968). Adv. Biol. Skin 10:231.

Epstein, J. H. (1970). In Photophysiology, A. C. Giese (Ed.), Vol. 5. Academic Press, New York.

Epstein, W. L., and Maibach, H. I. (1965). Arch. Dermatol. 92:462.

Esplin, D. W. (1970). In The Pharmacological Basis of Therapeutics, L. S. Goodman and A. Gilman (Eds.), 4th ed. Macmillan, New York, p. 1032.

Feldmann, R. J., and Maibach, H. I. (1970). J. Invest. Dermatol. 54:399.

Fitzpatrick, T. B. (1965). Trans. St. John's Hosp. Dermatol. Soc. 51:1.

Fleischmajer, R., and Fishman, L. (1965). Nature 205:264.

Flynn, G. L. (1979). In Modern Pharmaceutics, G. S. Banker and C. T. Rhodes (Eds.), Dekker, New York, p. 263.

Foldi, M. (1969). Diseases of Lymphatics and Lymph Circulation. Thomas, Springfield, Ill.

Forslind, B. (1970). Acta Derm. Venereol. (Stockh.) 50:161.

Forslind, B., and Thyresson, N. (1975). Arch. Dermatol. Forsch. 251:199.

Freedberg, I. M., and Baden, H. P. (1962). J. Invest. Dermatol. 38:277.

Gallop, P. M. (1964). Biophys. J. 4 (Suppl.):79.

Gerber, R., and Nowak, J. (1976). In Staphylococci and Staphylococcal Diseases: Proceedings of the 3rd International Symposium on Staphylococci and Staphylococcal Infection, J. Jeljaszewicz (Ed.). Fischer-Verlag, Stuttgart, p. 1131.

Giacometti, L. (1965). Adv. Biol. Skin 6:97.

Gilbert, I. H. (1966). J. Am. Med. Assoc. 196:253.

Goldschmidt, H., and Kligman, A. M. (1964). Arch. Dermatol. 88:709.

Gordon, R. S., and Cage, G. W. (1966). Lancet i:1246.

Grice, K., and Verbov, J. (1977). Rec. Adv. Dermatol. 4:173.

Hall, D. A. (1971). In Biophysical Properties of the Skin, H. R. Elden (Ed.). Wiley (Interscience), New York, p. 187.

Halprin, K. M. (1972). J. Invest. Dermatol. 86:14.

Hamilton, J. B. (1950). Ann. N.Y. Acad. Sci. 53:461.

Hashimoto, K. (1972a). J. Anat. 111:99.

Hashimoto, K. (1972b). J. Invest Dermatol. 58:381.

Hashimoto, K., and Lever, W. (1970). Arch. Dermatol. 101:287.

Higuchi, T. (1960). J. Soc. Cosmetic Chemists 11:85.

Higuchi, T., and Stella, V., Eds. (1975). Pro-drugs as Novel Drug Delivery Systems, ACS Symposium Ser., No. 14. American Chemical Society, Washington, D.C.

Holt, S. B. (1968). The Genetics of Dermal Ridges. Thomas, Springfield, Ill.

Horhota, S. T., and Fung, H.-L. (1978). J. Pharm. Sci. 67:1345.

Horhota, S. T., and Fung, H.-L. (1979). J. Pharm. Sci. 68:608.

Huber, C., and Christophers, E. (1977). Arch. Dermatol. Res. 257:293.

Hunter, J., McVittae, E., and Comaish, J. (1974). Br. J. Dermatol. 90:481.

Hurley, H. J., and Shelley, W. B. (1960). The Human Apocrine Sweat Gland in Health and Disease. Thomas, Springfield, Ill.

Hyman, A. B., and Guiducci, A. A. (1963). Adv. Biol. Skin 4:78, 110.

Ive, A., and Comaish, S. (1980). Rec. Adv. Dermatol. 5:285.

Jackson, D. S. (1965). Adv. Biol. Skin 6:219.

Jarrett, A. (1964). In Histochemistry of Keratinization, Zool. Soc. Symposia, London, No. 12. Academic Press, New York, p. 55.

Jarrett, A. (1967). J. Invest. Dermatol. 49:443.

Jarrett, A. (1968). Arch. Biochim. Cosmetol. 115:11.

Jarrett, A. (1973). The Physiology and Pathophysiology of the Skin, Vol. 1: The Epidermis. Academic Press, New York.

Jarrett, A. (1974). In The Physiology and Pathophysiology of the Skin, Vol. 3: The Dermis and the Dendrocytes. Academic Press, New York.

Jarrett, A., and Spearman, R. I. C. (1964). Histochemistry of the Skin: Psoriasis. English Universities Press, London.

Jarrett, A., and Spearman, R. I. C. (1967). Dermatol. Dig. 6:43.

Jeanrenaud, B. (1963). Helv. Med. Acta 30:1.

Jensen, H., and Moffet, N. (1970). J. Cell Sci. 6:511.

Kahl, F., and Pearson, R. (1967). J. Invest. Dermatol. 49:616.

Karsh, D. L., Umbach, R. E., Cohen, L. S., and Langou, R. A. (1978). Am. Heart J. 96:587.

Katz, M., and Poulsen, B. J. (1971). In Handbook of Experimental Pharmacology, B. B. Brodie and J. Gillette (Eds.), Vol. 28, Pt. 1. Springer-Verlag, New York, p. 103.

Kinmonth, J. B. (1972). The Lymphatics: Diseases, Lymphography and Surgery. Arnold, London.

Kligman, A. (1963). Adv. Biol. Skin 4:110.

Kligman, A. M. (1964). In The Epidermis, W. Montagna and W. C. Lobitz (Eds.). Academic Press, New York, p. 387.

Kligman, A. M. (1969). J. Am. Med. Assoc. 210:2377.

Kligman, A. M. (1974). In Sunlight and Man, T. B. Fitzpatrick (Ed.). University of Tokyo Press, Tokyo.

Kligman, A. M., and Shehadek, N. (1964). Arch. Dermatol. 89:461.

Kuno, Y. (1956). Human Perspiration. Thomas, Springfield, Ill.

Kûstala, U., and Mustakallio, K. K. (1967). J. Invest. Dermatol. 48:466.

Lacey, R. W. (1968). J. Clin. Pathol. 21:564.

Lacey, R. W. (1969). Br. J. Dermatol. 81:435.

Lewis, T. (1927). The Blood Vessels of the Human Skin and Their Responses Shaw, London.

Lewis, M. S., and Piez, K. A. (1963). Proc. Am. Chem. Soc., New York Meeting, Sept. 9-13.

Lowe, L. B., and Van der Leun, J. C. (1968). J. Invest. Dermatol. 50:308.

Lubowe, I. I. (1959). Ann. N.Y. Acad. Sci. 83:539.

Lubowe, I. I. (1963). New Hope for Your Skin. Dutton, New York.

Lund, H. Z., and Sommerville, R. L. (1957). Am. J. Clin. Pathol. 27:183.

Lyne, A. G., and Short, B. F. (1965). Biology of the Skin and Hair Growth. Angus & Robertson, Sydney.

McKenzie, A. W., and Wilkinson, D. S. (1977a). Rec. Adv. Dermatol. 4:285.

McKenzie, A. W., and Wilkinson, D. S. (1977b). Rec. Adv. Dermatol. 4:291.

McKenzie, A. W., and Wilkinson, D. S. (1977c). Rec. Adv. Dermatol. 4:???.

MacKenzie, I. C. (1972). In Epidermal Wound Healing, H. I. Maibach and D. T. Rovee (Eds.). Year Book Med. Publs., Chicago, p. 5.

MacKenzie, I. C. (1974). J. Invest. Dermatol. 62:80.

MacLeod, T. M., and Frain-Bell, W. (1971). Br. J. Dermatol. 84:266.

MacLeod, T. M., and Frain-Bell, W. (1975). Br. J. Dermatol. 92:417.

Matoltsy, A. G., and Matoltsy, M. (1962). J. Invest. Dermatol. 38:231.

Menton, D. N., and Eisen, A. Z. (1971). J. Ultrastruct. Res. 35:247.

Mercer, E. H. (1958). In The Biology of Hair Growth, W. Montagna and
R. A. Ellis (Eds.), Academic Press, New York, p. 113.

Mercer, E. H. (1961). Keratin and Keratinization. Pergamon Press,
Elmsford, N.Y.

Mier, P. D., and Cotton, D. W. K. (1976). The Molecular Biology of Skin.
Blackwell Sci. Publns., Oxford, England.

Montagna, W. (1963). Adv. Biol. Skin 4:19.

Montagna, W. (1964). J. Invest. Dermatol. 42:119.

Montagna, W., and Dobson, R. L. (1969). Adv. Biol. Skin 9:1.

Montagna, W., and Ellis, R. A. (1958). The Biology of Hair Growth.
Academic Press, New York.

Montagna, W., and Parakkal, P. F. (1974). The Structure and Function of
Skin, 3rd ed. Academic Press, New York.

Monthly Index of Medical Specialities (1978). 20(5):206.

Muller, S. A. (1971). J. Invest. Dermatol. 56:1.

Munger, B. L. (1965). J. Cell Biol. 26:79.

Munro, D. D., and Wilson, L. (1976). Br. J. Dermatol. 94(Suppl. 12).

Mustakallio, K. K., and Küstala, U. (1967). Acta Derm. Venereol. (Stockh.)
47:323.

Niebauer, G. (1968). Dendritic Cells of Human Skin. Karger, Basel.

Niebauer, G., Krawczyk, W. S., Kidd, R. L., and Wilgram, G. F. (1969).
J. Cell Biol. 43:80.

Nikkari, T. (1974). J. Invest. Dermatol. 62:257.

Noble, W. C., and Somerville, D. A. (1974). Microbiology of Human Skin.
Saunders, Philadelphia.

Noonan, P. K., and Wester, R. C. (1980). J. Pharm. Sci. 69:365.

Odland, G. F. (1964). In The Epidermis, W. M. Montagna and W. L.
Lobitz (Eds.). Academic Press, New York, p. 237.

Page, C. O., and Rimington, J. S. (1967). J. Lab. Clin. Med. 69:634.

Parish, W. E. (1979). In Textbook of Dermatology, A. Rook, D. S. Wilkinson, and F. J. G. Ebling (Eds.), 3rd ed., Vol. 1. Blackwell Sci.
Publns., Oxford, England, p. 249.

Parker, J. O., Augustine, R. J., Burton, J. P., West, R. O., and
Armstrong, P. W. (1976). Am. J. Cardiol. 38:162.

Partridge, S. M. (1970a). In Chemistry and Molecular Biology of the Intercellular Matrix, E. A. Balazs (Ed.), Vol. 1. Academic Press, New
York, p. 593.

Partridge, S. M. (1970b). Adv. Biol. Skin 10:357.

Peachy, R. D. G. (1971a). Br. J. Dermatol. 84:435.

Peachy, R. D. G. (1971b). Br. J. Dermatol. 84:447.

Pearson, R., Potter, B., and Strauss, F. (1974). Arch. Dermatol. 109:
349.

Peck, S. M., and Russ, W. R. (1947). Arch. Dermatol. Syphilol. 56:601.

Piez, K. A. (1967). In Treatise on Collagen, G. M. Ramachandran (Ed.),
Vol. 1. Academic Press, New York, p. 207.

Pinkus, H. (1951). J. Invest. Dermatol. 16:383.
Pinkus, H. (1952). J. Invest. Dermatol. 19:431.
Plewig, G., and Kligman, A. M. (1975). Acne: Morphogenesis and Treatment. Springer-Verlag, New York.
Plewig, G., and Marples, R. (1970). J. Invest. Dermatol. 54:13.
Pluechahn, V. D. (1973). Med. J. Aust. 1:860.
Polano, M. K. (1952). Skin Therapeutics. Elsevier, New York.
Polano, M. K. (1973a). Rec. Adv. Dermatol. 3:291.
Polano, M. K. (1973b). Rec. Adv. Dermatol. 3:372.
Polano, M. K. (1973c). Rec. Adv. Dermatol. 3:399.
Porter, K. R. (1964). Biophys. J. 4(Suppl.):167.
Potten, C. S. (1975). J. Invest. Dermatol. 65:488.
Prunieras, M. (1968). J. Invest. Dermatol. 52:1.
Ramsay, C. A. (1979). In Textbook of Dermatology, A. Rook, D. S. Wilkinson, and F. J. G. Ebling (Eds.), 3rd ed., Vol. 1. Blackwell Sci. Publns., Oxford, England, p. 523.
Reaven, E. P., and Cox, A. J. (1965). J. Invest. Dermatol. 45:422.
Reddish, G. F. (1957). Antiseptics, Disinfectants, Fungicides and Chemical and Physical Sterilization. Lea & Febiger, Philadelphia.
Renold, A. E., and Cahill, G. F. (1965). Adipose tissue. In Handbook of Physiology, Sec. 5. Churchill Livingstone, Edinburgh and London.
Riley, P. A. (1974). In The Physiology and Pathophysiology of the Skin. Vol. 3: The Dermis and the Dendrocytes, A. Jarrett (Ed.). Academic Press, New York, pp. 1104, 1219.
Robinson, S., and Robinson, A. H. (1954). Physiol. Rev. 34:202.
Rook, A. (1965). Br. Med. J. i:609.
Rook, A. (1979). In Textbook of Dermatology, A. Rook, D. S. Wilkinson, and F. J. G. Ebling (Eds.), 3rd ed., Vol. 2. Blackwell Sci. Publns., Oxford, England, p. 911.
Rook, A., Wilkinson, D. S., and Ebling, F. J. G., Eds. (1979). Textbook of Dermatology, 3rd ed., 2 vols. Blackwell Sci. Publns., Oxford, England.
Ross, R., and Bernstein, P. (1969). J. Cell Biol. 40:366.
Rothberg, S., Crounse, R. G., and Lee, J. L. (1961). J. Invest. Dermatol. 37:497.
Rothman, S. (1954). Physiology and Biochemistry of the Skin. Univ. of Chicago Press, Chicago.
Rubin, L. (1949). J. Invest. Dermatol. 47:456.
Rudall, K. M. (1964). In Progress in the Biological Sciences in Relation to Dermatology, A. Rook and R. H. Champion (Eds.), Vol. 2. Cambridge Univ. Press, New York, p. 355.
Rushmer, R. F., Buettner, K. J. K., Short, J. M., and Odland, G. F. (1966). Science 154:343.
Samman, P. D. (1979). In Textbook of Dermatology, A. Rook, D. S. Wilkinson, and F. J. G. Ebling (Eds.), 3rd ed., Vol. 2. Blackwell Sci. Publns., Oxford, England, p. 1825.

Sandberg, L. B., Weissman, N., and Gray, W. R. (1971). Biochemistry 10:52.
Sanderson, K. V., and Mackie, R. (1979). In Textbook of Dermatology, A. Rook, D. S. Wilkins, and F. J. G. Ebling (Eds.), 3rd ed., Vol. 2. Blackwell Sci. Publns., Oxford, England, p. 2129.
Sato, K. (1977). Rev. Physiol. Biochem. Pharmacol. 79:51.
Schellander, F., and Marks, R. (1973). Br. J. Dermatol. 88:563.
Scheuplein, R. J. (1967). J. Invest. Dermatol. 48:79.
Scheuplein, R. J., and Blank, I. H. (1971). Physiol. Rev. 51:702.
Schmidt-Nielsen, K. (1964). Desert Animals: Physiological Problems of Heat and Water. Oxford Univ. Press, New York.
Schmitt, F. O., Gross, J., and Highberger, J. H. (1955). Symp. Soc. Exp. Biol. 9:148.
Schreiner, E., and Wolff, K. (1969). Arch. Clin. Exp. Dermatol. 235:78.
Selwyn, S. (1975). Br. J. Dermatol. 93:487.
Selwyn, S., Marsh, P. D., and Sethna, T. N. (1976). In Chemotherapy, J. D. Williams and A. M. Geddes (Ed.), Vol. 5. Plenum Press, New York, p. 391.
Sevitt, S. (1957). Burns: Pathology and Therapeutic Applications. Butterworths, London, p. 321.
Shelley, W. B., and Hurley, H. J. (1958). Br. J. Dermatol. 70:45.
Shelley, W. B., and Hurley, H. J. (1975). Acta Derm. Venereol. (Stockh.) 55:241.
Smith, J. G., and Finlayson, G. R. (1965). J. Soc. Cosmetic Chemists 16:527.
Spearman, R. I. C. (1966). Biol. Rev. 41:59.
Squier, C. A. (1973). J. Ultrastruct. Res. 43:160.
Stoughton, R. B. (1974). Clin. Pharmacol. Ther. 16:869.
Sulzberger, M. B. (1952). Arch. Dermatol. Syphilol. 66:172.
Szabo, G. (1962). Adv. Biol. Skin 3:1.
Szabo, G. (1967). Phil. Trans. R. Soc. London, Ser. B 252:447.
Szabo, G. (1968). Adv. Biol. Skin 9:33.
Taplin, D. (1972). Adv. Biol. Skin 12:315.
Thayson, J. H., and Schwartz, I. L. (1953). J. Exp. Med. 98:261.
Thiele, F. A. J., Mier, P. D., and Reay, D. A. (1974). Bibl. Radiol. 6:140.
Thomas, J., Elsden, D. F., and Partridge, S. M. (1963). Nature 200:651.
Tregear, R. T. (1966). Physical Functions of Skin. Academic Press, New York.
Van der Leun, J. C., Lowe, L., and Beerens, E. (1974). J. Invest. Dermatol. 62:42.
Verbov, J. (1968). Br. J. Clin. Pract. 22:257.
Verbov, J. (1970). J. Invest. Dermatol. 54:261.
Verzar, F. (1964). Int. Rev. Connect. Tissue Res. 2:244.
Wade, A., and Reynolds, J. E. F., Eds. (1977). Martindale: The Extra Pharmacopoeia, 27th ed. Pharmaceutical Press, London.

Weiner, N. (1948). Cybernetics. Chapman & Hall, London.

Weinstein, G. D. (1972). Adv. Biol. Skin. 12:287.

Weinstein, G. D., and Frost, P. (1971). In Dermatology in General Medicine Replacement Kinetics, T. B. Fitzpatrick, K. A. Arndt, W. D. Clark, A. Z. Eisen, E. J. Van Scott, and J. H. Vaughan (Eds.), McGraw-Hill, New York, p. 78.

Weinstein, G. D., and Van Scott, E. J. (1965). J. Invest. Dermatol. 45: 257.

Wells, F. V., and Lubowe, I. I. (1964). Cosmetics and the Skin. Van Nostrand Reinhold, New York.

Wilkes, G. L., Brown, I. A., and Wildnauer, R. H. (1973). CRC Crit. Rev. Bioeng. p. 453.

Wilkinson, D. S. (1979a). In Textbook of Dermatology, A. Rook, D. S. Wilkinson, and F. J. G. Ebling (Eds.), 3rd ed., Vol. 1. Blackwell Sci. Publns., Oxford, England, p. 485.

Wilkinson, D. S. (1979b). In Textbook of Dermatology, A. Rook, D. S. Wilkinson, and F. J. G. Ebling (Eds.), 3rd ed., Vol. 2. Blackwell Sci. Publns., Oxford, England, p. 2293.

Wilson, L., and Marks, R. (1976). Mechanisms of Topical Corticosteroid Activity. Churchill Livingstone, Edinburgh and London.

Winkelmann, R. K. (1961). J. Soc. Cosmetic Chemists 12:80.

Winkelmann, R. K. (1969). Br. J. Dermatol. 81(Suppl. 4):11.

Wolff, H. H. (1973). Arch. Dermatol. Forsch. 247:145.

Wolff, K., and Honigsmann, H. (1971). J. Ultrastruct. Res. 36:176.

Wood, G. C. (1964). Int. Rev. Connect. Tissue Res. 2:1.

Woodburne, R. T. (1965). Essentials of Human Anatomy. Oxford Univ. Press, New York.

Yoffey, J. M., and Courtice, F. C. (1970). Lymphatics, Lymph and the Lymphomyeloid Complex. Academic Press, New York.

Zaias, N. (1963). Arch. Dermatol. 87:37.

Zubroid, C. G. (1967). Arch. Dermatol. 96:560.

— 2 —

BASIC PRINCIPLES OF DIFFUSION
THROUGH MEMBRANES

I. THE DIFFUSION PROCESS

A. Introduction

Passive diffusion is the process whereby matter moves from one region of a system to another, down a concentration gradient, following random molecular motions. We may conveniently illustrate it by the simple experiment of the diffusion of a dye from a solution into a pure solvent. If we carefully pour water on top of an aqueous solution in a cylinder so that no convection currents form, we observe the following: Initially, the colored solution is separated from the water by a well-defined boundary. However, with time, the supernatant colors as the bottom layer fades. Eventually the entire solution becomes uniformly tinted. The transfer of dye molecules from the lower layer to the upper regions of the cylinder is the process of diffusion.

At the molecular level, the phenomenon is one of intense movement. Molecules of dye and water travel randomly among each other with the approximate velocities of rifle bullets. Each molecule constantly collides elastically with other molecules so that it sometimes moves toward a zone of lower concentration and sometimes toward a region of higher concentration. The "random walk" nature of its movement means, however, that the molecule has no preferred direction one way or the other. If we consider a horizontal section in the solution together with two neighboring thin, equal elements of volume one just above and one just below the section, we can explain how the dye molecules move from a region of high concentration to one of low concentration. In any finite interval of time, on average a definite fraction of the molecules in the lower element of volume will cross the section from below. The same fraction of molecules in the upper element will traverse the section from above. However, as there are more dye molecules in the lower element than in the upper one, random molecular movements provide a net transfer of dye molecules from the lower to the upper side of the section. The same holds true for solvent molecules but in the reverse direction. There is thus a steady net transfer of molecules which finally form a homogeneous solution.

Such interdiffusion of miscible materials, characterized by molecular migration down a concentration gradient, is thermodynamically a spontaneous, irreversible process. As such, the individual components of an equilibrated system cannot be separated without doing work on the system. For such a spontaneous process, the free energy of the system decreases under isothermal conditions and we can write

$$\Delta G = \Delta H - T \, \Delta S \tag{2.1}$$

where ΔG is the free-energy change, ΔH is the enthalpic change, T is the absolute temperature, and ΔS is the entropic change. For ideal solutions, ΔH is zero and the change in free energy of diffusive mixing arises from increased entropy, i.e., increased disorder. For all real situations there will be a small contribution from enthalpic change, but we usually neglect this and regard diffusion as an entropy driven process.

In the foregoing discussion we are concerned with the interdiffusion of at least two substances, and therefore we require at least two diffusion equations to describe the movement of each species present. However, if there is no net volume change across the plane of reference, the interpenetration rates are equal in magnitude but opposite in sign. Then we need only one of the equations to describe the diffusional process, and we need not consider explicitly the second equation. Thus the diffusion coefficients for each species are mutually dependent. This fact has important implications when the molecules involved differ markedly in size, e.g., water and protein. Then the larger molecules may be limiting and make the diffusive current for each species low.

B. Diffusion in an Isotropic Medium: Fick's First Law

The basic hypothesis underlying the mathematical theory of diffusion in isotropic materials is that the rate of transfer of diffusing substance through unit area of a section is proportional to the concentration gradient measured normal to the section. This is expressed as Fick's first law of diffusion (Fick, 1855):

$$J = -D \frac{\partial C}{\partial x} \tag{2.2}$$

where J is the rate of transfer per unit area of surface (the flux), C is the concentration of diffusing substance, x is the space coordinate measured normal to the section, and D is the diffusion coefficient. The negative sign indicates mathematically that the flux is in the direction of decreasing concentration, i.e., down the concentration gradient. In many situations, D can be considered as a constant, e.g., diffusion in simple dilute solutions. In other circumstances, e.g., diffusion in high polymers, D depends markedly on concentration. Variable values for D arise from the same factors which lead to deviations at high concentrations from osmotic pressure laws, ideal gas laws, etc., as well as in situations where the diffusant directly affects the properties of the diffusion medium. These include concentration-dependent and time-dependent effects in polymeric films. In some experiments, e.g., with membranes, an average integral diffusion coefficient, $\bar{D}$, may be derived which relates to the differential coefficient by

$$\bar{D} = \frac{1}{C_0 - C_h} \int_{C_0}^{C_h} D \, \partial C \qquad (2.3)$$

where $x = 0$ to $x = h$ defines the thickness of the various regions making up the membrane; $\bar{D} = D$ when the diffusion coefficent is independent of concentration.

The units of D are (length)^2 (time)$^{-1}$, usually specified as $cm^2 \, sec^{-1}$. We can convert this to a velocity by using the equation for a "random walk," $\bar{x} = (2Dt)^{1/2}$, where $\bar{x}$ represents the mean displacement of a molecule from its original position, along the x axis (Einstein, 1926).

The concentration gradient is usually taken as the driving force for diffusion, but more correctly the activity differential or chemical potential differential is the fundamental parameter which determines the rate and direction of the flux. However, for most situations of pharmaceutical and medical interest, we are limited to low concentrations because of the pharmacological and physicochemical properties of drugs. In such situations, activity coefficients remain within a narrow range in a given isotropic medium and concentration differentials may be used to characterize permeation phenomena. It is also important to realize that Fick's first law applies for an isotropic medium, i.e., one whose diffusional and structural properties in the region of each point within the material are the same for all three coordinates in space. The flow of diffusing substance at any point, for such a symmetrical situation, is along the normal to the surface of constant concentration through this point. For substances in which the material properties are not identical for each direction in space, i.e., anisotropic media, diffusion properties depend on the direction in which they are measured.

1. Differential equation of diffusion: Fick's second law

Fick's first law contains three variables, J, C, and x, of which J is additionally a multiple variable. As such the law is not readily usable in most experimental situations, so we employ Fick's second law. This expression, which reduces the number of variables by one, is readily derived and provides us with the fundamental mathematical statement of diffusion in a form most useful in resolving many diffusional problems (Crank, 1975). For an isotropic medium in which D is independent of concentration and direction, for a rectangular volume element we arrive at

$$\frac{\partial C}{\partial t} = D\left(\frac{\partial^2 C}{\partial x^2} + \frac{\partial^2 C}{\partial y^2} + \frac{\partial^2 C}{\partial z^2}\right) \tag{2.4}$$

where x, y, and z are the space coordinates.

For the usual experimental situation in which diffusion is unidirectional i.e., the concentration gradient is only along the x axis, this equation reduces to the form normally known as Fick's second law:

$$\frac{\partial C}{\partial t} = D\frac{\partial^2 C}{\partial x^2} \tag{2.5}$$

This differential diffusion equation states that the rate of change in concentration with time at a point within a diffusional field is proportional to the rate of change in concentration gradient at that point. Other formulations of the foregoing equations arise if we consider elements of volume of different shapes, such as a cylinder or sphere, or if we transform the coordinates. For each experimental design we need an exact solution of Eq. (2.5) and each derivation depends on the boundary conditions of the diffusion problem. Only those solutions relevant to percutaneous absorption, either in vivo or in vitro, or as simulated with artificial membranes and models, or which relate to drug release from topical vehicles will be considered here. For readers wishing to expand the necessarily condensed treatments presented here, full details are given in several excellent sources (Crank, 1975; Jost, 1960; Carslaw and Jaeger, 1959; Jacobs, 1935; Barrer, 1941).

2. Simple "zero-order" flux case

Many experimental designs used in studies of pharmaceutical and medicinal interest employ a membrane which separates two compartments, with a concentration gradient operating during a run and "sink" conditions (essentially zero concentration) prevailing in the receptor compartment. Daynes (1920) and Barrer (1939) provided a solution for this unidimensional experimental situation where the diffusive flow begins at x = 0, the high concentration surface of the membrane, and continues toward the other membrane surface where x = h. For boundary conditions C = C_0 (constant) at x = 0 for all t (time), C = 0 at all x > 0 for t = 0 (initial condition), C = 0 at x = h for all values of t (sink condition), and a constant diffusion coefficient D, the concentration at any point in a plane perpendicular to the flux vector at x, is provided in the form of a trigonometrical series

$$C = C_0 \frac{x}{h} + \frac{2}{\pi} \sum_{n=1}^{\infty} \frac{C_0}{n} \cos{(n\pi)} \sin{\left(\frac{n\pi x}{h}\right)} \exp{\left(-\frac{Dn^2 \pi^2 t}{h^2}\right)} \tag{2.6}$$

As t approaches infinity, the terms involving the exponentials vanish and we achieve a linear concentration gradient. Thus, to an experimental approximation, after a sufficient time a steady state is reached in which the concentration remains constant at all points in the membrane. Barnes (1934) considered the errors that are introduced if one assumes that a linear gradient exists across the membrane during the entire time course of diffusion.

In practice, Eq. (2.6) is solved for M, the cumulative mass of diffusant which passes per unit area through the membrane in time t. The expression is differentiated with respect to x to yield the instantaneous concentration gradient, the flux dM/dt is determined at x = h, and this is integrated from t = 0 to t = t. We then obtain the total amount of diffusing substance which has passed through the membrane in time t from

$$M = \frac{DC_0 t}{h} - \frac{hC_0}{6} - \frac{2hC_0}{\pi^2} \sum_{n=1}^{\infty} \frac{(-1)^n}{n^2} \exp\left(-\frac{Dn^2\pi^2 t}{h^2}\right) \tag{2.7}$$

3. Lag-time method

As t in Eq. (2.7) approaches infinity, this expression approaches the straight line

$$M = \frac{DC_0}{h}\left(t - \frac{h^2}{6D}\right) \tag{2.8}$$

If we differentiate Eq. (2.8), we obtain the steady state flux dM/dt, which is the slope of the straight line

$$\frac{dM}{dt} = \frac{DC_0}{h} \tag{2.9}$$

If a steady state plot is extrapolated to the time axis, the intercept so obtained at M = 0 is the lag time L:

$$L = \frac{h^2}{6D} \tag{2.10}$$

To within the accuracy of plotting (within 1% error) the steady state is achieved after about 2.7 times the lag time (Fig. 2.1). From Eq. (2.10), D is easily estimated, provided that the membrane thickness h is known. Thus L, together with the steady state flux, provide estimates of the other diffusion parameters which control permeation, since the solute concentration at the membrane surface C_0 can be calculated.

In most diffusion experiments one measures not C_0, which is the concentration existing within the first layer of the membrane, but C_0', the concentration in the donor phase which bathes the membrane. Under many conditions, the surface layers of the membrane rapidly equilibrate with the adjacent phases. These equilibria can be expressed in terms of distribution

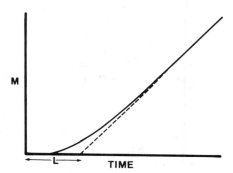

FIG. 2.1 The time course for absorption for the simple zero-order flux case obtained by plotting M, the cumulative amount of diffusant crossing unit area of membrane, as a function of time. Steady state is achieved when the plot becomes linear; extrapolation of the linear portion to the time axis yields the lag time L.

or partition coefficients when the adjacent phases are liquid, semisolid, and solid, or solubility coefficients for the gaseous phase. Thus, concentrations are typically related by

$$C_0 = C_0' K \tag{2.11}$$

where K is the partition coefficient of the solute between membrane and bathing solution. Substitution in Eq. (2.9) yields

$$\frac{dM}{dt} = \frac{DC_0' K}{h} \tag{2.12}$$

Thus the partition coefficient for a system can be determined from steady state data in a diffusion run. This procedure should give comparable results to independent measurements obtained by equilibrating a piece of the membrane with the donor solution and analyzing directly the concentrations in each phase (Van Amerongen, 1955).

It is worth noting that work which uses skin as the membrane often obtains a pseudo-steady-state plot from which flux values may be calculated. However, the linear portion of the plot may not always be compatible with the full curve illustrated in Fig. 2.1.

Equation (2.12) shows why this simple permeation process is referred to as a zero-order process. By analogy with chemical kinetic processes, Eq. (2.12) represents a zero-order process with a rate constant of DK/h (Flynn et al., 1974).

Sometimes with biological membranes it may prove difficult or impossible to measure K by either of the aforementioned methods. When this happens we often employ a composite parameter of permeability which includes both K and D. Some confusion arises in the literature because of the dual definition of this permeability coefficient P which may be defined as $P = KD$ or $P = KD/h$. The latter definition is often used when the magnitude of h, the membrane thickness, is uncertain, e.g., diffusion through cadaver skin.

If we investigate the relative permeabilities of a series of compounds under conditions where only the permeability coefficients can be measured, and not D and K individually, then we cannot separate differences arising from diffusive contributions to the flux (affecting D) from those provided by partitioning contributions (which modify K).

4. Short time approximation

An alternative approach for evaluating diffusion coefficients is that of Rogers et al. (1954) and Short et al. (1970), although the latter group appears to have used an incorrect time interval in the experimental work. This short time method is designed for situations where an inconveniently long time is required to establish the steady state condition, e.g., for slowly diffusing penetrants in cadaver skin when days may be required for steady state induction. Thus we have problems when solutes have very low diffusivities or membranes are very thick, or these two factors combine. Such difficulties as analytical instrument instability, membrane degradation, and problems in maintaining sink conditions make a short time method an attractive proposition. By integrating a Fourier transformation of Eq. (2.7), an expression valid at small t is obtained

$$\log\left(\frac{M}{t^{3/2}}\right) = \log\left(\frac{8C_0' K}{h^2 \pi^{3/2}}\right) + \frac{3}{2} \log D - \frac{h^2}{2.3(4)Dt} \tag{2.13}$$

A plot of $\log(M/t^{3/2})$ versus $1/t$ has a gradient of $-h^2/9.2D$, which provides an estimate of D if the membrane thickness is known. The intercept on the $\log(M/t^{3/2})$ axis is equivalent to $\log(8C_0' KD^{3/2}/h^2 \pi^{1/2})$, which yields estimates of the remaining parameters. The short time method is valid up to 2.7 times the lag time. In our experience, the main drawback to this method is analytical. At very short times, receptor solutions are very dilute and membranes do not "behave" well, passing more material than would be predicted from theoretical considerations.

5. Full curve analysis

In many experimental situations, we gather data both during the short time period and in the steady state. Depending on which of the aforementioned methods we use to calculate permeability coefficients or diffusion coefficients, we discard a portion of these data. An alternative approach is to use all experimental readings and to fit the data to Eq. (2.7) by an iterative least-squares computer program. Foreman and Kelly (1976) have done this with some success for the diffusion of nandrolone through hydrated human cadaver skin. A significant danger in this method arises from possible inaccuracies in the transient flow data, as discussed before; forcing the equation to give the best fit to all the data will give equal weight to those points of questionable precision and may degrade the accuracy of the diffusional parameters deduced.

Another approach accepts that there exists an actual discrepancy between the experimentally determined steady state diffusivity of a drug in the skin and the non-steady-state value. This discrepancy can be reconciled by using a model which includes dissolved mobile molecules in equilibrium with immobile molecules bound to skin sites (Chandrasekaran et al., 1976, 1978, 1980). Section III.D.4 of Chap. 4 discusses this theory in more detail

6. Dimensional analysis

It is useful to present diffusion equations in terms of dimensionless parameters so that solutions for all values of the diffusion coefficient, the membrane thickness, and time can be obtained from graphs or tabulated values which cover these dimensionless parameters (Crank, 1975; Carslaw and Jaeger, 1959; Henry, 1939; McKay, 1930; Olson and Schultz, 1942). Thus, if we rewrite Eq. (2.7) in such a form and incorporate the partition coefficient and the donor phase concentration, we have

$$\frac{M}{hKC_0'} = \frac{Dt}{h^2} - \frac{1}{6} - \frac{2}{\pi^2} \sum_{n=1}^{\infty} \frac{(-1)^n}{n^2} \exp\left(-\frac{Dt}{h^2} \pi^2 n^2\right) \qquad (2.14)$$

All the terms in the equation are either dimensionless or numerical constants. The dimensionless terms M/hKC_0' and Dt/h^2 are plotted in Fig. 2.2

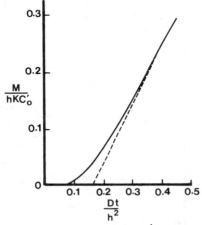

FIG. 2.2 Plot of M/hKC_0' versus Dt/h^2. The graph allows calculation of the total amount of material which penetrates unit area of a membrane (M) as a function of time. (From Dugard, 1977.)

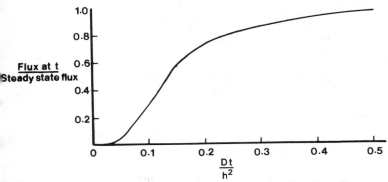

FIG. 2.3 Plot of the ratio of flux at time t to steady state flux as a function of Dt/h^2. The graph allows calculation of the rate of material penetrating unit area of a membrane as a function of time. (From Dugard, 1977.)

which is effectively a graph of total amount penetrated as a function of time (Dugard, 1977). The graph may be used to predict the total amount penetrated up to a particular time by the following procedure: The value of Dt/h^2 at the set time is calculated, and the corresponding value of M/hKC_0' is read from the graph. Knowing hKC_0', we can thus find M.

The absorption rate may be particularly relevant in toxicological studies (Dugard, 1977). If we differentiate Eq. (2.14) with respect to time, we arrive at the absorption rate, or flux at time t:

$$\frac{dM}{dt} = \frac{DKC_0'}{h} \left[1 - 2 \sum_{n=1}^{\infty} (-1)^{n+1} \exp\left(- \frac{Dt}{h^2} \pi^2 n^2\right) \right] \qquad (2.15)$$

This equation may be expressed graphically by plotting the dimensionless parameters, ratio of flux at time t to final steady state flux, against Dt/h^2 (Fig. 2.3). To determine the flux at a given time, Dt/h^2 is calculated and the flux ratio is read from the graph. As we know the steady state absorption rate, the unknown rate may be readily calculated.

It is useful to be able to calculate the amount of penetrant which is dissolved in the membrane for any time of contact with the bathing solution. If Q is the amount of diffusing substance in the membrane at time t, and Q_∞ the corresponding amount at infinite time then (Crank, 1975)

$$\frac{Q}{Q_\infty} = 1 - \frac{8}{\pi^2} \sum_{n=0}^{\infty} \frac{1}{(2n + 1)^2} \exp\left[- \frac{Dt}{h^2} \pi^2 (2n + 1)^2 \right] \qquad (2.16)$$

For an ideal membrane, at steady state the concentration gradient is linear (Fig. 2.4), and thus

$$Q_\infty = \frac{C_0' Kh}{2} \qquad (2.17)$$

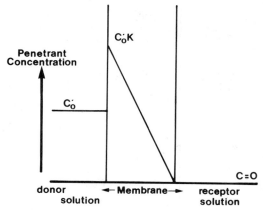

FIG. 2.4 Concentration profile across ideal membrane at steady state: simple zero-order flux case.

Figure 2.5 represents a plot of Q/Q_∞ against Dt/h^2. As before, the value of Dt/h^2 may be calculated for the time of interest and the corresponding value of Q/Q_∞ may be read from the graph. Since Q_∞ is known from Eq. (2.17), Q may be deduced.

7. Effect of temperature on diffusion

Variables in a diffusion experiment such as the partition coefficient and the membrane thickness tend to be relatively unaffected by temperature

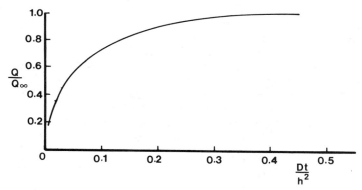

FIG. 2.5 Plot of the ratio of amount of penetrant dissolved in a membrane to the amount dissolved at infinite time as a function of Dt/h^2. The graph allows calculation of the amount of material in unit area of membrane as a function of time. (From Dugard, 1977.)

change. The diffusion coefficient, however, varies exponentially with temperature by the Arrhenius-type relationship

$$D = D_0 \exp\left(-\frac{E_D}{RT}\right) \quad \text{or} \quad \ln D = \ln D_0 - \frac{E_D}{RT} \tag{2.18}$$

where D_0 is the hypothetical diffusivity at infinite temperature, which may be obtained as the intercept of a plot of $\ln D$ versus $1/T$; R is the gas constant; T is the absolute temperature; E_D is the energy of activation for diffusion and is markedly influence by the environment presented to the diffusing molecule. Barrie (1968) quotes values of about 5 kcal mol^{-1} for the diffusion of low molecular weight nonelectrolytes in solution, with up to 15 to 20 kcal mol^{-1} for diffusion of similar materials in some polymers. In polymers in which the polymer molecules interlink, the solute diffuses only if the pore spaces are larger than the diffusant particles and if the pore shape is suitable. The transfer of material across such polymers is sometimes distinguished from "true" diffusion and may then be called "permeation." If we define the permeability or permeability coefficient as the product of the partition coefficient and the diffusion coefficient, we can write the analogous equation as

$$P = P_0 \exp\left(-\frac{E_p}{RT}\right) \quad \text{or} \quad \ln P = \ln P_0 - \frac{E_p}{RT} \tag{2.19}$$

where for the permeability P the energy of activation for permeation is E_p. Here, E_p is a measure of the energy needed for the net transfer of a mole of solute through the amorphous regions of a polymer, and it is the sum of the activation energy for diffusion and the heat of solution.

If a polymeric membrane has a transition point, the foregoing equations may not be valid. One advantage of cellulose acetate is that it has no glass transition temperature, permitting us to study permeation over a wide range of temperatures.

II. COMPLEX DIFFUSIONAL BARRIERS

A. Barriers in Series

So far we have dealt only with the simple situation in which diffusion occurs in a single isotropic medium. Skin, however, is a heterogeneous multilayer tissue consisting of stratum corneum, viable epidermis, and dermis, and within each layer we may recognize strata of different physicochemical properties. In percutaneous absorption, therefore, the concentration gradients develop over many strata in a multilayered barrier. It is thus necessary to consider the diffusional properties in general of laminates, i.e., multilayers sandwiched together, with each layer behaving as an isotropic field.

Each layer of the laminate contributes a diffusional resistance R: R is directly proportional to the layer thickness h and is indirectly proportional to the product of the layer diffusivity D and the partition coefficient K with respect to the external phases, which we assume to be of the same composition. For the ith layer

$$R_i = \frac{h_i}{D_i K_i} = \frac{1}{P_i} \tag{2.20}$$

where P_i is the thickness-weighted permeability coefficient. The total diffusional resistance of all the layers R_T is given by the summation expression

$$R_T = \sum R_i = \frac{h_1}{D_1 K_1} + \frac{h_2}{D_2 K_2} + \frac{h_3}{D_3 K_3} + \cdots + \frac{h_n}{D_n K_n} = \frac{1}{P_T} \tag{2.21}$$

In situations where resistances in all sections of the field are independent of diffusant concentration, the order of arrangement of the laminate layers does not influence the net steady state flux across the entire barrier.

For a three-ply membrane (and skin is often treated as such a material) the overall complex permeability is given by

$$P_T = \frac{(D_1 D_2 D_3)(K_1 K_2 K_3)}{h_1 D_2 D_3 K_2 K_3 + h_2 D_1 D_3 K_1 K_3 + h_3 D_1 D_2 K_1 K_2} \tag{2.22}$$

If one segment has a much greater resistance than the other segments (e.g., that of the stratum compared with that of the viable epidermis or dermis), then the single high-resistance phase determines the composite barrier property. Then $P_T = K_i D_i / h_i$, where i refers to the resistant phase.

When we perform a typical diffusional experiment and plot the total amount which has penetrated a barrier with respect to time, the profile obtained with a series barrier will be qualitatively the same as that with a single isotropic membrane. If we do not have detailed knowledge of the diffusional mechanism operating within the experimental membrane, then we must be careful how we interpret our results, e.g., the calculation of diffusion coefficients by the lag-time method (Eqs. 2.7-2.12).

After we have defined a laminate in terms of its complex permeability coefficient, this term may be used in place of the simple permeability coefficient in a flux equation based on steady state conditions.

For non-steady-state conditions, the situation is more complicated (Barrie et al., 1963). However, once again, when only one of the layers provides nearly all the diffusional resistance, then besides determining the steady state flux this layer also controls the lag time, i.e., $L = h_i^2 / 6 D_i$ in zero-order diffusion.

1. Diffusion layer control

For the common situation of a membrane in contact with a fluid donor phase and a fluid receptor phase, we vigorously stir the liquids so as to reduce the thickness of the stationary layers. However, although the thickness of such layers will be controlled by the rate of stirring, unstirred solvent layers will always form at stationary surfaces. Thus, when permeation is from an aqueous phase through a lipid (nonpolar) membrane into a receptor aqueous phase of lesser concentration, an unstirred aqueous layer will exist at each membrane surface. This trilaminar system has been analyzed for steady state flux under zero-order boundary conditions (Stehle and Higuchi, 1967; Flynn and Yalkowsky, 1972; Flynn et al., 1972) to give

$$\frac{dM}{dt} = \left[\frac{KD_M D_{AQ}}{h_M D_{AQ} + (h_{AQ(I)} + h_{AQ(II)})KD_M} \right] (C_0' - C_R') = P_T \, \Delta C \qquad (2.23)$$

where K is the membrane-water partition coefficient and subscripts M and AQ refer to membrane and aqueous phases, respectively; $h_{AQ(I)}$ is the thickness of the donor diffusion layer and $h_{AQ(II)}$ is the thickness of the receptor diffusion layer; C_0' is the donor concentration and C_R' is the receptor concentration.

In most instances, $h_M D_{AQ} \gg KD_M (h_{AQ(I)} + h_{AQ(II)})$ and P_T will reduce, as before, to KD_M/h_M. The concentration gradient exists entirely within the membrane; both the flux and the lag time are membrane controlled, and the lag time is $h_M^2/6D_M$. However, for diffusants with very large partition coefficients (i.e., those which are very lipid soluble), or for very thin membranes, or, in particular, when both factors combine, then in the rare situation when D_M is similar in magnitude to D_{AQ}, P_T may become equal to $D_{AQ}/(h_{AQ(I)} + h_{AQ(II)})$. This shows that the diffusion layers provide almost the entire diffusional resistance, i.e., diffusion layer control operates. Equation (2.23) indicates that, if the partition coefficient goes on ever increasing, then the permeation process becomes diffusion layer controlled when it is insensitive to further increase in the value of the partition coefficient.

From Eq. (2.23) for the trilaminar system, we see that $1/P_T = h_M/KD_M + (h_{AQ(I)} + h_{AQ(II)})/D_{AQ}$. We can follow the method of Zwolinski et al. (1949) and plot the reciprocals of the permeability coefficients as a function of the membrane-water partition coefficients. Equation (2.23) requires that such a plot for a series of compounds should give rise to a straight line passing through the origin when diffusion in the membrane is the rate-limiting step. When diffusion in the boundary layers is rate limiting, a horizontal line results. Roberts et al. (1978) have done this for a series of phenolic compounds diffusing through human skin in vitro. They find that their plots suggest that diffusion through the aqueous boundary layers is rate limiting for solutes with large stratum corneum-water partition coefficients.

When permeation is under diffusion layer control, for ultrathin membranes the lag time will be given by $(h_{AQ(I)} + h_{AQ(II)})^2/6D_{AQ}$. When the nonpolar membrane is thick and K is sufficiently large to ensure diffusion layer control, the lag time is (Flynn et al., 1972)

$$L = \frac{h_M h_{AQ(I)} h_{AQ(II)} K}{(h_{AQ(I)} + h_{AQ(II)}) D_{AQ}} \qquad (2.24)$$

When the diffusion layers are equal in thickness (h_{AQ})

$$L = \frac{h_M L_{AQ} K}{2D_{AQ}} \qquad (2.25)$$

Thus, under these conditions, the lag time will increase with increase in the magnitude of the partition coefficient.

2. Effect of temperature in series diffusion

When the activation energies of the diffusion coefficients in the various layers of the laminate are very different and no one layer is dominant with respect to diffusional resistance, then the temperature dependence is complex. In principle at least, a plot of log P against $1/T$ can provide valuable information about the nature of a series barrier and the mechanics of transport. If over the temperature range considered one layer only provides most of the diffusional resistance, the activation energy will depend only on the diffusion coefficient in that layer. If activation energies for the different layers are already known and are different, then an experimental determination of the dominant activation energy will indicate which is the rate-controlling layer (Flynn et al., 1974).

B. Barriers in Parallel

Human skin is pierced by shunts and pores such as hair follicles and sweat glands. We may idealize this complex structure and consider the simple situation in which the diffusional medium consists of two or more diffusional pathways linked in parallel. Then the total diffusional flux per unit area of composite, J_T, is the sum of the individual fluxes through the separate routes (Crank, 1975; Scheuplein, 1966). Thus, for transient or steady state diffusion

$$J_T = f_1 J_1 + f_2 J_2 + \cdots + f_n J_n \qquad (2.26)$$

where f_1, f_2, etc. denote the fractional areas for each diffusional route. Thus, for any boundary conditions operating, we may determine the total flux of solute by solving Fick's laws for each route. We then adjust for the relative areas of the various routes and sum over all the diffusional pathways. As an example, we can take the simple but useful model of two parallel, linear routes of equal length through a membrane. Applying the usual zero order conditions $C = C_0$ (constant) at $x = 0$ for all t, $C = 0$ at all $x > 0$ for $t = 0$, $C = 0$ at $x = h$ for all t with constant diffusion coefficients, we simply combine two solutions of Eq. (2.7), weighted for the fractional areas

$$M = f_1 \left[\frac{D_1 K_1 C_0' t}{h} - \frac{h K_1 C_0'}{6} - \frac{2h K_1 C_0'}{\pi^2} \sum_{n=1}^{\infty} \frac{(-1)^n}{n^2} \exp\left(-\frac{D_1 n^2 \pi^2 t}{h^2}\right) \right]$$

$$+ f_2 \left[\frac{D_2 K_2 C_0' t}{h} - \frac{h K_2 C_0'}{6} - \frac{2h K_2 C_0'}{\pi^2} \sum_{n=1}^{\infty} \frac{(-1)^n}{n^2} \exp\left(-\frac{D_2 n^2 \pi^2 t}{h^2}\right) \right] \quad (2.27)$$

where $C_0 = C_0' K_i$. As before, as t approaches infinity, the cumulative mass which has crossed the complex membrane is given by

$$M = f_1 \frac{D_1 K_1 C_0'}{h} \left(t - \frac{h^2}{6D_1} \right) + f_2 \frac{D_2 K_2 C_0'}{h} \left(t - \frac{h^2}{6D_2} \right) \quad (2.28)$$

The steady state flux through the combined parallel routes is then

$$J_T = \frac{dM}{dt} = C_0' \left(f_1 \frac{D_1 K_1}{h} + f_2 \frac{D_2 K_2}{h} \right) \quad (2.29)$$

In general, for independent, linear parallel pathways during steady state

$$J_T = C_0' (f_1 P_1 + f_2 P_2 + \cdots + f_n P_n) \quad (2.30)$$

where P_i represents thickness-weighted permeability coefficients.

In the same way as for the single barrier membrane (cf. Eqs. 2.9 and 2.10) we obtain the lag time given by the intercept of a plot of M against t by putting $M = 0$ in Eq. (2.28), from which

$$L = \frac{h^2}{6} \left(\frac{f_1 K_1 + f_2 K_2}{f_1 K_1 D_1 + f_2 K_2 D_2} \right) \quad (2.31)$$

If only one of the routes allows diffusant to pass, i.e., the other route is impervious, then the solution reduces to the simple membrane model with the steady state flux determined by the fractional area and the permeation rate through the open channel.

The presence of parallel pathways for diffusion may be revealed in some instances in the plot of M against t. For a membrane composed of two routes for which the transient periods are experimentally separable, the diffusion plot first appears regular as diffusant passes through the more permeable pore. However, when material then starts issuing from the resistant pathway, the total flux suddenly increases and further time is required to reestablish a new steady state line with an increased slope. Scheuplein et al. (1969) provide an example of this for human skin.

If a pore is either not straight or is orientated at an angle to the plane of the membrane (and thus to the assumed direction of the diffusional field), then the effective diffusional path length will be greater than the membrane thickness. The effective membrane thickness H is given by

$$H = \tau h \tag{2.32}$$

where τ is the so called tortuosity factor. All parameters which depend on membrane thickness will have to be modified, e.g., to calculate D from the lag time we need

$$D = \frac{\tau^2 h^2}{6L} \tag{2.33}$$

A second mechanical complication arises when the diameter of the solute molecule approaches that of the pore. This phenomenon of hindered diffusion will be considered subsequently (Beck and Schultz, 1972; Pappenheimer, 1953; Renkin, 1954; Higuchi and Higuchi, 1960).

Effect of temperature in parallel pathways

As for the series barrier model, the temperature dependency for parallel routes is complex. Scheuplein (1966) analyzed the situation for two independent routes. If we make use of the Arrhenius-type relationship of Eq. (2.18), we can rewrite Eq. (2.29) as

$$J_T = C'_0 \left[f_1 \frac{K_1 D_{01}}{h} \exp\left(-\frac{E_{D1}}{RT}\right) + f_2 \frac{K_2 D_{02}}{h} \exp\left(-\frac{E_{D2}}{RT}\right) \right] \tag{2.34}$$

Scheuplein (1966) showed that an investigation of temperature effects on the diffusion of water through human skin provided valuable evidence relating to the structure of the stratum corneum.

C. Barriers with Dispersed Phases

Another type of heterogeneity in practical materials exist when discrete particles of one phase disperse in a continuum of another phase (Barrer, 1968). In general, to describe fully the properties of a composite material of this kind we need to consider:

1. The composition, state of matter, and other properties of the continuous phase and the dispersed phase

2. The overall concentration or relative volume of the dispersed phase and its interaction with the diffusing species
3. The geometry of the dispersed phase (shape, size, and size distribution; spatial distribution; orientation and topology)

Crank (1975) discussed in some detail the mathematical problems of a two-phase system, particularly for arrays of spheres, cylinders, and ellipsoids, and provided some key references. Higuchi and Higuchi (1960) dealt with the subject from a pharmaceutical standpoint, discussing the application of the theory to the passage of drugs through biological membranes, the design of protective ointments, and drug release from semisolid dispersed systems (creams and ointments).

For simplicity, we will deal here only with those systems in which the diffusional field is at least isotropic at the macroscopic level, although molecularly anisotropic. We therefore assume that randomly oriented immobile particles are uniformly dispersed in a continuum and are small compared with the thickness of the barrier; for emulsions, the particles are spherical. We may recognize three separate conditions; where the dispersed phase is inert, where the dispersed phase sorbs the diffusant, and there the dispersed phase is both sorptive and permeable.

1. Inert dispersed phase

Dispersed phases (gases, liquids, or solids) in polymer membranes are often referred to as fillers. When the filler is inert, i.e., diffusionally inactive, it may influence the diffusional pattern by the combined effect of the following mechanisms:

1. The internal phase decreases the available diffusional pathway by occupying a finite fraction of the barrier volume.
2. The filler increases the average diffusional pathlength by forcing the diffusant to stream around the inclusion.

The relative volumes of matrix and filler may be defined by their volume fractions, ϕ_1 and ϕ_2, respectively, where $\phi_1 = 1 - \phi_2$. For a random dispersion, the relative cross sectional area of each phase is equal to its relative volume. Just as for pores (Eq. 2.32), the average pathlength for the solute is given by τh. For a zero-order process with receptor sink (cf. Eq. 2.12), the steady state flux equation becomes

$$J = \frac{dM}{dt} = C_0' \left(\frac{KD}{h} \frac{\phi_1}{\tau} \right) = C_0' \left(\frac{KD(1 - \phi_2)}{H} \right) \tag{2.35}$$

where K and D refer to the continuous phase.

The filler volume fraction does not affect the lag time, but the tortuosity factor does:

$$L = \frac{h^2 \tau^2}{6D} = \frac{H^2}{6D} \tag{2.36}$$

2. Adsorptive dispersed phase

An active filler is one which sorbs the diffusant, either by adsorption or absorption. The former process is less complicated and thus more easily considered. When the adsorption process follows Langmuir's isotherm, there are two distinct mechanisms (Flynn et al., 1974).

Case I (Finger et al., 1960; Flynn and Roseman, 1971) In this formulation, the amount of permeant adsorbed depends directly on concentration. For the standard zero-order permeation process, the steady state flux is given by Eq. (2.35). Therefore J is only influenced by the changes in the effective area for diffusion and the effective path length. The lag time, however, depends on the filler adsorptive constant z, the filler volume fraction, and the square of the tortuosity and is given by

$$L = \frac{H^2}{6D}(1 + z\phi_2) \tag{2.37}$$

A plot of L/H^2 against ϕ_2 will have a slope of $z/6D$ and an intercept of $1/6D$. One can therefore estimate D and z. An example of the use of these relationships involves the permeation of ethyl p-aminobenzoate through silicone rubber membranes which contain a silica filler (Most, 1970; Flynn and Roseman, 1971).

Case II (Higuchi and Higuchi, 1960) This case represents the condition in which the filler adsorbs a fixed amount of solute, i.e., at the isotherm plateau. The steady state equation is the same as for the Case I mechanism (Eq. 2.35), but the lag time is given by

$$L = \frac{H^2}{D}\left(\frac{1}{4} + \frac{Z\phi_2}{2KC_0'}\right) \tag{2.38}$$

where Z is the saturation adsorptive capacity of the filler. The lag time in a Case II mechanism depends on the donor phase concentration. Thus the lag time may be very long at low applied phase concentrations, e.g., when the permeant is irreversibly bound to the filler in chemisorption. Equation (2.38) is only approximate as L reduces to $H^2/4D$ instead of $H^2/6D$ as $Z\phi_2$ approaches zero.

3. Absorptive, permeable dispersed phase

In biphasic or multiphasic systems such as emulsions, the dispersed phase may absorb some of the diffusant. The permeable droplets will permit diffusional flow within themselves, and such diffusion will affect both steady state and transient processes. The situation then becomes complex and difficult to analyze. For steady state and spherical particles, Higuchi and Higuchi (1960) deduced an expression for the effective permeability coefficient P_T:

$$P_T = \frac{2P_1^2(1 - \phi_2) + P_1P_2(1 + 2\phi_2) - GP_1[(P_2 - P_1)/(2P_1 - P_2)]^2(2P_1 + P_2)(1 - \phi_2)}{P_1(2 + \phi_2) + P_2(1 - \phi_2) - G[(P_2 - P_1)/(2P_1 + P_2)]^2(2P_1 + P_2)(1 - \phi_2)} \tag{2.39}$$

where P_1 and P_2 are the individual permeabilities for the planar case, and G is a constant ranging from about 0.4 to 0.8.

D. Time Variable Boundaries

There are various experimental arrangements in which the barrier's dimensions or its diffusional properties, or both, change during the mass transport process. The release of drugs suspended in a stationary matrix, such as an ointment, is a relevant problem of the "moving boundary" type (Higuchi, 1960, 1961). We can consider the following simplified model. The drug particles are small compared with the average distance of diffusion. They are uniformly distributed in an isotropic homogeneous matrix, and sink conditions prevail in the receptor phase. Then, when the concentration gradient is established (a quasi-steady state exists), the amount of drug M released to the sink per unit area in the planar geometry is

$$M = (2A - C_s) \left\{ \frac{D_v t}{1 + [2(A - C_s)/C_s]} \right\}^{1/2} \tag{2.40}$$

where A is the total concentration of drug, soluble and suspended, in the vehicle matrix; C_s is the saturation concentration (the solubility) of the drug in the matrix; and D_v is the diffusion coefficient in the vehicle matrix.

When the solubility of the drug in the vehicle is very small and A is appreciable (i.e., $A \gg C_s$), we can write

$$M \simeq (2AD_v C_s t)^{1/2} \tag{2.41}$$

and

$$\frac{dM}{dt} \simeq \left(\frac{AD_v C_s}{2t} \right)^{1/2} \tag{2.42}$$

The amount released is thus directly related to the square root of time.

As free drug diffuses from the vehicle into the sink, the region containing solid particles gradually recedes from the vehicle-sink interface. This is why the situation is referred to as a "moving boundary" type of diffusion. When the matrix contains an inert filler, then the volume fraction of the matrix continuum and the tortuosity must be taken into account (Higuchi, 1963; Chandrasekaran and Hillman, 1980). (See also Chap. 4, Section III.D.2.)

III. INFLUENCE OF MATERIAL PROPERTIES ON DIFFUSION

In this section we will briefly review the fundamental physicochemical principles that control the most important properties of both solute and barrier phase as these properties affect the process of diffusion. We will consider such mass transport properties as subdivided into diffusant solubility, partition coefficients, effective concentrations, and factors which affect diffusivity.

A. Diffusant Solubility

In all the diffusant equations discussed previously, we see that the flux of solute is proportional to the concentration gradient across the entire barrier phase. Thus, for any mass transport situation, one requirement for maximal flux is that the solute should be in saturated solution in the donor phase. In studying solubility with respect to percutaneous absorption, we will generally be interested in how solubility changes for either an experimental homologous series or for a range of pharmacologically active analogs in a given solvent. Alternatively, we may wish to optimize the solubility of an active drug, such as a topical corticosteroid, by controlling the solvent composition of the vehicle. Thus, a saturated solution may be obtained at a selected concentration of the drug by experimenting with a series of solvents or, more usually, by blending two liquids to form a miscible binary mixture with suitable solvent properties. For such investigations we do have some general guidelines, and these are discussed below.

In a homologous series, for most solvents the solubilities of members of the series decrease exponentially with increase in chain length. Numerous workers have investigated the effect on solubility of progressively adding CH_2 groups to the molecule (for references, see the extensive review by Davis et al., 1974). A satisfactory equation which represents the data is of the form

$$\log S_n = \log S_0 - Bn \qquad\qquad (2.43)$$

where S_n is the solubility of a homolog of chain length n; S_0 is the solubility of the reference homolog containing zero CH_2 groups (often this is a hypothetical value which may be obtained from the intercept on the ordinate of the log S versus n plot); and the constant B is the CH_2 group contribution to solubility. For water as the solvent, values for nonelectrolytes range between about 0.24 for long-chain alkanoic acids (n = 9 and above) and 0.73 for alkanols, with most substances providing values in the region of 0.5 to 0.7 (Sarraco and Spaccamela Marchetti, 1958). The group contribution B depends on the chemical nature and physical state (solid or liquid) of the pure solute. For most substances investigated, the solubility in water thus decreases by a factor of 3 to 5 for each methylene group added. For hydrocarbon solvents, B may be close to zero. Sarraco and Spaccamela Marchetti (1958; also Spaccamela Marchetti and Sarraco, 1958) compiled an extensive list of the solubilities of homologous aliphatic substances in various solvents.

When in any homologous or congeneric series of compounds the pure
solute changes from a liquid to the solid state, the plot of solubility against
chain length often shows a discontinuity or change in gradient. This occurs
at the chain length of the liquid-to-solid transition. In addition, solid homologs often show odd-even effects in solubility which are associated with
alternating melting points (Ralston, 1948; Breusch and Kirkali, 1968;
Breusch, 1969). It is the differences in the energetics of crystal packing of
odd and even chains, leading to alternations in the heats of fusion, that provide these variations. Furthermore, the first few homologs in a series may
behave differently from the remainder, with regard both to odd-even effects
and the B value. Thus, Yalkowsky et al. (1972) showed that the solubilities
of alkyl p-aminobenzoates in water cannot be described by the simple logarithmic relationship of Eq. (2.43) but that the plot of log S_n versus n provided two intersecting straight lines. Short-chain and long-chain homologs
behaved differently, because in the former group the nonchain portion of
the molecule exerts a disproportionate influence on crystal structure. If a
homologous series of solid solutes all have similar heats of fusion, then
the group contribution to solubility is about the same as for liquid homologs
(Kakovsky, 1957).

Aqueous solubilities of nonpolar organic compounds depend on their
molecular surface areas, which are essentially hydrophobic in nature (Davis
et al., 1972). Thus, the affinity for water decreases exponentially as molecular hydrophobic surface area increases, and it is this, not the absolute
lipid affinity, which governs the increase in lipid-water partition coefficients
in a series of homologs or analogs.

Fuller reviews of solubility theory are provided by Hildebrand and
Scott (1950, 1962), McBain and Hutchinson (1955), Ralston (1948), Yalkowsky
et al. (1962), and Davis et al. (1974).

B. Partition Coefficient

The important role that the partition coefficient may play in establishing the
flux rate has been emphasized previously (Eq. 2.12). In particular, when
the membrane provides the sole—or by far the major—source of diffusional
resistance, then the magnitude of the partition coefficient (bathing solution
to membrane) is very important. This is often the situation with percutaneous absorption, in which the resistance of the stratum corneum to the passage of the diffusant is usually the rate-limiting step in the overall absorption process. The stratum corneum to vehicle partition coefficient is then
crucially important in establishing a high initial concentration of diffusant
in the first layer of the tissue.

The relationship between partitioning behavior, chemical structure,
and biological activity is a pervasive theme in modern pharmaceutical

literature. Collander made the first extensive study of group contributions
to partition coefficients, although this approach is now usually associated
with the publications of Hansch and his co-workers [Davis et al. (1974) provide an extensive reference list, together with a detailed discussion; Hansch
and Leo (1979) recently published a monograph on correlation analysis in
chemistry and biology]. In such work, simple immiscible solvents have
been used, often pure water or buffers for the aqueous phase, with the
nonaqueous solvent being vegetable oils, diethyl ether, chloroform, iso-
butanol, octanol, oleyl alcohol, hexane, heptane, cyclohexane, or isopropyl
myristate. Nonaqueous polar solvents are advocated by many workers who
have attempted to correlate biological activity with physicochemical properties of drug molecules (e.g., Burton et al., 1964; Flynn, 1971; Hansch and
Dunn, 1972). However, Beckett and Moffat (1969), Bickel and Weder (1969),
and Shibab (1971) provide evidence that partition coefficients obtained with
heptane or hexane and water or aqueous buffer correlate biological data
better than do coefficients obtained with polar solvents. The most popular
solvent for general work has been octanol. Isopropyl myristate is recommended for work related to skin diffusion, as its blend of polar and nonpolar
properties is supposed to mimic to some extent the complex lipid/polar
nature of the stratum corneum.

In related fields, Harris et al. (1973) have performed detailed work on
group contribution to partitioning and related thermodynamic parameters,
for ion pairs in chloroform-water partition systems. Tomlinson (1975) has
reviewed how group contribution values may be related to chromatographic
data; McCall (1975) and Mirrlees et al. (1976) have discussed methods
whereby data may be obtained rapidly by liquid-liquid chromatographic
techniques. Diamond and Katz (1974) have listed group values for the transfer of solutes into liposomes.

In the group contribution approach to partitioning, a functional group in
the solute molecule is presumed to provide a set contribution to the overall
partition coefficient of the entire molecule. Thus, in the simple situation of
a homologous series we can write an equation of the form

$$\log K_n = \log K_0 + \pi n \qquad (2.44)$$

where K_n is the partition coefficient of the homolog of chain length n; K_0 is
the partition coefficient of the reference homolog of chain length zero; and
π is the group contribution. For the more general case in which we compare
the partition coefficient of a substituted compound (K_{RX}) with that of the
unsubstituted parent compount (K_{RH}),

$$\log K_{RX} = \log K_{RH} + \pi_X \qquad (2.45)$$

Thus, for a partitioning system of immiscible liquids, if we know the
partition coefficient of a reference compound, the logarithm of the partition
coefficient of the homolog or analog of interest may be calculated. We simply

add the sum of the π values (group contributions) of the substituent groups to the log (partition coefficient) of the reference chemical. It is fortunate that results obtained with one partitioning system very often parallel those obtained with an alternative system. Thus Collander (1951) found that for a homologous series of compounds partitioned between water and two different solvent systems (i, j)

$$\log K_i = a \log K_j + b \qquad (2.46)$$

where a and b are constants. It appears that this equation is valid for a wide range of polar and semipolar solvents (Leo and Hansch, 1971; Leo et al., 1971) but that the fit is poorer for polar-nonpolar comparisons. It is thus usually possible to assess, at least qualitatively, the effect that a molecular modification of a drug will have in one partitioning system if its effect in another is known. Thus, one can with reasonable confidence extrapolate a trend obtained from, say, an octanol/water or an isopropyl myristate/ water system to an aqueous vehicle/stratum corneum partitioning system such as may operate in an in vivo percutaneous absorption process. Thus, one assumes that an equation of the type

$$\log K_{SC} = a' \log K_i + b' \qquad (2.47)$$

is valid, where K_{SC} is the partition coefficient for stratum corneum and K_i is the partition coefficient for a simple solvent.

The dramatic effect which the partition coefficient plays in controlling the flux of a solute through a membrane is most easily illustrated with a series of alkyl homologs. If we take the π value for a methylene group for biological membranes as 0.3 (Yalkowsky and Flynn, 1973), then for a variation in chain length of 10 units, the partition coefficient will increase 1,000-fold (in Eq. 2.44, $\pi n = 3$). For solvents such as hexane, $\pi = 0.6$ (Davis et al., 1972) and the partition coefficient will increase by 10^6 ($\pi n = 6$). When we consider that for most homologous series the diffusivities in water or in artificial membranes will only decrease by a factor of 2 or 3 when the chain length increases by 10 methylene units, we see that partitioning dominates permeation effects. When the membrane provides the rate-limiting step in the diffusion process, the steady state flux of the homologs as measured from solutions of equivalent concentrations will increase in proportion to the increase in the partition coefficient. However, there is a limit to this increase in flux with increase in partition coefficient. For all lipid-like membranes, as the partition coefficient increases it reaches a value at which the system crosses over to diffusion layer control (see Sec. II.A.1). When in diffusion layer control the permeation process becomes insensitive to partition coefficient, and then the flux reaches a plateau (Stehle and Higuchi, 1967). Recent excellent treatments concerning the influence that partition coefficients (and solubilities) have on membrane diffusion are those of Valvani and Yalkowsky (1980) and Yalkowsky and Morozowich (1980).

Although written primarily with reference to gastrointestinal absorption, these reviews contain much material directly relevant to skin absorption. Sec. III. F. 2 of Chap. 4 reviews other aspects of partition coefficient theory which are directly relevant to skin permeation.

C. Effective Concentrations

Although the concentration differential is usually considered to be the driving force for diffusion, it is the chemical potential gradient or activity gradient which is the fundamental parameter. As discussed previously, in many situations for practical purposes the distinction is negligible, but in other circumstances we must take it into account. Thus, the thermodynamic activity of the penetrant in either the donor phase or the membrane may be radically altered by such phenomena as pH change, complex formation, or the presence of surfactants, micelles, or cosolvents. Such factors also modify the effective partition coefficient, since K is a ratio of the activity coefficients in each phase.

1. pH variation

According to the simple form of the pH-partition hypothesis, only un-ionized molecules pass across lipid membranes in significant amounts (Shore et al., 1957). Ionized species do not have favorable free energies for transfer to lipid phases. Now weak acids and weak bases are dissociated to different degrees, depending on the pH and the pK_a or pK_b of the diffusant. Thus, the fraction of the un-ionized drug in the applied phase determines the effective membrane gradients, and this fraction is a function of pH (Aguiar and Fifelski, 1966; Kakemi et al., 1967; Grouthamel et al., 1971; Benet, 1973; Wagner and Sedman, 1973).

2. Cosolvents

Polar solvent mixtures such as water and propylene glycol are used in topical therapy to produce saturated solutions of the drug in the vehicle and so to maximize the concentration gradient across the stratum corneum membrane. However, in general, the partition coefficient of a drug between a membrane and a solvent mixture falls as the drug solubility in the solvent system rises. Thus, these two factors—increase in solubility in the vehicle and magnitude of the partition coefficient with reference to the membrane—work in opposition with regard to promoting flux through the membrane. Hence, it is important not to oversolubilize a drug in a vehicle if the aim is to promote penetration through the stratum corneum. One should aim to produce a saturated solution of the diffusant. The biopharmaceutical importance of cosolvents is discussed in more detail in Chap. 4, Sec. III. E.

3. Surface activity and micellization

Micelles form when surfactant monomers associate to produce particles of colloidal dimensions; the concentration at which this occurs is called the critical micelle concentration (CMC). Above the CMC, as the concentration of surfactant increases, the micelles multiply with negligible change in the monomer concentration. Micelles differ from other colloids in that they are in dynamic equilibrium with nonassociated surfactant.

We can recognize two main arrangements—one in which the diffusant under investigation is surface active and forms micelles; the other where a surfactant is present in addition to the diffusant. When the diffusant associates into micelles, the total apparent solubility of the agent in the aqueous phase can increase dramatically, with a consequent decrease in the apparent partition coefficient, as discussed previously. However, the concentration of free monomer remains essentially constant, as does the true (monomer) partition coefficient. Then, if the rate controlling membrane is impermeable to the micelle, this aggregate will have little effect on the permeation process other than by providing a reservoir to replace monomers which have left the donor phase. Then the micelles deaggregate to maintain constant donor concentration of the monomer. However, micelles can have a significant effect on mass transport when the aqueous diffusion layer provides the rate-limiting step in permeation (Gibaldi et al., 1970; Short et al., 1970; Courchene, 1964).

When the drug and the surfactant are not the same (which is the usual situation), then the part played by the surfactant in the transport of the drug across membranes is more complicated. The effect of surfactants upon the absorption and biological activity of drugs is important, as they are widely used in solubilized systems in pharmaceutical formulations. The topic of solubilization and its relevance to pharmacy has been the subject of many review articles, notably by Mulley (1964), Swarbrick (1965), Elworthy (1967), Sjoblom (1967), and Elworthy et al. (1968). The literature contains many reports which clearly demonstrate that surfactants can influence the rate and extent of absorption of drugs (see reviews by Blanpin, 1968, and Swisher, 1968). The pharmacological activity may be enhanced or retarded [e.g., surfactants reduce the intestinal absorption of glucose and methionin in the rat (Nissim, 1960; Taylor, 1963) and retard the rectal absorption of triiodophenol (Riegelman and Crowell, 1958)]. Lish and Weikel (1959) reported that drug absorption was enhanced when surfactants were included in a medication. As Levy (1963) noted, much of the difficulty in interpreting some of these observations has arisen because of the different types of effects which surfactants can exert. These influences include interactions with synthetic and biological membranes, interaction with the drug, and interaction with the dosage form.

Gibaldi and Feldman (1970) proposed a model to rationalize the effect of a surfactant on the transport rate of a drug. In this scheme, the drug in the surfactant solution partitions between the micellar and the aqueous (nonmicellar) pseudophases, with a partition ratio which is independent of drug concentration. This partition coefficient is additional to the partition coefficient of nonmicellar drug referred to the membrane. The absorption of the drug in the micellar phase is considered to be negligible. Since the micellar drug is unavailable for absorption, the effective concentration of the unassociated diffusing species will be lowered and the flux will drop proportionally. In an extreme case, the concentration of free drug may be so low that transport becomes limited by the micellar diffusion rate in the donor solution or by the energy requirements for removal of the drug from the micelle when the colloidal particle reaches the membrane surface. The interfacial barrier mechanism operates for some steroid molecules in the presence of bile acid-lecithin micelles when the nonaqueous phase is hexadecane (Surpuriya and Higuchi, 1972). Barry and El Eini (1976a,b) showed that the flux rates for hydrocortisone, dexamethasone, testosterone, and progesterone through cellulose acetate membrane decreased in the presence of supramicellar concentrations of an alkyl polyoxyethylene surfactant because of the partitioning behavior of the steroids into the micelles. However, when allowance was made for this partitioning, it was found that the permeability coefficients of the unsolubilized drugs increased compared to those from water. Similarly, for submicellar concentrations of nonionic surfactants, the permeation rates for these four steroids also increased compared to water. It seems that monomeric surfactant molecules can enhance the adsorption of steroid on to the donor side of the cellulose acetate membrane (thus increasing the membrane-donor solution partition coefficient), possibly by reducing the surface tension between the membrane and the aqueous solution. Kesting et al. (1968) showed that surfactant adsorption at a membrane/water interface allowed faster permeation rates for hydrogen bonding solutes than for non-hydrogen-bonding solutes. The absorption rate of barbiturates across goldfish membranes increased in the presence of submicellar concentrations of polysorbate 80 (Levy et al., 1966). Levy and Anello (1968) demonstrated that the increased absorption rate of secobarbital when dissolved in the same solution of polysorbate 80 arose from an increase in the permeability of the biological membrane, rather than from the formation of a more rapidly absorbed nonmicellar polysorbate-secobarbital complex. Yasuda (1968) suggested that the surfactant causes the membrane to swell and thus increases the diffusion of the drug across the barrier. Again, in this context, Nogami et al. (1969) considered that adsorption of the drug molecules onto the membrane could be the rate-determining step of drug transfer. The surfactant must, therefore, in some way modify the rate of adsorption. Bikhazi and Higuchi (1970) and Goldberg and Higuchi (1969) have discussed the importance of the interfacial barrier in many biopharmaceutical situations. Juni et al. (1978) analyzed the permeation profiles of local anesthetics dissolved in surfactant solutions, using silicone and ethylene-vinyl acetate copolymer membranes.

     In addition, surfactants have specific effects on skin which relate to interfacial tension lowering in hair follicles and changes in protein conformation in the stratum corneum. These features will be dealt with in Chap. 4, Sec. III. C. 3. h.

3. Complexation

Complex formation is in many ways analogous to micellar solubilization in the manner in which it affects drug permeation through membranes. Thus, when complexes form, the apparent solubility and the apparent partition coefficient change. If complexes only assemble in the aqueous donor phase, then they influence transport through the membrane in a way similar to micellization, i.e., they decrease the flux rate because the concentration of free drug falls. However, if the complex is also stable in the membrane and can diffuse therein, then both free drug and complexed drug can pass across the membrane. In essence we have two parallel pathways available for transport, and for a complete analysis of the mechanism we must deduce (1) the stability constants for the complexes, (2) the diffusion coefficients of the drug and complex in the donor phase, (3) their diffusion coefficients in the membrane, and (4) the partition coefficients for the free and complexed drug between the phases. Permeability may increase, decrease, or remain unchanged, depending on the relative magnitudes of these factors.

An example of how to separate these features was provided by Nakano and Patel (1970) when they studied the passage of p-nitrophenol across silicone rubber membranes as affected by alkylamides. They found that dimethylpropamide, diethylacetamide, and diethylpropamide increased the apparent permeability to the phenol but dimethylacetamide produced no effect. Similarly, some caffeine-drug complexes reduced the apparent permeabilities to the drugs, because the complexes had lower partition coefficients than the respective free drugs (Bates et al., 1970). However, because the caffeine-drug complexes were more hydrophobic than free caffeine and thus their partition coefficients into a lipid phase were increased compared to free caffeine, the apparent permeability to the caffeine increased.

D. Factors Which Affect Diffusivity

The speed with which materials diffuse depends first and foremost on the state of matter of the diffusing medium. In gases and air, typical diffusion coefficients are large (on the order of 0.05–1.00 cm^2 sec^{-1}) because the free volume or void space available to the molecules is large compared to their size and the mean free path between molecular collisions is great. In liquids, the void space is much smaller, mean free paths are decreased, and diffusivities are much reduced. Thus, for an aqueous lotion on the skin, diffusion coefficients within the vehicle would be in the region of 10^{-5} to 10^{-6} cm^2 sec^{-1}. Diffusivities progressively drop as the consistency of the material increases until, for a true crystalline solid with no free volume, molecules other than small gas molecules are stopped completely.

The diffusion coefficient of a drug, either in a topical vehicle or in the skin, depends on the properties of the drug and the diffusion medium and on the extent of interaction between them. The diffusivity D is related to the frictional resistance f experienced by the diffusing particle, the gas constant R, the absolute temperature T, and Avogadro's number N by the following equation (Jost, 1960):

$$D = \frac{RT}{fN} \tag{2.48}$$

Following Flynn et al. (1974), we will examine the variations which arise from Eq. (2.48) for some idealized situations relevant to skin therapy, i.e., diffusion in homogeneous liquids, in aqueous and nonaqueous solutions, in gels, and in polymers.

1. Diffusivity in homogeneous liquids

When a particle diffuses through a homogeneous liquid, the frictional resistance to its passage depends mainly upon the particle's size and shape, as well as on the type of solvent. No single equation relating D and f is valid for all circumstances (Sutherland, 1905; Li, 1955; Edward, 1970; Bretsznajder, 1971). A widely used relationship (Tanford, 1961) was derived by Sutherland (1905) for situations in which spherical particles are in sufficiently dilute solutions so that solute-solute interactions can be neglected:

$$f = 6\pi\eta r \left(\frac{2\eta + r\beta}{3\eta + r\beta}\right) \tag{2.49}$$

Here η is the solvent viscosity, r is the hydrodynamic radius of the diffusing particle (which may include contributions from material adsorbed or entrapped by the particle), and β is a "slip" factor. The slip factor measures the tendency of solvent molecules to adhere to the diffusing species. When the diffusing particles are large compared with the solvent molecules, the small molecules tend to be dragged along with the diffusant and β approaches infinity. When the slip factor is sufficiently large, the parenthesized term in Eq. (2.49) approaches unity and we have then the Stokes' expression:

$$f = 6\pi\eta r \tag{2.50}$$

When solute and solvent sizes become comparable, there is little resistance to slip, β approaches zero, and Eq. (2.49) becomes

$$f = 4\pi\eta r \tag{2.51}$$

The ideal situation for applying Eq. (2.51) is in self-diffusion when the diffusant and solvent are identical. The frictional resistance can even fall below that given by Eq. (2.51) when the diffusant is smaller than the solvent (Tanford, 1961).

However, large molecules and colloidal particles in solution will adopt a wide variety of configurations which deviate from a simple sphere. To deal with this situation it is necessary to select suitably idealized shapes which can be used as approximations for such configurations. Ellipsoids of revolution are selected to represent these diffusants because it is easy to write equations for ellipsoidal boundaries. For an ellipse with major semi-axis a and minor semiaxis b, a prolate ellipsoid is obtained by revolution about the major axis and an oblate ellipsoid is formed by revolution about the minor axis. When a/b becomes large, the prolate ellipsoid represents a long thin rod and the oblate ellipsoid approaches the shape of a flat circular disk. We then allow for the greater resistance a nonspherical particle experiences as its surface area increases relative to that of a sphere (Herzog et al., 1934; Perrin, 1936). We can write an expression which is the ratio F of the frictional resistance of the ellipsoid f_e to that which would operate on a sphere of the same volume f as given by Eq. (2.50). For an oblate ellipsoid (semiaxes a, a, b)

$$F = \frac{f_e}{6\pi\eta r} = \frac{(a^2/b^2 - 1)^{1/2}}{(a/b)^{2/3} \tan^{-1}(a^2/b^2 - 1)^{1/2}} \tag{2.52}$$

where r is the radius of a sphere of equal volume to the ellipsoid, i.e., $4\pi r^3/3 = 4\pi a^2 b/3$. For a prolate ellipsoid (semiaxes a, b, b)

$$F = \frac{f_e}{6\pi\eta r} = \frac{(1 - b^2/a^2)^{1/2}}{(b/a)^{2/3} \ln\dfrac{1 + (1 - b^2/a^2)^{1/2}}{b/a}} \tag{2.53}$$

where $4\pi r^3/3 = 4\pi ab^2/3$. Tanford (1961) provides graphic representations for F as a function of a/b and shows that log F is linearly related to log (a/b) at high values of a/b.

From the above, we can usefully discuss two extreme situations—one in which the diffusing particles are approximately spherical and of a size similar to the solvent molecules; the other in which large, asymmetric particles diffuse through a liquid. In the former situation, in which the molar volume of the solute v is equal to that of the solvent, then, combining Eqs. (2.48) and (2.51),

$$D = \frac{kT}{4\pi\eta r} \tag{2.54}$$

as R/N = k. As $v = 4\pi r^3 N/3$, then

$$D = \frac{kT}{4\pi\eta} \left(\frac{4\pi N}{3v}\right)^{1/3} \tag{2.55}$$

For large, asymmetric particles, combining Eqs. (2.48) and (2.50),

$$D = \frac{kT}{6\pi\eta F} \left(\frac{4\pi N}{3v}\right)^{1/3} \tag{2.56}$$

To estimate D, we then proceed as follows:

1. The viscosity is either known or is readily measured and therefore provides no problem.
2. The frictional ratio can be obtained by solving Eq. (2.52) or (2.53). The axial ratio can be estimated from bond distances and group radii (Yalkowsky and Zografi, 1972) or from space-filling molecular models. Unless the particles are very elongated, the frictional ratio correction contributes less than 10% to the estimate of D and may thus be ignored to a first approximation.
3. Again, for an approximate value of D, we need only estimate the molecular or molar volume. This cannot be measured directly, but the experimentally measured partial molal volume is a reasonable approximation to the true value (Stigter, 1967). One can calculate the Van der Waals volume of the diffusant (Edward, 1970) or employ space-filling molecular models (Beck and Schultz, 1972; Goldstein and Solomon, 1960). As the molar volume of a substance is an additive property of the constituent atoms and functional groups, values for partial molal volumes of large drug molecules such as the steroids may be estimated from published values of the individual atoms or groups (for examples, see Flynn et al., 1974). It is true that simply adding group contributions provides only an approximate value for the partial molal volume, except possibly in ideal solutions; in practice, the partial molal volume depends on temperature as well as the nature and mole fraction of other components in the mixture (Tanford, 1961). However, for approximate estimations the procedure appears to be satisfactory, and it has been widely used.

When the concentration increases sufficiently, solute-solute interactions become significant and the thermodynamic activity coefficient of the diffusant, γ, alters. If the solution viscosity remains the same as that of the solvent, then in general (Stein, 1967):

$$D = D_{C=0}\left[1 + C\left(\frac{\partial \ln \gamma}{\partial C}\right)\right] \tag{2.57}$$

Thus, D depends on C at high concentrations but is independent of C at low concentrations. When C is sufficiently high, the viscosity can increase and this additional effect on diffusivity may be accounted for by modifying Eq. (2.57):

$$D = D_{C=0}\left[1 + C\left(\frac{\partial \ln \gamma}{\partial C}\right)\right]\frac{\eta}{\eta_{C=0}} \tag{2.58}$$

Materials which complex with the diffusant decrease D, as do the phenomena of self-aggregation and, in particular, micellization.

Increasing the temperature of a homogeneous solution alters the diffusivity in several ways. The higher the temperature, the greater is the thermal motion of the diffusant and D increases proportionally, as indicated by Eq. (2.48). More important, however, is the effect on solvent viscosity. Thus, raising the temperature of water from 20°C to 30°C decreases the viscosity by 20% compared with a change of only 3.4% in kT; the viscosity change has a greater effect than the increased thermal motion (Eqs. 2.54 and 2.56). A temperature increase can also disrupt complexes and micelles and affect molecular activity coefficients. It is only if such indirect effects of temperature on diffusivity are negligible and D is related to T by Eq. (2.48) and its modifications that the energy of activation for diffusion in a solvent is a constant for that solvent.

2. Diffusivity in aqueous solutions

Flynn et al. (1974) applied the principles discussed in the previous subsection to diffusion in water at 25°C. Calculated values of diffusivity of solutes in water, D_{calc}, as obtained from Eqs. (2.54) and (2.56), then become

$$D_{calc} = \frac{4.95 \times 10^{-5}}{v^{1/3}} \qquad (2.59)$$

and

$$D_{calc} = \frac{3.3 \times 10^{-5}}{v^{1/3}} \qquad (2.60)$$

For 68 compounds ranging in size from methane ($v = 22.4$ cm^3 mol^{-1}) to β-cyclodextrin (1,235 cm^3 mol^{-1}), they compared the calculated diffusivities as expressed by Eqs. (2.59) and (2.60) with experimentally determined values. For the small molecules methane and ethane, experimental diffusivities were slightly higher than D_{calc} from Eq. (2.59); for the large molecules tetrose, pentose, and hexose, experimental diffusivities were slightly lower than values calculated from Eq. (2.60). For the 63 remaining diffusants, the experimental values fell within the range of the diffusion coefficients calculated theoretically.

In general, the smaller solutes exhibit diffusivities close to those calculated from Eq. (2.59), while Eq. (2.60) provides a better approximation for larger diffusants. When a methylene group is added to a molecule the diffusivity decreases only slightly (D is proportional to $v^{1/3}$), and this effect is insignificant for a large molecule. This small decrement contrasts with the marked effect which group addition has on the partition coefficient (cf. Sec. III.B). It is usual, therefore, to ignore the effects of any change in diffusivity on ascending a homologous series in favor of the dramatic increase in partition coefficient which dominates the permeation process.

When we compare homologous series on the basis of diffusivity at a comparable molar volume, the order becomes alkanes > alcohols > amides > acids > amino acids > dicarboxylic acids. Thus, the more water molecules which are hydrogen-bonded to the polar group of the diffusant, the greater is the hydrodynamic volume of the solute and the slower the molecule diffuses. When molecules ionize, repulsive effects may produce a more elongated structure (Albery et al., 1967) or promote solvation (Longworth, 1936; Wendt and Gosting, 1959); both effects decrease diffusivity.

As discussed in the previous subsection, the diffusivity usually falls as the solute concentration increases; however, below a concentration of 0.1 M, diffusivities are generally within a few percent of the infinitely dilute values.

Above the CMC, surfactants micellize and the apparent diffusion coefficient drops as colloidal aggregates form. Materials which are solubilized by such micelles acquire the hydrodynamic properties of the micelle. Thus, highly polar materials such as cadmium ions adsorb onto the surface of nonionic micelles (Novodoff et al., 1972). Large anions, such as those of tartrazine, amaranth, carmoisine, and erythrosine, may interact with cationic surfactants such as the alkyltrimethylammonium bromides and may even form coacervates (Barry and Russell, 1972; Barry and Gray, 1974). Molecules which are asymmetric with distinct polar and nonpolar regions (such as testosterone, hydrocortisone, dexamethasone, progesterone, salicylamide, and salicylic and benzoic acids) may solubilize in the palisade layer of the micelle, aligning themselves with surfactant chains (Short et al., 1970; Short and Rhodes, 1971; Barry and El Eini, 1976a,b; Feldman et al., 1971; Gibaldi et al., 1970). Nonpolar molecules will dissolve in the hydrocarbon core of the micelle. Oppositely charged surfactants may form mixed micelles (Kolp et al., 1963) which may also coacervate, e.g., alkyltrimethylammonium bromides with bile salts (Barry and Gray, 1975a,b).

Temperature variation affects aqueous diffusivity according to Eq. (2.48) (Wilke, 1949; Benson and Gordon, 1945; Longsworth, 1954). Energies of activation derived from aqueous diffusion experiments generally range between 4.5 and 5.0 kcal mol^{-1}.

3. Diffusivity in nonaqueous solutions

When designing topical drug delivery systems or investigating percutaneous absorption, we are also concerned with the interactions which organic groups may undergo in nonaqueous solutions. Such groups may interact at several locations, e.g., within the vehicle, in nonpolar membranes which may be used as models representing the stratum corneum, in the lipid portion of the stratum corneal matrix, or even in nonpolar solvents used as receptor fluids in diffusion or release experiments. Carbon tetrachloride is such a nonaqueous solvent which has been well studied and which can serve as a model nonpolar phase in which the aggregation behavior of polar solutes may be investigated.

In ideal solutions, differences between diffusivities of a solute in various solvents arise only from the different solvent viscosities. However, in practical systems there are complications. A solute which is large compared with water ($v = 18$ cm^3 mol^{-1}) has its frictional resistance in water described by Eq. (2.50). In a solvent such as carbon tetrachloride ($v = 315$ cm^3 mol^{-1}), the solute molecule may be comparable in size and then Eq. (2.51) would describe its frictional resistance. In addition, interactions which take place in one solvent may be insignificant in another solvent.

In a manner similar to their treatment of the aqueous solution environment, Flynn et al. (1974) compared the calculated diffusivities of 17 compounds in carbon tetrachloride at 25°C as obtained from Eqs. (2.55) and (2.56) with experimental diffusion coefficients (Longsworth, 1966). Because water and carbon tetrachloride possess nearly identical viscosities at 25°C, Eqs. (2.59) and (2.60) could be used directly. Solutes such as the C$_5$ to C$_{12}$ normal alkanes, with molar volumes significantly less than that of carbon tetrachloride, exhibit experimental diffusivities greater than those deduced from Eq. (2.59). Diffusion coefficients of higher alkanes with sizes comparable to carbon tetrachloride are adequately represented by Eq. (2.59). Still larger solutes possess diffusivities lying within the range encompassed by Eqs. (2.59) and (2.60). However, when the molecule gains polar groups, its behavior deviates. The C$_{16}$ hexadecanoic acid has the same molar volume as hexadecane (265 cm^3 mol^{-1}), yet its apparent experimental diffusivity is similar to that of the C$_{32}$ alkane ($v = 525$ cm^3 mol^{-1}). This is because the long-chain acid exists as a dimer in carbon tetrachloride, with $v = 530$ cm^3 mol^{-1}. Shorter-chain acids, such as acetic acid, similarly dimerize. Alcohols such as methanol, ethanol, and hexadecanol show concentration-dependent diffusivities, with different values for the monomer and tetramer (Flynn et al., 1974).

There are several semiempirical methods for estimating diffusion coefficients in terms of solute and solvent properties and diffusivity data for many nonaqueous solvents have been compiled (Sutherland, 1905; Li, 1955; Edward, 1970; Bretsznajder, 1971; Longsworth, 1966).

4. Diffusivity in gels

We next deal with the type of gel that consists of a three-dimensional network of polymer which encloses and is interpenetrated by a liquid. We will concentrate on aqueous gels, but similar considerations apply to other systems. Gel is rather a broad term, which may be used to encompass several classes of systems. When the matrix is rich in liquid, the product may be termed a jelly. When most of the liquid is removed so that only the framework remains, the system becomes a xerogel. Thixotropic gels are those in which the structure breaks down on shearing so that the consistency decreases but in which the structure rebuilds on standing.

The gelling agent can modify the observed diffusivity of a solute by either mechanically impeding its movement or by adsorbing the solute on the polymer surface. Since the actual pathway for diffusion in gels is through the fluid phase, the factors which affect diffusivity in pure liquid phases similarly control diffusion within gels. Here we will only concern ourselves with how the presence of a solid phase further alters the diffusivity of solutes, concentrating first on situations in which the regions available for diffusion are very large compared with the hydrodynamic volume of the penetrant. For gels in which the solute also permeates the polymer network, we can employ the principles of parallel pathways, as discussed previously (Sec. II.B).

Because the diffusional pathway is through the entrapped fluid phase in the gel pores, the microscopic viscosity is relevant, not the bulk or macroviscosity. Thus, as T. Graham first pointed out, the diffusion rates of many crystalloids through dilute gels differ only slightly from the rates in the pure solvents. Classical experiments showed that the electrical mobility of the hydrogen ion in a gel was close to that calculated for water (see Alexander and Johnson, 1950); Taft and Malm (1939) showed that the diffusivities of salts in aqueous gelatin solutions before and after setting remained the same. Thus, the chain length of the polymer and its degree of cross-linking are important in controlling the overall consistency of a gel but not in influencing the diffusionally important microviscosity.

The polymer may modify the observed diffusivity of a solute by a mechanical obstruction effect, which depends on the size of the solute molecule and the volume fraction of the polymer, ϕ. In effect, the solute travels through fluid regions and collides with individual polymer segments. Then, the microscopic viscosity and the number of polymer segments present determine diffusivity. If the polymer exerts a purely obstructive effect, then for diffusion of small solutes through aqueous gels (Lauffer, 1961):

$$D_{pn} = \frac{D_w}{1 + 2\phi/3} \qquad (2.61)$$

where D_w and D_{pn} are the diffusion coefficients of the solute in water and in the (nonabsorbing) aqueous polymer gel, respectively. In calculating ϕ, one may have to allow for the volume of water immobilized by the polymer, e.g., as water of hydration. The larger the diffusant, the greater is its collision diameter and the more likely it is to collide with a polymer segment. Thus, large diffusants are more affected by polymeric materials than are small ones. If the polymer only exerts an obstructive effect, polar and nonpolar diffusants should be affected similarly, i.e., there should be no specific structural effects.

If, in addition to obstructing the solute, the polymer interacts with or adsorbs the penetrant, then it can be shown (Schantz and Lauffer, 1962) that

$$D_{pa} = \frac{D_w}{1 + A\phi} \qquad (2.62)$$

where D_{pa} is the diffusivity in the presence of adsorbing polymer and A is the adsorption constant of the diffusant per unit volume of gel. Equation (2.62) applies below saturation; when the diffusant saturates the gel we have

$$D'_{pa} = \frac{D_w}{1 + A\phi/k}$$ (2.63)

where k is a constant.

The chemical nature of the penetrant strongly influences the magnitude of the adsorption effect. For a given solute, A depends on the number of adsorptive sites per unit volume of polymer and on the relative strengths of attraction of these sites and the solvent for the diffusant. The sites available may be specific to particular functional groups. Thus, a particular polymer may have many sites capable of interacting with amide groups but few which will bind carboxylates. Competitive adsorbants may release bound diffusant and thus increase the apparent diffusivity. Thus, bovine serum albumin reduces the apparent diffusivity of chloramphenicol, but submicellar amounts of sodium lauryl sulfate counteract this effect (Alhaigne et al., 1972).

For a particular polymer and a homologous series of compounds, the values of A would be expected to increase exponentially as we ascend the series. This is because the solubility usually decreases exponentially with chain length (see Sec. III.A).

As ϕ increases, it becomes more useful to characterize the gel, which is often in a membranous form at high polymer concentrations, by its porosity and a tortuosity factor (see Secs. II.B and II.C). When the hydrodynamic radius of the diffusant approaches the pore radius, the penetrant can no longer freely diffuse. For mathematical simplicity, the pores in the membrane are assumed to be uniform cylinders oriented at right angles to the diffusant flow, and the diffusant molecules are assumed spherical. Geometrical idealizations other than cylindrical pores are possible (Bjerrum and Mangold, 1927) but are not necessary for most work.

There are two main factors which contribute to the observation that the solute flux through a small aqueous pore is less than the value calculated from the geometry of the pore and the solute's aqueous diffusivity (Renkin, 1954). For a molecule to pass into a pore, it must enter through the opening without striking the edge (Ferry, 1936). The center of the solute molecule (radius r_s) must pass through a circle of radius $(r_p - r_s)$, where r_p is the radius of the pore. Then A, the effective area of the opening, is

$$A = A_p\left(1 - \frac{r_s}{r_p}\right)^2$$ (2.64)

in which A_p is the total cross sectional area of the pore. The second factor corrects for the friction between a molecule moving within a pore and its walls (Renkin, 1954; Lane, 1950).

$$\frac{A}{A_p} = 1 - 2.104 \frac{r_s}{r_p} + 2.09 \left(\frac{r_s}{r_p}\right)^3 - 0.95 \left(\frac{r_s}{r_p}\right)^5 \qquad (2.65)$$

The total restriction to diffusion, arising from the combined effects of steric hindrance at the entrance to the pores and frictional resistance within the pores, may be expressed by combing Eqs. (2.64) and (2.65) in the form

$$\frac{D_p}{D_f} = \left(1 - \frac{r_s}{r_p}\right)^2 \left[1 - 2.104 \left(\frac{r_s}{r_p}\right) + 2.09 \left(\frac{r_s}{r_p}\right)^3 - 0.95 \left(\frac{r_s}{r_p}\right)^5\right] \qquad (2.66)$$

where D_p/D_f gives the ratio of diffusivity within the pore D_p to the diffusivity in free solution D_f.

According to Eq. (2.66), as r_s becomes very small compared to r_p ($r_s/r_p \rightarrow 0$), D_p approaches D_f. As $r_s \rightarrow r_p$, D_p/D_f approaches zero, i.e., $D_p \rightarrow 0$ and the solute movement is blocked. For $r_s/r_p < 0.2$, Eq. (2.66) can be simplified to

$$\frac{D_p}{D_f} = \left(1 - \frac{r_s}{r_p}\right)^4 \qquad (2.67)$$

Beck et al. (1972) found that such equations held for solutes of different molecular volumes diffusing through right cylindrical pores ranging from 45 to 300 Å in diameter. Barry and Brace (1977) measured the permeation of estrone, estradiol, estriol, and dexamethasone across cellulose acetate membrane. They analyzed their results in the light of the partial molal volume approach expressed by Eqs. (2.59) and (2.60), as modified by Eqs. (2.61) to (2.67).

Equations (2.66) and (2.67) show that the size of the diffusant molecule can have a dramatic effect on the diffusion rate; this principle underlies the mechanism of size segregation in the technique of differential dialysis (Craig and Pulley, 1962; Craig, 1964).

This relationship between solute radius, solute diffusivity, and pore radius can be used to calculate an "equivalent pore radius" for biological membranes. Such calculations suggest values between 3.5 and 6 Å (Solomon, 1968; Sha'afi et al., 1971; Solomon and Gary-Bobo, 1972; Stein, 1967). Most drugs have radii similar to or greater than the equivalent pore radii of biological membranes and thus do not undergo pore transport. Additionally, of course, many drug species are sufficiently hydrophobic to ensure that they are not constrained to aqueous diffusional routes within the biological membrane.

5. Diffusivity in amorphous isotropic polymers

In polymers above the glass transition temperature, it is not possible to relate diffusivity to molecular size by simple relationships such as Eqs. (2.54) and (2.55). Therefore, for the purposes of this book, only a very brief account of the more important generalizations which may be made is given here; for further details, the interested reader is referred to Crank and Park (1968), Barrer (1941), Glasstone et al. (1941), Lieb and Stein (1969), and Mears (1971).

In general, diffusivity in polymers is more sensitive to molecular size or weight compared with homogeneous liquids and decreases with molecular size. However, diffusivity becomes less sensitive to size as size increases; this is especially apparent for increases in length within a homologous series. Molecular shape has a greater effect in polymers than in liquids. Whereas in polymers a sphere usually has a lower diffusivity than an ellipsoid of equivalent volume, in a liquid the diffusion coefficient decreases as the solute deviates from a spherical shape (Eqs. 2.55 and 2.56). Branched compounds possess lower diffusivities than their linear isomers. Functional groups are important when interactions produce aggregates whose geometry differs significantly from that of the monomer or when the groups interact with fixed sites on filler surfaces.

The effect of temperature on diffusion in polymers is usually described by Eq. (2.18). The energy of activation tends to increase linearly with diffusant size until we reach a plateau value characteristic of the polymer. Values range from 7 to 20 kcal mol^{-1}; they are thus larger than those in homogeneous liquids. Below the glass transition point, crystallites form. Since these are essentially unavailable as diffusional pathways, they act as impermeable inclusions within the polymer.

Diffusivities in polymers are almost always related to diffusant concentration by

$$D = D_{C=0} \exp(kC) \tag{2.68}$$

where k is a constant at a given temperature in a particular polymer and is independent of size for most solutes (Aitken and Barrer, 1955). Deviations occur if the diffusant self-associates, e.g., as occurs with fatty acids and alcohols.

Above about 1% concentration, the diffusant can dilute or solvate the polymer. The polymer matrix may expand and loosen, so that secondary effects on the solute's diffusivity lead to significant deviations in Eq. (2.68) (Horowitz and Fenichel, 1964; Fenichel and Horowitz, 1964).

If we consider that the stratum corneum is similar in diffusional properties to a soft polymer, then we may expect that the structured nature of the medium will lead to a steep molecular weight dependence of the diffusion coefficient. How this concept can be developed for biological membranes in general has been examined by Stein (1981).

SYMBOLS

A	adsorption constant of polymer in aqueous gel; total concentration of drug; effective cross sectional area of pore opening
A_p	cross-sectional area of pore
B	CH_2 group contribution to solubility
C	concentration
C_s	saturation concentration (solubility) of drug in matrix
C_0, C_h	concentration at $x = 0$, $x = h$ in membrane, respectively
C_R'	receptor concentration
C_0'	donor concentration
D	diffusion coefficient, diffusivity
$\bar{D}$	average integral diffusion coefficient
D_{AQ}	diffusion coefficient in aqueous phase
D_M	diffusion coefficient in membrane
D_f	diffusion coefficient in free solution
D_i	diffusion coefficient in ith layer in laminate
D_p	diffusion coefficient within a pore
D_{pa}	diffusion coefficient in absorbing aqueous polymer gel
D_{pa}'	diffusion coefficient in absorbing aqueous polymer gel above saturation
D_{pn}	diffusion coefficient in nonabsorbing aqueous polymer gel
D_v	diffusion coefficient in vehicle matrix
D_w	diffusion coefficient in water
D_0	hypothetical diffusion coefficient at infinite temperature
D_{01}	hypothetical diffusion coefficient at infinite temperature—route 1
D_{02}	hypothetical diffusion coefficient at infinite temperature—route 2
E_D	energy of activation for diffusion
E_{D1}	energy of activation for diffusion—route 1
E_{D2}	energy of activation for diffusion—route 2

E_p	energy of activation for permeation
F	ratio of frictional resistance of ellipsoid to equivalent sphere in diffusion
G	constant
H	effective membrane thickness
J	flux of diffusant
J_T	total flux in a composite membrane
J_1, J_2, etc.	fluxes through areas 1, 2, etc.
K	partition coefficient
K_{RH}	partition coefficient of unsubstituted parent compound
K_{RX}	partition coefficient of substituted compound
K_i	partition coefficient for a single solvent; partition coefficient for ith layer in a laminate
K_n	partition coefficient of homolog of chain length, n
K_{SC}	partition coefficient for stratum corneum
K_0	partition coefficient of reference homolog with n = 0
L	lag time
M	cumulative mass of diffusant penetrated per unit area
M_∞	cumulative mass of diffusant penetrated per unit area at infinite time
N	Avogadro's number
P	permeability coefficient, permeability
P_T	total thickness-weighted permeability coefficient of all layers of a laminate; complex permeability; effective permeability coefficient when adsorptive, permeable disperse phase is present
P_i	thickness-weighted permeability coefficient of ith layer
P_0	hypothetic permeability coefficient at infinite temperature
P_1	permeability coefficient of continuous phase
P_2	permeability coefficient of disperse phase
Q	amount of diffusant in membrane per unit area
Q_∞	amount of diffusant in membrane per unit area at infinite time

R	gas constant; diffusional resistance (laminates)
R_T	total diffusional resistance of all layers of a laminate
R_i	diffusional resistance of ith layer in laminate
S_n	solubility of homology of chain length n
S_0	solubility of reference homolog with n = 0
T	absolute temperature
Z	saturation adsorptive capacity of filler
a	constant; major semiaxis of ellipse and ellipsoid
a'	constant
b	constant; minor semiaxis of ellipse and ellipsoid
b'	constant
f	frictional resistance of diffusing particle (sphere)
f_e	frictional resistance of ellipsoid in diffusion
f_1, f_2, etc.	fraction areas available for diffusion
h	thickness of membrane
$h_{AQ(I)}$	thickness of donor diffusion layer
$h_{AQ(II)}$	thickness of receptor diffusion layer
h_i	thickness of ith layer in laminate
k	constant; Boltzmann constant
n	integer
r	hydrodynamic radius of diffusing particle; radius of sphere
r_p	radius of pore
r_s	radius of solute molecule
t	time
v	molar volume
x, y, z	space coordinates
$\bar{x}$	mean displacement of a molecule in diffusion
z	filler adsorptive constant

β	slip factor in frictional resistance of diffusing particles
η	coefficient of viscosity; solvent viscosity
π	3.142; group contribution to partition coefficient
π_x	group contribution of x group to partition coefficient
τ	tortuosity factor
ϕ	volume fraction of polymer in gel
ϕ_1	volume fraction of matrix of continuous phase
ϕ_2	volume fraction of filler or dispersed phase
ΔG	free-energy change
ΔH	enthalpy change
ΔS	entropy change
∞	infinity

REFERENCES

Aguiar, A. J., and Fifelski, R. J. (1966). J. Pharm. Sci. 55:1387.

Aitken, A., and Barrer, R. M. (1955). Trans. Faraday Soc. 51:116.

Albery, W. J., Greenwood, A. R., and Kibble, R. F. (1967). Trans. Farady Soc. 63:360.

Alexander, A. E., and Johnson, P. (1950). Colloid Science. Oxford Univ. Press, New York.

Alhaigne, F., Marchetti, M., Riccieri, F. M., and Santucci, E. (1972). Farmaco 27:145.

Barnes, C. (1934). Physics 5:4.

Barrer, R. M. (1939). Trans. Faraday Soc. 35:368.

Barrier, R. M. (1941). Diffusion in and Through Solids. Macmillan, New York.

Barrer, R. M. (1968). In Diffusion in Polymers, J. Crank and G. S. Park (Eds.). Academic Press, New York, p. 165.

Barrie, J. A. (1968). In Diffusion in Polymers, J. Crank and G. S. Park (Eds.). Academic Press, New York, p. 280.

Barrie, J. A., Levine, J. D., Michaels, A. S., and Wong, P. (1963). Trans. Faraday Soc. 59:869.

Barry, B. W., and Brace, A. R. (1977). J. Pharm. Pharmacol. 29:397.

Barry, B. W., and El Eini, D. I. D. (1976a). J. Pharm. Pharmacol. 28:210.

Barry, B. W., and El Eini, D. I. D. (1976b). J. Pharm. Pharmacol. 28:219.

Barry, B. W., and Gray, G. M. T. (1974). J. Pharm. Sci. 63:548.

Barry, B. W., and Gray, G. M. T. (1975a). J. Colloid Interface Sci. 52: 314.

Barry, B. W., and Gray, G. M. T. (1975b). J. Colloid Interface Sci. 52: 327.

Barry, B. W., and Russell, G. F. J. (1972). J. Pharm. Sci. 61:502.

Bates, T. R., Galownia, J., and Johns, W. H. (1970). Chem. Pharm. Bull. 18:656.

Beck, R. E., Schultz, J. S., and Jerome, S. (1972). Biochem. Biophys. Acta 255:273.

Beckett, A. H., and Moffat, H. C. (1969). J. Pharm. Pharmacol. 21 (Suppl.):239S.

Benet, L. Z. (1973). In Drug Design, E. J. Ariens (Ed.), Vol. 4. Academic Press, New York, p. 26.

Benson, G. C., and Gordon, A. R. (1945). J. Phys. Chem. 13:490.

Bickel, M. H., and Weder, H. J. (1969). J. Pharm. Pharmacol. 21:160.

Bikhazi, A. B., and Higuchi, W. I. (1970). J. Pharm. Sci. 59:744.

Bjerrum, N., and Mangold, E. (1927). Kolloid Z. 43:5.

Blanpin, O. (1968). Prod. Pharm. 13:425.

Bretsznajder, S. (1971). Prediction of Transport and Other Physical Properties of Fluids, Chap. 8. Pergamon Press, Elmsford, N.Y.

Breusch, F. L. (1969). Fortschr. Chem. Forsch. 12:119.

Breusch, F. L., and Kirkali, A. (1968). Fette Seifen Anstrichmittel 70: 864.

Burton, D. E., Clark, K., and Gray, G. W. (1964). J. Chem. Soc. p. 1314.

Carslaw, H. S., and Jaeger, J. C. (1959). Conduction of Heat in Solids. Oxford Press, New York.

Chandrasekaran, S. K., and Hillman, R. (1980). J. Pharm. Sci. 69:1311.

Chandrasekaran, S. K., Michaels, A. S., Campbell, P., and Shaw, J. E. (1976). Am. Inst. Chem. Eng. 22:828.

Chandrasekaran, S. K., Bayne, W., and Shaw, J. E. (1978). J. Pharm. Sci. 67:1370.

Chandrasekaran, S. K., Campbell, P. S., and Watanabe, T. (1980). Polymer Eng. Science 20:36.

Collander, R. (1951). Acta Chem. Scand. 5:774.

Courchene, W. I. (1964). J. Phys. Chem. 68:1870.

Craig, L. C. (1964). Science 144:1093.

Craig, L. C., and Pulley, A. O. (1962). Biochemistry 1:89.

Crank, J. (1975). The Mathematics of Diffusion, 2nd ed. Oxford Univ. Press (Clarendon), New York.

Crank, J., and Park, C. S. (1968). Diffusion in Polymers. Academic Press, New York.

Davis, S. S., Higuchi, T., and Rytting, J. H. (1972). J. Pharm. Pharmacol. 24:30P.

Davis, S. S., Higuchi, T., and Rytting, J. H. (1974). Adv. Pharm. Sci. 4:73.

Daynes, H. A. (1920). Proc. R. Soc. Lond. A97:286.

Diamond, J. M., and Katz, Y. (1974). J. Membrane Biol. 17:121.

Dugard, P. H. (1977). Adv. Mod. Toxicol. 4:525.

Edward, J. T. (1970). J. Chem. Educ. 47:261.

Einstein, A. (1926). Investigations on the Theory of Brownian Motion. Dover, New York, 1956.

Elworthy, P. H. (1967). Pharm. J. 199:107.

Elworthy, P. H., Florence, A. T., and MacFarlane, C. B. (1968). Solubilization by Surface Active Agents. Chapman & Hall, London.

Feldman, S., Gibaldi, M., and Reinhard, M. (1971). J. Pharm. Sci. 60: 1105.

Fenechel, I. R., and Horowitz, S. B. (1964). Ann. N.Y. Acad. Sci. 125: 290.

Ferry, J. D. (1936). J. Gen. Physiol. 20:95.

Fick, A. (1855). Poggendorff's Ann. 94:59.

Finger, K. F., Lemberger, A. P., Higuchi, T., Busse, L. W., and Wurster, D. E. (1960). J. Am. Pharm. Assoc., Sci. Ed. 49:569.

Flynn, G. L. (1971). J. Pharm. Sci. 60:345.

Flynn, G. L., and Roseman, T. J. (1971). J. Pharm. Sci. 60:1788.

Flynn, G. L., and Yalkowsky, S. H. (1972). J. Pharm. Sci. 61:838.

Flynn, G. L., Carpenter, O. S., and Yalkowsky, S. H. (1972). J. Pharm. Sci. 61:312.

Flynn, G. L., Yalkowsky, S. H., and Roseman, T. J. (1974). J. Pharm. Sci. 63:479.

Foreman, M. I., and Kelly, I. (1976). Br. J. Dermatol. 95:265.

Gibaldi, M., and Feldman, S. (1970). J. Pharm. Sci. 59:579.

Gibaldi, M., Feldman, S., and Weiner, N. D. (1970). Chem. Pharm. Bull. 18:715.

Glasstone, S., Laidler, K. J., and Eyring, H. (1941). The Theory of Rate Processes. McGraw-Hill, New York.

Goldberg, A. H., and Higuchi, W. I. (1969). J. Pharm. Sci. 58:1341.

Goldstein, D. A., and Solomon, A. K. (1960). J. Gen. Physiol. 44:1.

Grouthamel, W. G., Tan, G. H., Dittert, L. W., and Doluisio, J. T. (1971). J. Pharm. Sci. 60:1160.

Hansch, C., and Dunn, W. J. (1972). J. Pharm. Sci. 61:1.

Hansch, C., and Leo, A. (1979). Substituent Constants for Correlation Analysis in Chemistry and Biology. Wiley, New York.

Harris, M. J., Higuchi, T., and Rytting, J. H. (1973). J. Phys. Chem. 77:2694.

Henry, P. S. H. (1939). Proc. R. Soc. Lond. A171:215.

Herzog, R. O., Illig, R., and Kudar, H. (1934). Z. Physik. Chem. (Leipzig) A167:329.

Higuchi, T. (1960). J. Soc. Cosmetic Chemists 11:85.

Higuchi, T. (1961). J. Pharm. Sci. 50:874.

Higuchi, T. (1963). J. Pharm. Sci. 52:1145.

Higuchi, W. I., and Higuchi, T. (1960). J. Am. Pharm. Assoc., Sci. Ed. 49:598.

Hildebrand, J. H., and Scott, R. L. (1950). The Solubility of Nonelectrolytes. Van Nostrand Reinhold, New York.

Hildebrand, J. H., and Scott, R. L. (1962). Regular Solutions. Prentice-Hall, Englewood Cliffs, N.J.

Horowitz, S. B., and Fenichel, I. R. (1964). J. Phys. Chem. 68:3378.

Jacobs, M. H. (1935). Diffusion Processes. Springer-Verlag, New York.

Jost, W. (1960). Diffusion in Solids, Liquids, Gases. Academic Press, New York.

Juni, K., Tomitsuka, T., Nakano, M., and Arita, T. (1978). Chem. Pharm. Bull. 26:837.

Kakemi, K., Arita, T., Hori, R., and Konishi, R. (1967). Chem. Pharm. Bull. 15:1534.

Kakovosky, I. A. (1957). In Proc. 2nd Int. Congr. Surface Activity, Vol. 4, Butterworths, London, p. 225.

Kesting, R. E., Subcasky, W., and Paton, J. (1968). J. Colloid Interface Sci. 28:156.

Kolp, D. G., Laughlin, R. G., Krause, F. P., and Zimmerman, R. E. (1963). J. Phys. Chem. 67:51.

Lane, J. A. (1950). In Chemical Engineer's Handbook, J. H. Perry (Ed.), Sect. II. McGraw-Hill, New York, p. 753.

Lauffer, M. (1961). Biophys. J. 1:205.

Leo, A., and Hansch, C. (1971). J. Org. Chem. 36:1539.

Leo, A., Hansch, C., and Elkins, D. (1971). Chem. Rev. 71:525.

Levy, G. (1963). Prescription Pharmacy. Pitman Med. Publ., London.

Levy, G., and Anello, J. A. (1968). J. Pharm. Sci. 57:101.

Levy, G., Miller, K. E., and Reuning, R. H. (1966). J. Pharm. Sci. 55:394.

Li, J. C. M. (1955). J. Chem. Phys. 23:518.

Lieb, W. R., and Stein, W. D. (1969). Nature 224:240.

Longsworth, L. G. (1936). In American Institute of Physics Handbook. AIP, New York, p. 2.

Longsworth, L. G. (1954). J. Phys. Chem. 67:51.

Longsworth, L. G. (1966). J. Colloid Interface Sci. 22:3.

McBain, M., and Hutchinson, E. (1955). Solubilization and Related Phenomena. Academic Press, New York.

McCall, J. M. (1975). J. Med. Chem. 18:549.

McKay, A. T. (1930). Proc. Phys. Soc. 42:547.

Mears, P. (1971). Polymers: Structure and Bulk Properties. Van Nostrand Reinhold, New York, Chap. 12.

Mirlees, M. S., Moulton, S. J., Murphy, C. T., and Taylor, P. J. (1976). J. Med. Chem. 19:615.

Most, C. F. (1970). J. Appl. Polymer Sci. 11:1019.

Mulley, B. A. (1964). Adv. Pharm. Sci. 1:86.

Nakano, M., and Patel, N. K. (1970). J. Pharm. Sci. 59:77.

Nissim, J. A. (1960). Nature 187:308.

Nogami, H., Nagai, T., and Uchida, H. (1969). Chem. Pharm. Bull. 17: 176.

Novodoff, J., Rosano, H. L., and Hoyer, H. V. (1972). J. Colloid Interface Sci. 38:424.

Olson, F. C., and Schultz, O. T. (1942). Ind. Eng. Chem. 34:875.

Pappenheimer, J. R. (1953). Physiol. Rev. 33:387.

Perrin, F. (1936). J. Phys. Radium 7:1.

Ralston, A. W. (1948). Fatty Acids and Their Derivatives. Wiley, New York.

Renkin, E. M. (1954). J. Gen. Physiol. 38:225.

Riegelman, S., and Crowell, W. J. (1958). J. Pharm. Sci. 47:127.

Rodgers, W. A., Buritz, R. S., and Alpert, D. (1954). J. Appl. Phys. 25:868.

Sarraco, G., and Spaccamela Marchetti, E. (1958). Ann. Chim. (Rome) 48:1357.

Schantz, E. J., and Louffer, M. A. (1962). Biochemistry 1:658.

Scheuplein, R. J. (1966). Biophys. J. 6:1.

Scheuplein, R. J., Blank, I. H., Brauner, G. J., and MacFarlane, D. J. (1969). J. Invest. Dermatol. 52:63.

Sha'afi, R. I., Gary-Bobo, C. M., and Solomon, A. K. (1971). J. Gen. Physiol. 58:238.

Shibab, A. A. (1971). Ph.D. Thesis, University of London.

Shore, P. A., Brodie, B. B., and Hogben, C. A. M. (1957). J. Pharmacol. Exp. Ther. 119:36.

Short, P. M., and Rhodes, C. T. (1971). J. Pharm. Pharmacol. 23:239S.

Short, P. M., Abbs, E. T., and Rhodes, C. T. (1970). J. Pharm. Sci. 59:995.

Sjoblom, L. (1967). In Solvent Properties of Surfactant Solutions, K. Shinoda (Ed.). Dekker, New York.

Solomon, A. K. (1968). J. Gen. Physiol. 58:335.

Solomon, A. K., and Gary-Bobo, C. M. (1972). Biochim. Biophys. Acta 255:1019.

Spaccamela Marchetti, E., and Saracco, G. (1958). Ann. Chim. (Rome) 48:1371.

Stein, W. D. (1967). The Movement of Molecules Across Cell Membranes. Academic Press, New York.

Stein, W. D. (1981). In Membrane Transport, S. L. Bonting and J. J. H. H. M. de Pont (Eds.). Elsevier/North-Holland Biomed. Press, New York, p. 1.

Stehle, R. G., and Higuchi, W. I. (1967). J. Pharm. Sci. 56:1367.

Stigter, D. (1967). J. Colloid Interface Sci. 23:397.

Surpuriya, V., and Higuchi, W. I. (1972). J. Pharm. Sci. 61:375.

Sutherland, G. B. B. M. (1905). Phil. Mag. 9:781.

Swarbrick, J. (1965). J. Pharm. Sci. 54:1229.

Swisher, R. D. (1968). Arch. Environ. Health 17:232.

Taft, R., and Malm, L. E. (1939). J. Phys. Chem. 43:499.

Tanford, C. (1961). Physical Chemistry of Macromolecules. Wiley, New York.

Tanquary, A. C., and Lacey, R. E. (1974). Controlled Release of Biologically Active Agents (Adv. Exp. Med. Biol. 47). Plenum Press, New York.

Taylor, C. B. (1963). J. Physiol. 165:199.

Tomlinson, E. (1975). J. Chromatogr. 113:1.

Valvani, S. C., and Yalkowsky, S. H. (1980). In Physical Chemical Properties of Drugs, S. H. Yalkowsky, A. A. Sinkula, and S. C. Valvani (Eds.). Dekker, New York, p. 201.

Van Amerongen, G. J. (1955). Rubber Chem. Technol. 28:821.

Wagner, J. G., and Sedman, A. J. (1973). J. Pharmacokinetics Biopharm. 1:23.

Wendt, R. P., and Gosting, L. G. (1959). J. Phys. Chem. 63:1287.

Wilke, C. R. (1949). Chem. Eng. Progr. 45:218.

Wish, P. M., and Weikel, J. H. (1959). Toxicol. Appl. Pharmacol. 1:501.

Yalkowsky, S. H., and Flynn, G. L. (1973). J. Pharm. Sci. 62:210.

Yalkowsky, S. H., and Morozowich, W. (1980). In Drug Design, E. J. Ariens (Ed.), Vol. 9. Academic Press, New York, p. 121.

Yalkowsky, S. H., and Zografi, G. (1972). J. Pharm. Sci. 61:793.

Yalkowsky, S. H., Flynn, G. L., and Slunik, T. G. (1972). J. Pharm. Sci. 61:852.

Yasuda, M. (1968). Encyclopedia Polymer Sci. Technol. 9, N. M. Bikales, J. Conrad, A. Ruks, and J. Pereman (Eds.). Interscience, New York, p. 794.

Zwolinski, B. J., Eyring, H., and Reese, L. E. (1949). J. Phys. Colloid Chem. 53:1426.

— 3 —

SKIN TRANSPORT

I. INTRODUCTION

The skin is particularly effective as a selective barrier to the penetration (or elimination) of a diverse range of substances. The epidermis is the major element in this control as illustrated by the evidence that most small, water-soluble nonelectrolytes can diffuse into the capillary system a thousand times more rapidly when the epidermis is absent, damaged, or diseased than when it is present and intact. Furthermore, in the intact skin the penetration rates of different substances may differ by a factor of 10^5. How this selective permeability of the skin arises, and how we can predict and control it by relating the physiological and physicochemical attributes of the skin to the properties of the penetrant in a vehicle, is a fruitful field of study. However, it is only in recent years that experimental investigations have progressed from a descriptive approach to a fundamental correlation of the physicochemical and biological considerations inherent in the intricate process of percutaneous absorption. Scientists are now gathering data to relate the intrinsic properties of the skin barrier to the molecular requirements for breaching it, as modified by interactions with topical vehicles. The ultimate aim in dermatological biopharmaceutics is to design active drug molecules with selective permeability to be incorporated into vehicles which enable the medicament to arrive at the active site in the biophase at a controlled rate and there to maintain a sufficient concentration for the required time. In the future we may also expect this approach to be used more widely to provide systemic therapy via the percutaneous route (Shaw et al., 1975, 1977; Michaels et al., 1975; Chandrasekaran et al., 1976, 1978; see also Chap. 4, Sec. III.D.4).

The literature on skin transport published up to the middle of the 1960s was reviewed by Rothman (1954) and Tregear (1964, 1966a). Kligman (1964) provides a valuable account of the structure and function of the stratum corneum, and Malkinson (1964), together with Malkinson and Rothman (1963), review percutaneous absorption and provide extensive reference lists. More up-to-date work on skin permeability is discussed by Blank and Scheuplein (1969), Scheuplein and Blank (1971), and Scheuplein (1978a,b, 1980). Modern reviews which are notable for their emphasis on biopharmaceutical concepts include Idson (1971, 1975), Katz (1973), Katz and Poulsen (1971, 1972), Poulsen (1973), Higuchi (1977), Dugard (1977), and Flynn (1979). Other useful surveys are those of Wagner (1961), Barr (1962), Wells and Lubowe (1964), Stoughton (1965), Vinson et al. (1965), Vickers (1966), Reiss (1966), Winkelmann (1969), Barrett (1969), Schaefer (1974), Mershon (1975), Malkinson and Gehlmann (1977), and Wester and Maibach (1977).

II. ROUTES OF PENETRATION

When a molecule moves onto the intact skin, either from the external environment or from a vehicle, it first makes contact with the sebum, cellular debris, bacteria, and other exogenous materials which coat the skin. In

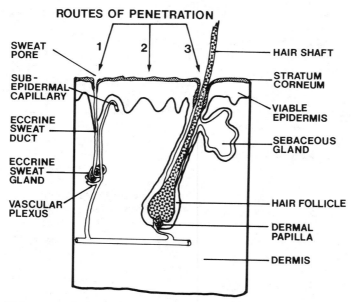

FIG. 3.1 The three potential routes of penetration of a diffusant into the subepidermal tissue of skin: (1) via the sweat ducts; (2) across the continuous stratum corneum; or (3) through the hair follicles with their associated sebaceous glands.

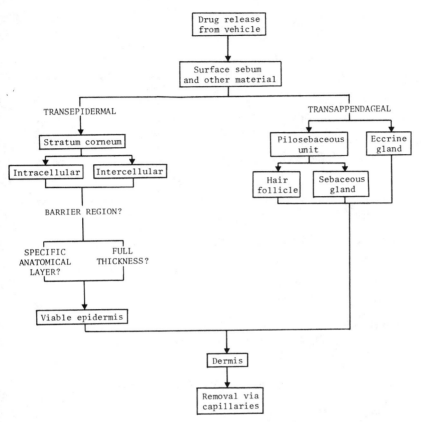

FIG. 3.2 Network of alternative pathways for percutaneous absorption. In Chap. 4, Sec. I and Fig. 4.1 deal with relevant additional aspects of the percutaneous absorption process. (Modified from Katz and Poulsen, 1971.)

general, the diffusant then has three potential routes of entry to the subepidermal tissue—through the hair follicles with their associated sebaceous glands, via the sweat ducts, or across the continuous stratum corneum between these appendages (Fig. 3.1). The actual pathway for penetration via the pilosebaceous apparatus could be through the hair fiber itself, through the outer root sheath of the hair into the viable cells of the follicle, or through the air-filled canal and into the sebaceous gland. The route for the sweat duct may be through either the lumen or the walls to below the epidermis and through the thin ring of keratinized cells. Dense capillary networks closely envelope the bases of both the sweat ducts and the hair follicles. Most molecules reaching these highly permeable vascular regions would immediately sweep into the systemic circulation.

Workers who favor the appendageal route as the premier mode of entry cite as evidence the rapid diffusion of charged dyes through sweat ducts when they apply a potential gradient (Abramson and Gorin, 1940), the formation of perifollicular wheals (Shelley and Melton, 1949; Cummings, 1969), and the preferential staining of hair follicles with dyes (MacKee et al., 1945; Rein, 1926; Rothman, 1954). Supporters of diffusion through the unbroken stratum corneum cite the small fractional surface area of the appendages (Scheuplein, 1967), the evidence that varying the number of appendages does not affect the steady state permeation (Treherne, 1956), and the very large activation energies measured, which would be improbable if the route was the relatively rapid appendageal pathway (Blank et al., 1967).

In a more detailed analysis, Katz and Poulsen (1971) have illustrated the various possibilities in the form of a network of alternative routes and they have cataloged the pros and cons of the relative importance of the different pathways (Fig. 3.2; see also Flynn, 1979). It is necessary to summarize these possible alternatives in the light of the available evidence before arriving at a general conclusion.

A. Sebum and Surface Material

Except for the palms of the hands and the soles of the feet, human skin possesses sebaceous glands which secrete a lipid mixture. Significant work on the composition of the surface fat of human skin has been performed by MacKenna et al. (1950, 1952), Wheatley (1953, 1954, 1956, 1957, 1963), James and Wheatley (1956), Boughton et al. (1957), Boughton and Wheatley (1959), Wheatley et al. (1964), Nicolaides and Rothman (1953), Nicolaides and Wells (1957), Rothman et al. (1947), Weitkamp et al. (1947), Wilkenson (1969), and Haahti (1961). Techniques for isolating human sebaceous glands and analyzing their contents allowed conclusions to be drawn regarding which components of the lipid mixture found on the skin surface originated in the sebaceous glands and which were produced in the ducts or on the surface by bacterial or endogenous enzymes (Kellum, 1967). Skin lipids are a complex mixture of free fatty acids and fatty acids esterified with glycerol, wax alcohols, and cholesterol, together with hydrocarbons, particularly squalene. Significant quantities of ferric chloride reducing substances have been reported, which may act as antioxidants in sebum, together with phospholipids and α-tocopherol (MacKenna et.al., 1950, 1952; Kvorning, 1949; Festenstein and Morton, 1952; Nicolaides, 1963). Sebum composition varies with age, sex, race, and site; there is a more striking species difference among mammals than for any other organ product (Wheatley, 1956).

The surface layer deposited when sebum mixes with sweat, bacteria, and dead cells is irregular, thin, and discontinuous, with estimates of thickness varying between 0.4 and 10 μm (Tregear, 1966a,b; Griesemer,

1960; Miescher and Schönberg, 1944; Kligman, 1963a, b). Mild swabbing with acetone or ether does not affect the rate of transepidermal water loss, and increasing the normal amount of sebum 10 times has only a slight effect (Kligman, 1963a, b). No correlation was found between the total amount of skin surface lipids, their composition, and the hydration state of stratum corneum (Gloor et al., 1980). Furthermore, sebum is miscible with water and allows water, polar, and nonpolar materials to penetrate (Rothman, 1955; Tregear, 1966a, b; Higuchi, 1960). This evidence, together with some additional minor points summarized by Scheuplein and Blank (1971), lead us to conclude that the presence of sebum is a negligible element in modifying percutaneous absorption. In a broader context, Kligman (1963a, b) is strongly of the opinion that human sebum is useless. He considers that claims for its ability to provide barrier function properties, to inhibit water loss, to regulate surface water by emulsion formation, to maintain an antibacterial and an antifungal cover, and to function as a precursor for vitamin D are unfounded.

B. Skin Appendages

The presence of skin appendages means that the epidermis behaves, in diffusion terms, as a complex parallel barrier (see Chap. 2, Sec. II. B), with three possible diffusional routes—intact stratum corneum, hair follicles, and sweat ducts. If we approximate each pathway to the same length h but with different diffusion coefficients D_i, we can approximate the rate of diffusion within each pathway by the finite simple membrane equation

$$\frac{M}{hKC_0'} = \frac{D_i t}{h^2} - \frac{1}{6} - \frac{2}{\pi^2} \sum_{n=1}^{\infty} \frac{(-1)^n}{n^2} \exp\left(-\frac{D_i n^2 \pi^2 t}{h^2}\right) \tag{3.1}$$

where M is the cumulative amount of material per unit area passing through the tissue of thickness h; K is the partition coefficient; C_0' is the applied concentration; t is time; and n is an integer with values from 1 to infinity. The equation is thus the simple zero-order flux case dealt with in Chap. 2 (cf. Eq. 2.14), and the conditions listed in that chapter apply.

Note that M is a different function of time for each pathway because of the different diffusion coefficients corresponding to each route. When considering the relative contributions which the different pathways make to flux of material, not only must we take into account the diffusivities of the solute within the separate routes, their effective areas, and their effective path lengths, but also the time scale of the permeation process.

1. Steady state flux

We can make a reasonable estimate of the effective diffusion volumes of potential pathways through the stratum corneum and also arrive at

TABLE 3.1 Fractional Diffusion Volumes and Diffusion Coefficients for Water or Simple Small Nonelectrolytes: Potential Pathways Through the Stratum Corneum

Diffusion route	Number per cm^2	Fractional diffusion volume	Diffusion coefficient, $cm^2 sec^{-1}$
Hair follicles (average)	40-70	$1-2 \times 10^{-3}$	$5-20 \times 10^{-8}$
Hair follicles (scalp)	200-1000	$5-25 \times 10^{-3}$	
Sweat ducts (average)	200-250	$3-5 \times 10^{-4}$	$1-20 \times 10^{-6}$
Sweat ducts (palms and soles)	500-800	$8-15 \times 10^{-4}$	
Stratum corneum: intercellular		0.05 (dry) 0.01 (wet)	
transcellular		0.95 (dry) 0.99 (wet)	$1-10 \times 10^{-11}$ $1-10 \times 10^{-10}$

Source: Scheuplein and Blank (1971).

approximate values for the diffusion coefficients of water or other simple, small nonelectrolytes through these routes (Table 3.1). The fractional area available for transappendageal absorption is small (about 0.1%). The diffusion coefficients of small nonelectrolytes moving by this route are larger than those for the stratum corneum pathway, but they are less than the self-diffusion coefficients of water and other liquids (Glasstone et al., 1941; Hammond and Stokes, 1953). Thus, for all molecules which diffuse at least as rapidly as water, the route through the appendages cannot contribute appreciably to the steady state flux, i.e., at large values of t when the exponential term controlling transient diffusion becomes negligible. This is illustrated in Fig. 3.3, which shows a plot of amount of material penetrating as a function of time for two routes. The curve labeled $D = 10^{-7}$ ($cm^2 sec^{-1}$) is appropriate for hair, that marked $D = 10^{-9}$ ($cm^2 sec^{-1}$) corresponds to hydrated stratum corneum. Although the diffusional flux through hair is initially much larger than that through stratum corneum, after 300 sec the stratum corneum route dominates.

In addition to such biophysical arguments, other evidence exists for route specificity in steady state flux. In particular, although material may

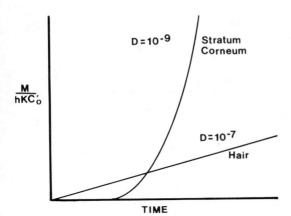

FIG. 3.3 Amount of material penetrating through hair and through hydrated unbroken stratum corneum as a function of time: D, the diffusion coefficient, is in units of $cm^2 \ sec^{-1}$. (From Scheuplein, 1972.)

enter the eccrine sweat ducts and glands, it then does not pass in significant amounts to the dermis (Witten et al., 1951, 1953, 1956). In anatomic sites where the stratum corneum is very thick and hairs are absent (the palms and the soles), the principal portal of entry might be expected to be the sweat glands. However, absorption of materials here, including histamine and allergens, is very poor (Herrmann, 1945; Shelley and Melton, 1949; Barr, 1962). From their anatomic nature, with orifices which are self-sealing slits and tortuous glands with an upward flow of sweat, one would not expect the eccrine sweat glands to provide a significant route of entry (Kligman, 1964; Malkinson, 1964). Additional extensive experimental evidence supports the general conclusion that the intra-appendageal route is insignificant (Blank, 1964; Blank et al., 1967; Treherne, 1956; Treagear, 1961).

Nonetheless, exceptions exist to the general observation that the shunt route (passage through the skin appendages) is insignificant in steady state penetration. This route may be important for ions (Tregear, 1966b) and for large polar molecules (see Sec. II.B.3). Of course, diseases which affect the stratum corneum (e.g., eczema and exfoliative dermatitis) damage the horny layer and may form extensive areas of artificial shunts, thus allowing materials to enter and to leave the epidermis more readily.

2. Transient diffusion

Skin appendages do act as diffusion shunts, and this mode of entry may be important at short times. During the early period of the diffusion process, passage through the shunts cannot be ignored even when the ultimate steady state flux through this pathway is small. Essentially, this is because of the nonlinear time dependency of transient diffusion, prior to the establishment of steady state conditions (Fig. 3.3). At short times (near the lag time applicable to the shunt route), the flux through the hair follicles is much larger than that through the stratum corneum. This is a consequence of the shorter lag time L for the pathway with the larger diffusion coefficient (L = $h^2/6D$). Moreover, since the transient flux depends exponentially on the diffusion coefficient rather than linearly as in the steady state [compare Eq. (3.1) with Eq. (3.2) for the steady state],

$$\frac{M}{hKC_0'} = \frac{D_i t}{h^2} - \frac{1}{6}$$ (3.2)

both local concentrations and fluxes for the respective routes may differ markedly shortly after the application of a penetrant. Thus, initial concentrations of penetrant in the living cells which surround the appendages can be much greater than the corresponding values in the bulk of the stratum corneum at the same time.

Transient diffusion through shunt pathways may be particularly important in bioassays which use pharmacological reactions. Phenomena such as erythema from nicotinates and blanching from topical steroids may be triggered by extremely small concentrations of potent molecules which penetrate relatively rapidly down the shunt route (see Stoughton, 1972).

An analogy which helps to clarify the interrelationship between shunt and membrane permeation is as follows (Scheuplein, 1976). Suppose that an army must traverse a difficult, muddy terrain and there are two methods available—either by walking across a few narrow footbridges which are widely separated (the shunt route) or by wading through the mud (the membrane pathway). The bridges obviously provide a faster, easier route, but because they are few and far apart, they are unavailable to most soldiers. After moving out, the first men across will arrive by the easier shunt route. But after a time (which represents the lag time for the low diffusivity pathway through the stratum corneum), the front ranks of the main body of men struggling through the mud finally reach the opposite bank.

3. Shunt diffusion of large, polar molecules

For the two competing routes of entry into the skin (the shunt path down the appendages and the transepidermal way), the two diffusion processes will become comparable at a precise time. This time will depend upon the effective fractional area for the appendages and the ratios of the diffusion coefficients of the penetrant for the shunt and the bulk processes. Ions and, in particular, large molecules such as the polar steroids have hydroxyl or other polar groups. These groups can bond with the hydrated keratin, which therefore impedes their movement. The resultant small membrane diffusion coefficients may ensure that the more easily penetrated skin appendages

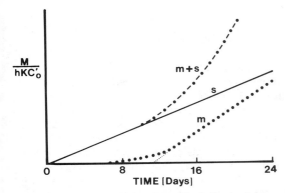

FIG. 3.4 Penetration of cortisol through separated epidermis. Key: m = unbroken membrane; s = shunts, i.e., follicles, ducts, and "holes"; m + s = the experimentally observed result. (From Scheuplein, 1972.)

provide the main portal of entry into the subepidermal layers of the skin, despite their small fractional area (Tregear, 1966b). Scheuplein (1972) has illustrated just such a situation for the penetration of cortisol (hydrocortisone) through separated epidermis in vitro. Figure 3.4 illustrates the experimentally observed result, labeled m + s. The curve is anomalous if we interpret it as representing a single diffusional process; the plot shows a considerable amount of early penetration and yet a long lag time and a relatively small steady state slope. The graph can be explained, however, as the sum of two diffusion processes. One route (m) has a small diffusion coefficient which operates over a large area of skin (the intact stratum corneum membrane). The alternate pathway (s) has a large diffusion coefficient, though only a small fractional area (the shunt route, consisting of follicles, ducts and "holes" formed in the skin when the tissue is mounted in the diffusion cell). If we compare the separate contributions of the two pathways to the total flux of penetrant, we see that such molecules as the polar steroids permeate so slowly through keratin that the limited amount which passes through the shunts constitutes almost the entire diffusional flux during many days of penetration (Scheuplein, 1976; Scheuplein et al., 1969; Wahberg, 1968; Dugard, 1977). Thus the anti-inflammatory topical steroids are anomalous in that both the vasoconstrictor (blanching) response (which is used as a marker in one of their bioassays) and their bulk permeation probably arise mainly from molecules which diffuse down the shunt route.

Recently, Wallace and Barnett (1978) used a pharmacokinetic compartmental analysis to suggest that at pH 6.5 methotrexate penetrates hairless mouse skin primarily by the shunt route. The effect of pH on the penetration of methotrexate through skin was correlated with solubility and partition coefficient determinations by Wallace et al. (1978).

C. Epidermal Route

   1. Barrier layer

   From considerations such as those just detailed, we conclude that in general the principal barrier function of the epidermis resides almost entirely in the stratum corneum. We can for the moment ignore shunt diffusion. But what of the other tissues which constitute skin? For a material absorbed percutaneously, the process is a sequence of deposition onto the stratum corneum, diffusion through it and through the living epidermis, and then passage through the upper part of the papillary dermis. The viable tissues may metabolize a drug, particularly the epidermis (which contains most of the catabolic enzymes that either render a topical drug inactive or activate a pro-drug). Thus, in the hairless mouse, oxygen consumption is five times greater in the epidermis than in the dermis (Laerum, 1969); in human skin, the activity of catechol O-methyltransferase is eightfold higher in the epidermis (Bamshad, 1969). The important role which living skin plays as an active metabolizing tissue and, in particular, how this process affects the topical bioavailability of a drug are subjects only now being treated fundamentally (Ando et al., 1977; see Chap. 4, Sec. II.D). The papillary layer of the dermis contains so many permeable capillaries that it is highly probable that most molecules enter the microcirculation soon after leaving the epidermis. Thus the average total residence time of a drug species in the dermal aqueous phase may only be of the order of a minute (Higuchi, 1977). The deeper layers of the dermis should not, in general, influence percutaneous absorption. However, Menczel and Maibach (1970, 1972) have shown that testosterone may be retained in the dermis; such tissue binding would affect the rate of removal by the capillaries. A further complication arises if the penetrant is very lipophilic. After the molecule passes the horny layer, it suddenly meets an aqueous interface in which it is poorly soluble. The thermodynamic activity of the diffusing species immediately below the barrier may then be relatively high and approach that in the barrier itself. The activity gradient from the stratum corneum to the viable tissues falls and consequently so does the flux. The rate-determining step may become the clearance rate from the barrier rather than the penetration of the barrier (Higuchi, 1977).

   For abdominal skin, we can approximate the thickness of the stratum corneum to 10 μm, the viable epidermis to 100 μm, and the upper portion of the dermis to 100 μm. We can then idealize the permeation process to the diffusion of a substance through a three-ply membrane, i.e., horny layer, viable epidermis, and dermis, with the microcirculation as an infinite sink (see Chap. 2, Sec. IIA). If we apportion separate diffusional resistances to the skin layers, the total diffusional resistance of the composite skin barrier in steady state permeation becomes

$$\sum R_i = \frac{h_{SC}}{D_{SC}K_{SC}} + \frac{h_E}{D_E K_E} + \frac{h_D}{D_D K_D} \qquad (3.3)$$

where R_i is the diffusional resistance of the ith layer and subscripts SC, E, and D refer to stratum corneum, viable epidermis, and papillary layer of the dermis, respectively. Using appropriate values for the parameters of Eq. (3.3), Scheuplein (1972) has calculated the resistance of the skin to the passage of water R_S from the sum of the tissue resistances

$$R_S = R_{SC} + R_E + R_D$$

$$= 9.1 \times 10^6 + 6.3 \times 10^3 + 6.3 \times 10^3 \qquad (3.4)$$

$$= 9.1 \times 10^6 \ sec \ cm^{-1}$$

The dermis and viable epidermis are extensively hydrated and diffusion coefficients are typical of liquid-state diffusion. In the dermis, molecules probably move within water-filled interstices. In contrast, the stratum corneum is a semifibrous structure which is characterized by a fiber or semisolid diffusivity. According to these calculations, the diffusional resistance of the stratum corneum to water is approximately 10^3 times that of either the viable epidermis or the superficial region of the dermis. Polar solutes (other than water) and larger molecules usually have smaller diffusion coefficients than that of water, and the stratum corneum becomes even more dominant in the total permeation process. In general, the conclusion that the horny layer provides the rate-limiting barrier for diffusion is true for the entire class of water-soluble substances.

For an example of a lipid-soluble molecule, Scheuplein (1972) chose octanol applied to cadaver skin as an aqueous solution. Comparing the result with that for water, he showed that the resistance of the skin had decreased dramatically and that this reduction arose from the more favorable distribution of the octanol into the stratum corneum (as measured by K_{SC}). The viable layers of the skin are relatively more significant barriers to the penetration of nonpolar molecules than of polar molecules, but they are still insignificant for in vivo percutaneous absorption (they represent only about 4% of the total diffusional resistance).

Thus, for polar and nonpolar molecules alike, the stratum corneum provides the rate-limiting barrier to percutaneous absorption.

In the past, suggestions have been advanced that a distinct barrier layer exists, located either within the stratum corneum or between the dry stratum corneum and the wet malpighian layer of the epidermis and sometimes identified with the stratum lucidum. Thus, Rein (1924) theorized that a negatively charged membrane existed which was impermeable to anions and which electrostatically trapped cations. Certain dyes were supposed to be stopped at this layer (MacKee et al., 1945). The "lucidum barrier" postulate persisted, even though Rosendal (1945) demonstrated that the entire bulk of the stratum corneum was the source of the high electrical resistance of the skin. (Electrical conductivity of the skin is an allied property to skin permeability to ions; both measure the ease with which ions penetrate the least permeable layer.) What may be taken as convincing evidence as to the presence or absence of a separate barrier zone within the stratum corneum comes from the technique of skin stripping (Wolf, 1939). This experimental procedure removes sequential layers of stratum corneum by repeated applications of adhesive cellophane tape. Blank (1953) measured the water permeability of excised full-thickness skin after stripping layers of the stratum corneum. An amended analysis of the results indicated that the data were consistent with the hypothesis that the horny layer functions as a homogeneous whole and no specific barrier stratum exists within the tissue (Blank, 1964; Scheuplein, 1972, 1976, 1978a,b). Other stripping experiments have confirmed this observation (Monash and Blank, 1958). Direct evidence that the horny layer is essentially uniformly impermeable comes from radiotracer studies which reveal the location of penetrants within the tissue some time after surface application. As expected for a homogeneous tissue, the largest amount has always been found in the outer layers, decreasing proportionally toward the deeper strata (Blank and Gould, 1962; Fredriksson, 1962; Matoltsy et al., 1962).

For certain materials, there may be a second barrier to absorption at or near the dermoepidermal junction, possibly in relation to the basement membrane (Marzulli, 1962; Ferguson and Silver, 1947; Menczel and Maibach, 1970; Fleischmajer and Witten, 1955). By autoradiography, certain electrolytes may be shown to stop almost completely at the dermoepidermal junction and not to penetrate into the dermis (Witten et al., 1951, 1953, 1956). Other studies have shown that inorganic phosphorus and chloride ions readily passed the basement membrane and that methylene blue and Evans blue failed to pass through the dermoepidermal junction but readily penetrated when the basement membrane was removed. Exposure to hyaluronidase or to collagenase enhances the penetrability of the basement membrane (Ohkubo and Sano, 1973). It has been suggested that urea or lactamide may be clinically useful for increasing basement membrane permeability (Handschumacher, 1974). Related to this is the fact that urea does seem to increase the permeability of stratum corneum to hydrocortisone by a moisturizing and keratolytic effect (see Chap. 4, Sec. III.B.1).

From the large volume of work on percutaneous absorption, there is little evidence on behalf of any active transport processes operating across the cells of the stratum corneum. Scheuplein (1972) has cataloged the experimental evidence which supports this view. For example, the permeability of the skin to water is the same whether it is measured in vivo or in vitro (Baker and Kligman, 1967; Burch and Winsor, 1946). Similar in vivo and in vitro correlations have been observed for ions and for nonelectrolytes (Sprott, 1965; Spruit and Malten, 1965, 1968; Dirnhuber and Tregear, 1960; Scheuplein et al., 1969). However, some investigators postulate that viable skin does possess an energy-producing pump which can actively transport water across the stratum corneum (Buettner and Holmes, 1958; Buettner, 1959; Beament, 1965).

Because stratum corneum is dead, it is usually assumed that there are no fundamental differences between in vivo and in vitro permeation processes. However, the possibility remains that minor differences exist in the way in which substances which penetrate skin with difficulty permeate excised skin and skin in vivo. The separation of the skin and its location in a diffusion apparatus may alter the physical state of the horny layer compared to the in vivo situation. In particular, the degree of hydration of the stratum corneum in nearly all laboratory experiments with aqueous solutions is artificially high compared to ambient conditions in most climates. The extent of swelling, the diameter of the sweat ducts, the degree of folding of the stratum corneum, and artificial holes formed during skin preparation may also modify the apparent permeability of the tissue to specific penetrants.

2. Mechanism of diffusion within the stratum corneum

a. Intercellular or transcellular diffusion   The stratum corneum is a multicellular membrane and electron microscopic evidence implies that the intercellular regions are filled with a lipid-rich amorphous material (Spearman and Riley, 1967; Matoltsy, 1976). In the dry membrane the intercellular volume may reach 5% of the total volume. In the hydrated tissue, the intracellular keratin primarily absorbs the water so that the ratio of intercellular to intracellular volume may drop to 1%. Thus, two possible pathways for diffusion exist—between or across the cells (Fig. 3.5). Although the intercellular volume is small, it is still sufficiently large to provide a significant route in theory, provided that the diffusion coefficient for this pathway is large enough. The situation is analogous to the comparison, already considered, of the appendageal route vis-à-vis the intact stratum corneum, where the fractional shunt volume available is at least 10 times less than the fractional intercellular volume and yet shunt diffusion may be significant.

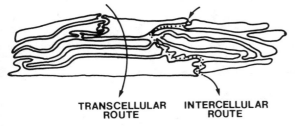

**TRANSCELLULAR   INTERCELLULAR
ROUTE   ROUTE**

FIG. 3.5 Representation of the stratum corneum membrane, illustrating two possible routes for diffusion. (From Scheuplein, 1972.)

TABLE 3.2 Thermodynamic Quantities Associated with the Diffusion of
Water and Alcohols Through Stratum Corneum, Corrected for
Desorption Energy[a]

	$E^{\ddagger}$, kcal mol^{-1}	$\Delta H^{\ddagger}$, kcal mol^{-1}	$\Delta S^{\ddagger}$, cal mol^{-1} deg^{-1}	$\Delta G^{\ddagger}$, kcal mol^{-1}
Water	15.6	14.9	16.6	9.95
Ethanol	16.4	15.8	17.7	10.5
Propanol	16.5	15.9	20.5	9.79
Butanol	16.7	16.7	23.0	9.84
Pentanol	16.5	16.9	24.1	9.72
Hexanol	10.9	11.7	9.26	8.94
Heptanol	9.9	11.3	6.42	9.34
Octanol	8.7	10.4	3.07	9.49

[a]Key: $E^{\ddagger}$ = experimental activation energy; $\Delta H^{\ddagger}$ = activation enthalpy for
diffusion; $\Delta S^{\ddagger}$ = activation entropy for diffusion; $\Delta G^{\ddagger}$ = free energy of activation, during formation of the transition state in diffusion (Glasstone et al.,
1941).
Source: Scheuplein (1978a, b).

However, on balance the available evidence indicates that for water-soluble
nonelectrolytes diffusion is not primarily intercellular. Thus, to account
for the observed permeability to polar alcohols and water, diffusion via the
intercellular route would have to be rapid, i.e., the diffusion coefficient
must be relatively large, which it is not. Furthermore, activation energies
(as derived from the temperature dependence of the permeability coefficient)
would need to be low, which they are not (Table 3.2). In fact, activation
energies for diffusion of these polar molecules through the stratum corneum
are high (of the order of 16 kcal mol^{-1}), as are the entropies of activation
(near 20 E.U.). If the molecules diffused through only a small fraction of
the membrane, low or negative activation entropies would be deduced. The
large values obtained in practice suggest strong chemical interactions between the tissue and the penetrant, and the thermodynamic values cannot be
correlated with rapid short-circuit diffusion between cells. Another objection
to a predominant intercellular route is that this would require that the cell
membranes should be extremely impervious to the solute, so confining the
diffusant to the extracellular pathway. Values of diffusivity for the cell walls

of the order of 10^{-11} cm^2 sec^{-1} would be required; this is very much smaller than can reasonably be expected (Harris, 1960; Scheuplein, 1965). Such arguments imply that molecules diffuse through intercellular regions, across cell walls, and through cells without discrimination, i.e., solutes penetrate by a transcellular mechanism (Scheuplein and Blank, 1971; Scheuplein, 1972, 1978a,b).

Under hydrated in vitro conditions, the stratum corneum swells intracellularly and sorbs about three to five times its own weight of water after 3 days of immersion (Scheuplein and Morgan, 1967). Under such conditions, the intracellular keratin binds large quantities of water. The partition coefficients for water-soluble substances released from an aqueous vehicle and absorbed intracellularly should then be close to unity. This has been observed in practice (see Table 3.3). If water and the polar alcohols were confined to the mainly lipid intercellular regions, then partition coefficients would be expected to increase markedly going from water to propanol. The nearly constant permeation data for water-soluble molecules support a diffusion mechanism which does not include lipid solubilization (Scheuplein, 1978a).

From chemical and permeation data, particularly the dependence of permeation on the partition coefficient (see Table 3.3: alcohols from butanol upward), it appears that lipid-soluble molecules segregate and diffuse through lipid regions in the stratum corneum. We cannot be certain of the exact location of the lipid in the horny layer, and we therefore cannot conclude unequivocally whether the morphological route for lipid-soluble penetrants is inter- or intracellular. However, Michaels et al. (1975) and Chandrasekaran and Shaw (1978), for their mathematical model of the stratum corneum, do assume a strict separation of protein and lipid. They postulate that the tissue consists of an essentially parallel array of thin plates (the stratum corneum cells), each consisting substantially of protein and separated from one another by thin layers of interstitial lipoidal material. In this view, the interstitial lipid phase is the continuous phase of the matrix and the large volume fraction of proteinaceous material is discontinuous. For any permeating species, there are two routes for penetration of the barrier. One requires transit solely through the intercellular lipid phase, and the other route employs alternate passage through cellular protein and intercellular lipid. Using the quantity σ to represent the lipid/protein partition coefficient, which can be approximated to the mineral oil/water partition coefficient, the aforementioned authors deduce

$$\bar{J} = 0.135\,\sigma\,\frac{D_L}{D_p}\left[\frac{1.16 + 0.0017(\sigma D_L/D_p)}{0.16 + (\sigma D_L/D_p)}\right] \qquad (3.5)$$

where $\bar{J}$ is the normalized flux, i.e., maximum transdermal flux divided by aqueous concentration (solubility); D_L is the lipid phase diffusion coefficient; and D_p is the protein phase diffusion coefficient.

TABLE 3.3 Average Permeability Data for Water and Aqueous Alcohol
Solutions Through Stratum Corneum and Dermis at 25°C[a]

Solute	Stratum corneum				Dermis		
	$P \times 10^7$	K	$D \times 10^{10}$	No.	$P \times 10^7$	$D \times 10^6$	No.
Water	1.4	0.88	4.2	45	170	6.9	10
Methanol	1.4	0.6	6.2	10	150	6.1	3
Ethanol	2.2	0.9	6.6	35	97	4.0	8
Propanol	3.3	1.1	8.0	21	86	3.6	9
Butanol	6.9	2.5	7.4	8	83	3.5	3
Pentanol	17	5.0	8.8	50	67	2.8	4
Hexanol	36	10	9.6	8	56	2.3	9
Heptanol	89	30	7.9	11	69	2.9	9
Octanol	140	50	7.7	13	72	3.0	3
Nonanol	170	—	—	3	—	—	—
Decanol	220	—	—	1	—	—	—

[a]Key: P = permeability coefficient (cm sec^{-1}); K = tissue-solvent partition
coefficient for the solute—taken as 0.6 for dermis; D = apparent membrane
diffusion coefficient for the solute (cm^2 sec^{-1}); No. = Number of experiments
averaged to provide the data.
Source: Scheuplein (1965, 1972, 1976); Scheuplein and Blank (1971);
Scheuplein and Ross (1970); Blank (1964); Blank et al. (1967). Data adjusted
for assumed thickness of hydrated stratum corneum = 26.6 μm (40 μm
usually accepted nowadays), dermis = 2.5 mm. Note that data quoted by
Scheuplein in his various papers differ somewhat depending on source,
assumed thickness of the membrane, number of experiments averaged,
error in recording cross-sectional areas of diffusional cells, and occasional
misprint; however, major trends are consistent.

The same authors tested this equation for ouabain, atropine, digitoxin,
scopolamine, diethyl carbamazine, chlorpheniramine, ephedrine, estradiol,
and nitroglycerin. They found that the best theoretical fit for the data was
when D_L/D_P was between 10^{-2} and 10^{-3} with an average value of 2×10^{-3}.
Fentanyl did not correlate as well. Based on this good agreement, they
concluded that their model for skin was valid, that the lipid-protein partition coefficients for the drugs could be approximated by their respective
mineral oil-water partition coefficients, and that the diffusion coefficients

of the drugs in the lipid phase of the tissue are about 500 times lower than in the protein phase.

There are other protagonists for the intercellular route in general (see Katz and Poulsen, 1971). In recent publications, Elias and co-workers have argued that previous work underestimated the fractional volume of the inter- cellular channels in the stratum corneum. From less destructive histological methods such as freeze fracture, etching, and substitution techniques, com- bined with electron microscopy, the latter group concludes that the volume of the intercellular regions of the stratum corneum may be three to seven times greater than was formerly thought. The volume may be even larger if we include intercellular dilatations. Elias and colleagues claim that this expanded, structurally complex and lipid-rich region may play a significant role in percutaneous transport and that junctional or intercellular speciali- zations may be important (see Elias and Friend, 1975; Elias et al., 1977a,b; Nemanic and Elias, 1980; Hashimoto, 1971; Squier, 1973; McNutt, 1973; Schreiner and Wolf, 1969).

Albery and Hadgraft (1979a,b) developed a mathematical treatment for percutaneous absorption which included interfacial barriers and which allowed for the depletion of the substance from the external phase. Equations were derived for continuous application and for pulse experiments. The authors tested their equations by timing the onset of erythema in man after the application of esters of nicotinic acid. They concluded that methyl nico- tinate penetrates stratum corneum via the intercellular route and that all solutes which are more soluble in the interstitial lipid phase than in the keratinized cells are also likely to follow the intercellular route.

b. Site of diffusional resistance   If we accept the idea that molecules migrate across cell walls of the stratum corneum, do we need to distinguish between the cell wall and the cell interior in providing the main diffusional barrier? There are several reasons for considering the cell wall. During keratinization, the walls were reported to double in thickness (increasing from 80 to 150 Å) and to incorporate chemically resistant material (Matoltsy and Parakkal, 1963). However, there is probably no true thickening of the membrane; instead, material simply deposits on its inner and outer surfaces (Breathnach et al., 1973). If we hydrolyze the stratum corneum with 5% NaOH for 12 hr, only the cellular membranes and their resistant extraneous coatings remain undigested. Furthermore, the permeability of the tissue increases dramatically after we remove the lipids with solvents (for this theory to apply it is assumed that lipid is removed only from cell walls). However, the view that the main resistance to diffusion resides in the cell walls requires the presence of a highly specialized dense lipid structure to provide diffusivities of the order of 5×10^{-12} cm^2 sec^{-1}. Such an ordered, close-packed structure would form with difficulty because of the mixture of bulky and straight-chain molecules which are present. There is no evi- dence from x-ray diffraction for such an organization. Moreover, the postu- late ignores the remaining 85% of the tissue which itself is semisolid and contains lipids that are similar, if not identical, to those incorporated within the cell walls. Finally, the concept is not supported experimentally, as it predicts a lower value for the permeability to water than is actually observed Water would be only slightly soluble in a lipid network in the cell walls. Its permeability coefficient would be at least 100-fold lower than the permeabilities of methanol and ethanol, which are appreciably soluble in oil. However, water and the polar alcohols possess very similar values for permeability coefficient, diffusion coefficient, and partition coefficient (Table 3.3). As such substances are completely miscible with water, the data suggest that these diffusants dissolve in an aqueous phase. Also, if we compare membrane-to-water partition coefficients with reference to whole stratum corneum (K_{SC}) with the corresponding values using an olive oil/water system (K_{OO}), we note the following: For the water-soluble primary alcohols, $K_{SC} > K_{OO}$, which implies that the stratum corneum is a better solvent for these molecules than is olive oil. For the lipid soluble alcohols of greater chain length, $K_{OO} > K_{SC}$, showing that the stratum corneum is a poorer solvent for such materials than is olive oil. Again, these results emphasize that the tissue must contain a significant aqueous component.

The overall conclusion is that probably the intracellular keratin structure, rather than the cell wall, is the main site of the membrane diffusional resistance (Scheuplein, 1965, 1972, 1978a,b; Scheuplein and Blank, 1971), although Yotsuyanagi and Higuchi (1972) contend that the thickened plasma membrane is the main diffusional barrier.

   c. Molecular diffusion pathways Electron micrographs of stratum corneum have been interpreted as indicating an extensive segregation of lipid between protein filaments, although there is no absolute proof of the presence of intracellular lipid (Brody, 1960; Scheuplein, 1978a,b). Thus the intracellular keratin forms a filament-matrix structure and presents a mosaic of polar and nonpolar regions, as illustrated diagrammatically in Fig. 3.6. In hydrated tissue, these separate lipid and polar regions provide parallel pathways for diffusion. Polar and nonpolar molecules will partition into one or other of the networks according to their relative affinities and will diffuse separately. This is implied by the solubility behavior of water-soluble and lipid-soluble molecules as discussed previously. Thermodynamic data for diffusion also support this view (Table 3.2). [For a useful discussion of the thermodynamics of diffusion in biological membranes, see Stein (1967).] The high values for the enthalpies and entropies of activation for water and the water-soluble alcohols indicate that the water structure within the hydrated membrane greatly hinders migrating molecules. Although polar molecules diffuse in the aqueous regions near the outer surface of the protein filament, rather than in the semicrystalline center, they are still impeded in their passage, particularly by hydrogen bonding. Nonpolar molecules which are sufficiently oil soluble tend to dissolve within the lipid material between the filaments, where hydrogen bonding is insignificant. As a conse-

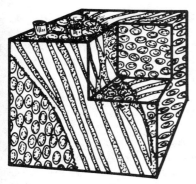

FIG. 3.6 Idealized representation of intracellular keratin in stratum corneum. (Modified from Scheuplein, 1972.)

quence of this, normal alcohols of six carbons and above have lower values of enthalpies and entropies.

A common feature for both polar and nonpolar permeation is the much higher free energy of activation for diffusion in the stratum corneum compared to diffusion in aqueous solution. Even for fully hydrated stratum corneum, the water is strongly bound, there are powerful solute-tissue interactions, the horny layer possesses a semisolid structure, and diffusion is much more difficult for all solutes than in aqueous solution.

Although the concept is widely accepted that penetrants partition into separate lipid and polar regions in the stratum corneum and then diffuse independently, some authors dispute this. From work on the permeation of phenolic compounds from aqueous solution through excised human skin, Roberts et al. (1978) deduce the following. For the more polar solutes, the main resistance to penetration is the lipid barriers in the horny layer. Diffusion of these phenols through the tissue appears to depend on the breaking of hydrogen bonds when the penetrant desolvates during permeation, together with the high consistency of the stratum corneum. Less polar solvates are retarded not only by the lipid barrier but also by a significant contribution of aqueous boundary layers to the overall diffusional resistance. As discussed in Chap. 2, Sec. II.A, with decreasing polarity of the penetrant the partition coefficient steadily rises until the permeation process becomes diffusion layer controlled.

From theoretical and experimental calculations on the partition coefficients of long-chain alcohols between water and oil, octanol, or stratum corneum, it appears that the horny layer behaves very similar to but somewhat more polar than butanol as regards its solubilizing ability for penetrants (Scheuplein and Blank, 1973; Scheuplein, 1978a). However, in hairless mouse skin, hydration effects the permeation of butanol and higher homologs, but not water, methanol, and ethanol; thus the mechanism of absorption of the very polar alcohols differs from that of the higher homologs. This suggests that small polar nonelectrolytes permeate through a pathway which is insensitive to normal chemical structure partitioning influences (Behl et al., 1980).

D. Speculations on Permeation Routes for Topical Drugs

Much of the preceding discussion as to the possible routes of penetration of molecules through intact skin has concentrated on two classes of penetrants—the alcohols and the steroids. The homologous series of alcohols provides an excellent range of molecules for fundamental physicochemical studies on skin permeation, but these simple compounds are of little interest as therapeutic agents in diseased states. Steroid studies, however, do have direct relevance to the treatment of inflammatory skin diseases by topical corticosteroids. We can use the results and conclusions of permeation experiments with these two groups of compounds, as discussed previously in this chapter to speculate as to the possible routes by which topically applied drugs reach the dermis (Scheuplein, 1978a).

Theoretically, because of their physicochemical nature, some topic medicaments should penetrate the bulk of the stratum corneum reasonably well. For these drugs it should be unnecessary to postulate any significant contribution to the steady state flux arising from shunt diffusion down the appendages. Small nonelectrolytes such as phenol, menthol, and salicylic and boric acids are in this class. Similarly, the antifungal agents haloprogin (MW 361) and undecenoic acid (MW 184) are relatively small lipid-soluble molecules without multiple polar groups to inhibit passage through the stratum corneum. Both agents should penetrate the horny layer well. Retinoid acid (vitamin A acid, tretinoin; MW 300), which is used to treat acne, should also penetrate readily. Other chemical forms and isomers of vitamin A, including retinyl acetate, penetrate mouse tail epidermis (Spearman and Jarrett, 1974).

On the other hand, many topical drugs may find that the stratum corneum provides too great an impediment to their diffusion and that the only significant route by which they may reach the dermis is via the appendages. For example, very large molecules should penetrate the stratum corneum with difficulty, although we have not yet established a critical size which restricts diffusion. It appears that electrolytes and polar molecules with three or more polar groups, particularly NH_2 and OH, require the shunt route to penetrate to any clinically significant extent.

Many topical therapeutic agents can be included as candidates for appendageal diffusion on the grounds of size and/or the presence of polar groups. Most anti-inflammatory topical steroids are probably too polar to penetrate significantly through intact stratum corneum, and this is probably true of hydrocortisone. Nystatin, a tetraene antifungal agent (approximate MW 926), has the amino sugar mycosamine in its structure. The antibiotic should therefore be a candidate for shunt diffusion, although Martindale: The Extra Pharmacopoeia (see Wade and Reynolds, 1977) states that nystatin is not absorbed through the skin and mucous membranes when applied topically. The polypeptide antibiotics gramicidin (approximate MW 2,000), bacitracin (MW 1,411), and polymyxin B (approximate MW 1,204) are large polar molecules with many polar NH_2 groups. The polyene antibiotics such as bacitracin and polymyxin B have two important components in their structures—a long polyhydroxylate chain which imparts water-soluble properties, and a lipophilic portion with conjugated double bonds. Gramicidin is a cyclic polypeptide, consisting of a large ring of amino acids joined by peptide bonds with side-chains. The aminoglycoside neomycin B (MW 615) contains amino groups and a disaccharide moiety. For all these antibiotics, any skin penetration should be limited to the shunt route. Similarly, tetracycline (MW 444) is very polar and even forms a trihydrate. Together with penicillin G and other polar antibacterials, it penetrates intact skin when applied in methanol (Knight et al., 1969). In the absence of a solvent such as methanol, which damages stratum corneum, any penetration of these agents would again probably be via the appendages.

From UV light fluorescence microscopy, Foreman et al. (1979) conclude that the hair follicle in hamster skin is an important route for skin penetration by components of coal tar.

References relevant both to skin permeation and to clinical efficacy of the aforementioned drugs may be found in the appropriate sections of Martindale: The Extra Pharmacopoeia (Wade and Reynolds, 1977).

It thus appears that a significant percentage of topical therapeutic agents may be included in the category of chemicals which should penetrate the skin by the shunt route. For these materials, the ultrastructure and chemistry of the bulk stratum corneum may be less relevant than the physicochemical nature of the material within the shunt pore (Scheuplein, 1978a). For sweat ducts, this substance approximates to saline; for follicular diffusion, it is hair or sebum. In these circumstances, values for diffusion coefficients and partition coefficients which were obtained from bulk stratum corneum measurements may not be strictly relevant. An exception to this concept would be when a formulator deliberately attempts to enhance skin penetration across the bulk of the stratum corneum by using accelerants. At the same time, the formulator could also promote appendageal absorption by employing surfactants.

An interpretation of an in vitro diffusion experiment may also be in error when in situ hydration of the stratum corneum membrane closes down the shunt routes. This may occur when, for example, relatively dry skin samples are clamped in a diffusion cell and then allowed to hydrate by water diffusing from donor or receptor solutions; the membrane swells, closing the shunt pores. Drugs which in vivo may well pass down the follicular route must then penetrate the bulk stratum corneum in the diffusion apparatus, with consequent anomalies in relating the data to the in vivo situation.

III. EPIDERMAL RESERVOIR

Malkinson and Ferguson (1955) originally postulated that topically applied agents may form a depot or reservoir within the stratum corneum; they based their theory on observations of the percutaneous absorption of radioactive glucocorticoids. Although in their experiment the applied material remained in contact with the skin throughout the test and thus the apparent reservoir could be explained by slow absorption from a surface film, subsequent work has amply demonstrated the validity of the depot postulate. In particular, Vickers (1963) demonstrated that a reservoir for potent fluorinated steroids existed in the horny layer. He applied to the skin small quantities of either triamcinolone acetonide or flucinolone acetonide in ethanol and occluded the area with a plastic film. Such occlusion hydrates the stratum corneum and promotes penetration of the steroids. When, after 16 hr, the film was removed, the sites blanched or vasoconstricted (MacKenzie and Stoughton, 1962). After the skin was washed, the blanching gradually diminished with time until it had disappeared. When the sites were reoccluded with the film at intervals as long as 12 to 14 days after the initial application of the steroids, the white areas reappeared, even though no more corticoid had been applied. Barry and Woodford, in a series of tests designed to determine the activities and bioavailabilities of a range of steroid formulations, showed that reservoir formation, as determined by the vasoconstrictor test, was a common phenomenon. For some 80 preparations covering the full spectrum of steroid potency and applied under occlusion for only 6 hr, just the weakest formulations (which were mainly hydrocortisone products) failed to produce blanching on subsequent reocclusion. When formulations were applied under nonoccluded conditions, reservoir formation was less marked (Woodford and Barry, 1974, 1977a, b; Barry and Woodford, 1974, 1975, 1976, 1977, 1978; Barry, 1976).

Further evidence for the reservoir effect has been obtained recently by Wickrema Sinha et al. (1978). These authors applied diflorasone diacetate cream to the skin of human volunteers, and 24 hr later 37.5% of the applied dose had penetrated below the surface of the skin and could not be wiped off. Since only 1.1% of the applied dose was excreted in the urine and the feces, it was concluded that 36.4% of the dose established a stratum corneum reservoir. Small but significant quantities of the steroid could still be recovered by skin swabbing as long as 22 days after the initial drug administration.

From such observations we conclude that a reservoir for steroids exists in the skin. Clinical and radiobiological studies suggest strongly that the depot resides in the stratum corneum and that it is not just a surface film (MacKenzie and Atkinson, 1964). Thus, an intact, normal horny layer is necessary to form a reservoir (Washitake et al., 1973). Intradermal injections of steroids (which thus bypass the stratum corneum) cannot establish a reservoir, nor do applications to stripped skin. After a depot forms in normal skin, it can be destroyed by stripping (Vickers, 1966, 1972). Sufficient potent steroid to influence epidermal mitosis may be retained within the depot (Munro, 1969).

The mechanism of reservoir formation most probably arises simply from the physicochemical nature of drug solubility and diffusion within the stratum corneum. It is not necessary to invoke special pharmacological reactions to explain the effect but simply to realize that the depot is prominent with a certain class of material, i.e., those substances with small diffusivities and low solubilities in the stratum corneum. In general, those factors that promote percutaneous absorption also potentiate reservoir formation. If the temperature and humidity above the horny layer increases (as, for example, under polythene occlusion), the steroid store increases. The longer the time for which the steroid is applied, the higher is its concentration; and the more protracted the period of occlusion, the greater is the depot. The higher the bioavailability of the drug from the vehicle, the more pronounced is the reservoir. In particular, certain solvents (known as accelerants, promoters, or penetration enhancers) induce superior reservoirs. Thus, dimethylsulfoxide functions as a potent solvent to promote the penetration of steroids and to enhance their depot formation, whereas dimethylacetamide and dimethylformamide are somewhat less active (Stoughton and Fritsch, 1964; Stoughton, 1965; Munro and Stoughton, 1965; for further details, see Chap. 4, Sec. III.C.3).

From facts such as these, we can deduce the mechanism which operates to lay down the depot. Treatments that enhance reservoir formation—such as occlusion or the use of accelerants—initially raise the steroid concentration in the upper layers of the stratum corneum to a relatively high level. When we remove the occlusive dressing, the moisture content of the stratum corneum soon returns to the usual physiological amount; if accelerants have been used to form the reservoir, they diffuse much quicker than the steroid and the systemic circulation removes them. In both instances, the stratum corneum quickly returns to normal, but it now contains a relatively high concentration of poorly diffusible, rather insoluble steroid. The upper strata of the horny layer may even be supersaturated with respect to the steroid, and some of the drug may precipitate. A fraction of the available molecules may bind to keratin or other tissue components, as the remainder diffuses slowly downward. Thus, a dynamic equilibrium establishes, for which insoluble and bound steroid serves as a source to replace molecules which slowly permeate to lower layers of the stratum corneum, the viable epidermis, and the dermis. Thus, ideal conditions exist for some steroid to remain in the horny layer for a protracted period of time (possibly even until the squames containing the drug are shed) and to provide a steady low flux of drug to the dermis. Thus, sensitive analytical methods can detect the presence of steroid in the horny layer for many days or even a few weeks after the initial application of the drug to the skin surface.

When we reocclude the application site some time after the initial deposition of drug, the physicochemical microenvironment of the stratum corneum alters as it again hydrates. Precipitated steroid may redissolve, and keratin-bound drug may be released. These diffusible steroid molecules permeate to the receptors in the biophase as a pulse in flux, the concentration of which is high enough to trigger once again the pharmacological response of blanching. This second activation of the vasoconstrictor effect provides the usual evidence for the steroid reservoir. The failure of steroid preparations of low potency (such as hydrocortisone formulations) to provide evidence of the steroid reservoir by means of the blanching test may relate simply to the low activity of the steroid in this bioassay. The low potency of hydrocortisone makes it difficult to measure the activity of its preparations in a normal blanching test, let alone upon reocclusion some days after the initial application of drug.

Thus, in some ways the stratum corneum behaves like a chromatography column toward penetrants, binding and releasing them according to changing conditions. However, the "stationary phase" of the horny layer is shed constantly. Topically applied steroids can decrease the mitotic rate of the basal layer of the epidermis and change the kinetics of stratum corneum proliferation and loss by desquamation. However, as far as the steroid reservoir effect is concerned, this partial inhibition of mitosis is a secondary effect and is not the cause of reservoir formation.

Substances other than steroids may form reservoirs. Dimethylacetamide (which is clinically more acceptable than dimethylsulfoxide) augments a hexachlorophane depot in the skin; this solution was more effective in reducing cutaneous bacterial counts than a commercial lotion of the same antiseptic concentration (Stoughton, 1966; Stoughton and Stoughton, 1968). This observation demonstrated for the first time a possible therapeutic value for a reservoir. It also appears that griseofulvin, sodium fusidate, and fusidic acid form depots in a manner analogous to the steroids (Munro and Stoughton 1965; Vickers, 1969, 1972). It is probably safe to conclude that many more materials form reservoirs but that such effects have not often been specifically investigated.

The therapeutic significance of such stratum corneum reservoirs is still unclear. Vickers (1972, 1980) believes that the depot is probably more preventative than truly therapeutic and that any pharmacological or therapeutic use must remain, at present, speculative.

Hadgraft (1979), in a theoretical approach, has derived mathematical expressions that describe the rates of release of drugs which form reservoirs in the stratum corneum.

IV. GENERAL CONCLUSION

In view of the complexities of the transport mechanisms discussed in the previous sections, it is worthwhile attempting to summarize our knowledge regarding the basics of percutaneous absorption. Such a summary must, of necessity, be in the form of a general conclusion applicable to most materials, with provisos and exceptions omitted for brevity and clarity.

The stratum corneum is a thin, tough, relatively impermeable membrane which provides the rate-limiting step in the process of percutaneous absorption. The entire horny layer, not just some specialized region, provides the main resistance to diffusion. The membrane allows no molecule to pass readily, but nearly all materials penetrate to some extent. Permeation is not primarily via the appendages nor via the intercellular route, but across the bulk of the stratum corneum. The intracellular keratin presents a mosaic of polar and nonpolar regions in which substances dissolve and diffuse according to their chemical affinities. As the tissue is dead, diffusion is a passive process governed by physicochemical laws in which active transport mechanisms play no part.

For electrolytes and large molecules with low diffusion coefficients, such as the polar steroids and antibiotics (and possibly some other topical drugs), shunt diffusion through the appendages may be significant. These appendages may provide the main route of entry through the skin under both transient and steady state conditions.

Once molecules pass the horny layer, they permeate rapidly through the living tissues of the epidermis and the dermis, thence to sweep readily into the systemic circulation.

SYMBOLS

C_0'	donor concentration
D	diffusion coefficient, diffusivity
D_E	diffusion coefficient in viable epidermis
D_D	diffusion coefficient in papillary dermis
D_L	lipid-phase diffusion coefficient
D_p	protein-phase diffusion coefficient
D_{SC}	diffusion coefficient in stratum corneum
$\bar{J}$	normalized flux
K	partition coefficient
K_D	partition coefficient for papillary dermis

K_E partition coefficient for viable epidermis

K_{OO} partition coefficient for olive oil

K_{SC} partition coefficient for stratum corneum

L   lag time

M   cumulative mass of diffusant penetrated per unit area

R_D diffusional resistance of papillary dermis

R_E diffusional resistance of viable epidermis

R_i diffusional resistance of ith layer in laminate

R_S diffusional resistance of skin

R_{SC} diffusional resistance of stratum corneum

h   thickness of membrane

h_D thickness of papillary dermis

h_E thickness of viable epidermis

h_{SC} thickness of stratum corneum

n   integer

t   time

σ lipid-protein partition coefficient

REFERENCES

Abramson, H. A., and Gorin, M. H. (1940). J. Phys. Chem. 44:1094.
Albery, J. W., and Hadgraft, J. (1979a). J. Pharm. Pharmacol. 31:129.
Albery, J. W., and Hadgraft, J. (1979b). J. Pharm. Pharmacol. 31:140.
Ando, H. Y., Ho, N. F. H., and Higuchi, W. I. (1977). J. Pharm. Sci. 66:1525.
Baker, H., and Kligman, A. M. (1967). Arch. Dermatol. 96:441.
Bamshad, J. (1969). J. Invest. Dermatol. 52:351.
Barr, M. (1962). J. Pharm. Sci. 51:395.
Barrett, C. W. (1969). J. Soc. Cosmetic Chemists 20:487.
Barry, B. W. (1976). Dermatologica 152(Suppl. 1):47.
Barry, B. W., and Woodford, R. (1974). Br. J. Dermatol. 91:323.
Barry, B. W., and Woodford, R. (1975). Br. J. Dermatol. 93:563.
Barry, B. W., and Woodford, R. (1976). Br. J. Dermatol. 95:423.
Barry, B. W., and Woodford, R. (1977). Br. J. Dermatol. 97:555.
Barry, B. W., and Woodford, R. (1978). J. Clin. Pharm. 3:43.
Beament, J. W. L. (1965). Symp. Soc. Exptl. Biol. 19:273.

Behl, C. R., Flynn, G. L., Kurihara, T., Harper, N., Smith, W., Higuchi, W. I., Ho, N. F. H., and Pierson, C. L. (1980). J. Invest. Dermatol. 75:346.

Blank, I. H. (1953). J. Invest. Dermatol. 21:259.

Blank, I. H. (1964). J. Invest. Dermatol. 43:415.

Blank, I. H., and Gould, E. (1962). J. Invest. Dermatol. 37:311.

Blank, I. H., and Scheuplein, R. J. (1969). Br. J. Dermatol. 81(Suppl. 4): 4.

Blank, I. H., Scheuplein, R. J., and MacFarlane, D. J. (1967). J. Invest. Dermatol. 49:582.

Boughton, B., and Wheatley, V. R. (1959). Biochem. J. 73:144.

Boughton, B., MacKenna, R. M. B., Wheatley, V. R., and Wormall, A. (1957). Biochem. J. 66:32.

Breathnack, A. S., Goodman, T., Stolinski, C., and Gross, M. (1973). J. Anat. 114:65.

Brody, I. (1960). J. Ultrastruct. Res. 4:264.

Buettner, K. J. K. (1959). J. Appl. Physiol. 14:269.

Buettner, K. J. K., and Holmes, F. F. (1958). J. Appl. Physiol. 14:261, 276.

Burch, G. E., and Winsor, T. (1946). Arch. Intern. Med. 74:437.

Chandrasekaran, S. K., and Shaw, J. E. (1978). Curr. Probl. Dermatol. 7:142.

Chandrasekaran, S. K., Michaels, A. S., Campbell, P., and Shaw, J. E. (1976). Am. Inst. Chem. Eng. 22:828.

Chandrasekaran, S. K., Bayne, W., and Shaw, J. E. (1978). J. Pharm. Sci. 67:1370.

Cummings, E. G. (1969). J. Invest. Dermatol. 54:64.

Dirnhuber, P., and Tregear, R. T. (1960). J. Physiol. (London) 152:58.

Dugard, P. H. (1977). Adv. Mod. Toxicol. 4:525.

Elias, P. M., and Friend. D. S. (1975). J. Cell Biol. 65:180.

Elias, P. M., Goerke, J., and Friend, D. S. (1977a). J. Invest. Dermatol. 69:535.

Elias, P. M., McNutt, N. S., and Friend, D. S. (1977b). Anat. Rec. 189: 577.

Feldman, R. J., and Maibach, H. I. (1974). Arch. Dermatol. 109:58.

Ferguson, R. L., and Silver, S. D. (1947). Am. J. Clin. Pathol. 17:35.

Festenstein, G. N., and Morton, R. A. (1952). Biochem. J. 52:168.

Fleischmajer, R., and Witten, V. H. (1955). J. Invest. Dermatol. 25:223.

Flynn, G. L. (1979). In Modern Pharmaceutics, G. S. Banker and C. T. Rhodes (Eds.). Dekker, New York, p. 263.

Foreman, M. I., Picton, W., Lukowiecki, G. A., and Clark, C. (1979). Br. J. Dermatol. 100:707.

Fredriksson, T. (1962). Acta Derm. Venereol. (Stockh.) 41:353.

Glasstone, G., Laidler, K. J., and Eyring, H. (1941). The Theory of Rate Processes. McGraw-Hill, New York, p. 529.

Gloor, M., Willebrandt, U., Thomer, G., and Kuperschmid, W. (1980). Arch. Dermatol. Res. 268:221.

Griesemer, R. D. (1960). J. Soc. Cosmetic Chemists 11:79.

Haahti, E. (1961). Scand. J. Clin. Lab. Invest. 13(Suppl. 59).

Hadgraft, J. (1979). Int. J. Pharmaceutics 2:265.

Hammond, B. R., and Stokes, R. H. (1953). Trans. Faraday Soc. 49:890.

Handschumacher, R. E. (1974). Clin. Pharmacol. Ther. 16:865.

Harris, E. J. (1960). Transport and Accumulation in Biological Systems. Butterworths, London, p. 39.

Hashimoto, K. (1971). J. Invest. Dermatol. 57:17.

Herrmann, F. (1945). Ann. Allergy 3:431.

Higuchi, T. (1960). J. Soc. Cosmetic Chemists 11:85.

Higuchi, T. (1977). In Design of Biopharmaceutical Properties Through Prodrugs and Analogs, B. Roche (Ed.). American Pharmaceutical Association, Washington, D.C., p. 409.

Idson, B. (1971). In Absorption Phenomena (Topics in Medicinal Chemistry, Vol. 4), J. L. Rabinowitz and R. M. Myerson (Eds.). Wiley (Interscience), New York, p. 181.

Idson, B. (1975). J. Pharm. Sci. 64:901.

James, A. T., and Wheatley, V. R. (1956). Biochem. J. 63:269.

Katz, M. (1973). In Drug Design (Medicinal Chemistry, Vol. 4), E. J. Ariens (Ed.). Academic Press, New York, p. 93.

Katz, M., and Poulsen, B. J. (1971). In Handbook of Experimental Pharmacology, B. B. Brodie and J. Gillette (Eds.), Vol. 28, Pt. 1. Springer-Verlag, Berlin, p. 103.

Katz, M., and Poulsen, B. J. (1972). J. Soc. Cosmetic Chemists 23:565.

Kellum, R. E. (1967). Arch. Dermatol. 95:218.

Kligman, A. M. (1963a). Adv. Biol. Skin 4:110.

Kligman, A. M. (1963b). Br. J. Dermatol. 75:307.

Kligman, A. M. (1964). In The Epidermis, W. Montagna and W. C. Lobitz (Eds.). Academic Press, New York, p. 387.

Knight, A. G., Vickers, C. F. H., and Percival, A. (1969). Br. J. Dermatol. 81(Suppl. 4):88.

Kvorning, S. A. (1949). Acta Pharmacol. 5:383.

Laerum, O. D. (1969). J. Invest. Dermatol. 52:63.

Laurberg, G. (1975). Dermatologica 151:30.

MacKee, G. M., Sulzberger, M. B., Herrmann, F., and Baer, R. L. (1945). J. Invest. Dermatol. 6:43.

MacKenna, R. M. B., Wheatley, V. R., and Wormall, A. (1950). J. Invest. Dermatol. 15:33.

MacKenna, R. M. B., Wheatley, V. R., and Wormall, A. (1952). Biochem. J. 52:161.

MacKenzie, A. W., and Atkinson, R. M. (1964). Arch. Dermatol. 89:741.

MacKenzie, A. W., and Stoughton, R. B. (1962). Arch. Dermatol. 86:608.

McNutt, N. S. (1973). J. Cell Biol. 59(2/Pt. 2):210a (abstr.).

Malkinson, F. D. (1964). In The Epidermis, W. Montagna and W. C. Lobitz (Eds.). Academic Press, New York, p. 435.

Malkinson, F. D., and Ferguson, E. H. (1955). J. Invest. Dermatol. 25: 281.

Malkinson, F. D., and Gehlmann, L. (1977). In Cutaneous Toxicity, V. A. Drill and P. Lazar (Eds.). Academic Press, New York, p. 63.

Malkinson, F. D., and Rothman, S. (1963). In Handbuch der Haut-und Geschlectskrankheiten: Normal und pathologische Physiologie der Haut J. Jadassohn (Ed.), Vol. 1, Pt. 3. Springer-Verlag, New York, p. 90.

Martindale: The Extra Pharmacopoeia, 27th ed. See Wade and Reynolds (1977).

Marzulli, F. N. (1962). J. Invest. Dermatol. 39:387.

Matoltsy, A. G. (1976). J. Invest. Dermatol. 67:20.

Matoltsy, A. G., and Parakkal, P. F. (1965). J. Cell. Biol. 24:297.

Matoltsy, A. G., Matoltsy, G., and Schrogger, A. (1962). J. Invest. Dermatol. 38:251.

Menczel, E., and Maibach, H. I. (1970). J. Invest Dermatol. 54:386.

Menczel, E., and Maibach, H. I. (1972). Acta Derm. Venereol. (Stockh.) 52:38.

Mershon, M. M. (1975). Applied Chemistry at Protein Interfaces, Adv. Chem. Ser. No. 145:41, Am. Chem. Soc., Washington, D.C.

Michaels, A. S., Chandrasekaran, S. K., and Shaw, J. E. (1975). Am. Inst. Chem. Eng. 21:985.

Miescher, G., and Schönberg, A. (1944). Bull. Schweiz. Akad. Med. Wiss. 1:101.

Monash, S., and Blank, H. (1958). Arch. Dermatol. 78:710.

Munro, D. D. (1969). Br. J. Dermatol. 81(Suppl. 4):92.

Munro, D. D., and Stoughton, R. B. (1965). Arch. Dermatol. 92:585.

Nemanic, M. K., and Elias, P. M. (1980). J. Histochem. Cytochem. 28: 573.

Nicolaides, N. (1963). Adv. Biol. Skin 4:167.

Nicolaides, N., and Rothman, S. (1953). J. Invest. Dermatol. 21:9.

Nicolaides, N., and Wells, G. C. (1957). J. Invest. Dermatol. 29:423.

Ohkubo, T., and Sano, S. (1973). Acta Derm. Venereol. (Stockh.) Suppl. No. 73:121.

Poulsen, B. J. (1973). In Drug Design (Medicinal Chemistry, Vol. 4), E. J. Ariens (Ed.). Academic Press, New York, p. 93.

Rein, H. (1924). Z. Biol. 81:125.

Rein, H. (1926). Haut Z. Biol. 84:41.

Reiss, F. (1966). Am. J. Med. Sci. 252:588.

Roberts, M. S., Anderson, R. A., Swarbrick, J., and Moore, D. E. (1978). J. Pharm Pharmacol. 30:486.

Rosendal, T. (1945). Acta Physiol. Scand. 9:39.

Rothman, S. (1954). Physiology and Biochemistry of the Skin. Univ. of Chicago Press, Chicago.

124   Dermatological Formulations

Rothman, S. (1955). J. Soc. Cosmetic Chemists 6:193.
Rothman, S., Smiljanic, A. M., and Shapiro, A. L. (1947). J. Invest.
    Dermatol. 8:81.
Schaefer, H. (1974). J. Soc. Cosmetic Chemists 25:93.
Scheuplein, R. J. (1965). J. Invest. Dermatol. 45:334.
Scheuplein, R. J. (1967). J. Invest. Dermatol. 48:79.
Scheuplein, R. J. (1972). Adv. Biol. Skin 12:125.
Scheuplein, R. J. (1976). J. Invest. Dermatol. 67:31.
Scheuplein, R. J. (1978a). In The Physiology and Pathophysiology of the
    Skin, A. Jarrett (Ed.), Vol. 5. Academic Press, New York, pp. 1669,
    1693, 1731.
Scheuplein, R. J. (1978b). Curr. Probl. Dermatol. 7:122.
Scheuplein, R. J. (1980). In Percutaneous Absorption of Steroids, P.
    Mauvais-Jarvis, C. F. H. Vickers, and J. Wepierre (Eds.). Academic
    Press, New York, p. 1.
Scheuplein, R. J., and Blank, I. H. (1971). Physiol. Rev. 51:702.
Scheuplein, R. J., and Blank, I. H. (1973). J. Invest. Dermatol. 60:286.
Scheuplein, R. J., and Morgan, L. G. (1967). Nature 214:456.
Scheuplein, R. J., and Ross, L. (1970). J. Soc. Cosmetic Chemists 21:
    853.
Scheuplein, R. J., Blank, I. H., Brauner, G. J., and MacFarlane, D. J.
    (1969). J. Invest. Dermatol. 52:63.
Schreiner, E., and Wolf, K. (1969). Arch. Klin. Exp. Dermatol. 235:78.
Shaw, J. E., Chandrasekaran, S. K., Michaels, A. S., and Taskovitch, L.
    (1975). In Animal Models in Human Dermatology, H. Maibach (Ed.).
    Churchill Livingstone, Edinburgh and London, p. 138.
Shaw, J. E., Chandrasekaran, S. K., Campbell, P. S., and Schmitt, L. G.
    (1977). In Cutaneous Toxicity, V. A. Drill and P. Lazar (Eds.). Aca-
    demic Press, New York, p. 83.
Shelley, W. B., and Melton, F. M. (1949). J. Invest. Dermatol. 13:61.
Spearman, R. I. C., and Jarrett, A. (1974). Br. J. Dermatol. 90:553.
Spearman, R. I. C., and Riley, P. A. (1967). Br. J. Dermatol. 79:31.
Sprott, W. E. (1965). Trans. St. John's Hosp. Dermatol. Soc. 51:56.
Spruit, D., and Malten, K. E. (1965). J. Invest. Dermatol. 45:6.
Spruit, D., and Malten, K. E. (1968). Berufsdermatosen 16:11.
Squier, C. A. (1973). J. Ultrastruct. Res. 43:160.
Stein, W. D. (1967). The Movement of Molecules Across Cell Membranes.
    Academic Press, New York.
Stoughton, R. B. (1965a). Arch. Dermatol. 91:657.
Stoughton, R. B. (1965b). Toxicol. Appl. Pharmacol. 7:1.
Stoughton, R. B. (1966). Arch. Dermatol. 94:646.
Stoughton, R. B. (1972). Adv. Biol. Skin 12:535.
Stoughton, R. B., and Fritsch, W. (1964). Arch. Dermatol. 90:512.
Stoughton, R. B., and Stoughton, G. (1968). J. Invest. Dermatol. 50:332.
Swanbeck, G. (1968). Acta Derm. Venereol. (Stockh.) 48:123.

Tregear, R. T. (1961). J. Physiol. (London) 156:303.

Tregear, R. T. (1964). In Progress in the Biological Sciences in Relation to Dermatology, A. Rook and R. H. Champion (Eds.), Vol. 2. Cambridge Univ. Press, New York, p. 275.

Treager, R. T. (1966a). Physical Functions of Skin. Academic Press, New York.

Treager, R. T. (1966b). J. Invest. Dermatol. 46:16.

Treherne, J. E. (1956). J. Physiol. (London) 133:171.

Vickers, C. F. H. (1963). Arch. Dermatol. 88:20.

Vickers, C. F. H. (1966). In Modern Trends in Dermatology, R. M. B. McKenna (Ed.), Vol. 3. Butterworths, London, p. 84.

Vickers, C. F. H. (1969). Br. J. Dermatol. 81:902.

Vickers, C. F. H. (1972). Adv. Biol. Skin 12:177.

Vickers, C. F. H. (1980). In Percutaneous Absorption of Steroids, P. Mauvais-Jarvis, C. F. H. Vickers, and J. Wepierre (Eds.). Academic Press, New York, p. 19.

Vinson, L. J., Masurat, T., and Singer, E. J. (1965). Basic Studies in Percutaneous Absorption: Final Comprehensive Report (Rep. No. 10). Army Chemical Center, Edgewood, Md.

Wade, A., and Reynolds, J. E. F., Eds. (1977). Martindale: The Extra Pharmacopoeia, 27th ed. Pharmaceutical Press, London.

Wagner, J. G. (1961). J. Pharm. Sci. 50:379.

Wahberg, J. E. (1968). Acta Derm. Venereol. (Stockh.) 48:549.

Wallace, S. M., and Barnett, G. (1978). J. Pharmacokinetics Biopharm. 6:315.

Wallace, S. M., Runikis, J. O., and Stewart, W. D. (1978). Can. J. Pharm. Sci. 13:66.

Washitake, M., Yajima, T., Anmo, T., Arita, T., and Hori, R. (1973). Chem. Pharm. Bull. 21:2414.

Weitkamp, A. W., Smiljanic, A. M., and Rothman, S. (1947). J. Am. Chem. Soc. 69:1936.

Wells, F. V., and Lubowe, I. I. (1964). Cosmetics and the Skin. Van Nostrand Reinhold, New York.

Wester, R. C., and Maibach, H. I. (1977). In Cutaneous Toxicity, V. A. Drill and P. Lazar (Eds.). Academic Press, New York, p. 63.

Wheatley, V. R. (1953). Biochem. J. 55:637.

Wheatley, V. R. (1954). Biochem. J. 58:167.

Wheatley, V. R. (1956). Am. Perfumer Aromat. 68:37.

Wheatley, V. R. (1957). J. Invest. Dermatol. 29:445.

Wheatley, V. R. (1963). Proc. Sci. Sec. Toilet Goods Assoc. 39:25.

Wheatley, V. R., Flesch, P., Esoda, E. C. J., Coon, W. M., and Mandol, R. (1964). J. Invest. Dermatol. 43:395.

Wickrema Sinha, A. J., Shaw, S. R., and Weber, D. J. (1978). J. Invest. Dermatol. 71:372.

Wilkenson, D. I. (1969). J. Invest. Dermatol. 54:339.

Winkelmann, R. K. (1969). Br. J. Dermatol. 81(Suppl. 4):11.

Witten, V. H., Ross, M. S., Oshry, E., and Hyman, R. B. (1951). J. Invest. Dermatol. 17:311.

Witten, V. H., Ross, M. S., Oshry, E., and Holmstrom, V. (1953). J. Invest. Dermatol. 20:93.

Witten, V. H., Brauer, E. W., Loeninger, R., and Holmstrom, V. (1956). J. Invest. Dermatol. 26:437.

Wolf, J. F. (1939). Z. Mikroskop. Anat. Forsch. 46:170.

Woodford, R., and Barry, B. W. (1974). Curr. Ther. Res. 16:338.

Woodford, R., and Barry, B. W. (1977a). J. Pharm. Sci. 66:99.

Woodford, R., and Barry, B. W. (1977b). Curr. Ther. Res. 21:877.

Yotsuyanagi, T., and Higuchi, W. I. (1972). J. Pharm. Pharmacol. 24:934.

— 4 —

PROPERTIES THAT INFLUENCE
PERCUTANEOUS ABSORPTION

I. INTRODUCTION

When we apply a drug preparation to a diseased skin, we do so with the usual intention of inducing a therapeutic response, even if the purpose is only to soothe the inflamed organ. This clinical response arises from a sequence of three drug-related processes: (1) release of the medicament from the vehicle, followed by (2) its penetration through the skin barriers and (3) its activation of the desired pharmacological response. Effective topical therapy optimizes these processes as they are affected by a trio of components—the drug, the vehicle, and the skin.

Some concept of the complexity of percutaneous absorption may be gained by considering Fig. 4.1. This diagram represents a simple idealization of the drug flux which may arise clinically following the common treatment in which we apply a drug to the skin as a solid suspension in a topical vehicle. Only permeation into the body is considered, and not back-diffusion.

The medicament may undergo any or all of the following events. The drug particles must first dissolve so that molecules may diffuse within the vehicle to reach the vehicle-stratum corneum interface. Interfacial effects are not usually considered important, but for the drug to move through the skin it must partition into the stratum corneum and diffuse within this very impermeable barrier. Some drug may bind at a so-called depot site; the remainder diffuses in the horny layer, meets a second interfacial barrier, and partitions into the viable epidermis. Whereas the initial partition process may have favored an increased flux (for example, when a lipophilic drug is released to the skin from an aqueous vehicle), the second partitioning will be unfavorable as the viable epidermis provides a more hydrophilic milieu compared with the stratum corneum. Any substance with a high

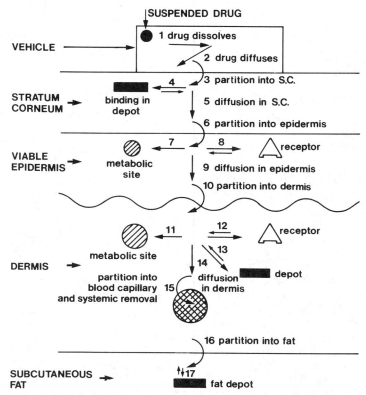

FIG. 4.1 Some stages in percutaneous absorption from a suspension ointment. Emulsion vehicles may include dissolution and partitioning processes
in the internal phase.

affinity for the horny layer and a very low water solubility may not be
absorbed percutaneously even though it may have penetrated the barrier
layer, particularly when it is applied in low concentrations. The thermodynamic activity of the diffusant in the viable epidermis immediately below
the barrier may approach that in the vehicle and in the top layer of the
stratum corneum. The rate-determining step will not now be the penetration
of the barrier but rather the clearance rate from the barrier (T. Higuchi,
1977). Metabolism may alter diffusion in the epidermis. The epidermis-to-
dermis partition coefficient may usually be assumed to be close to 1 and
may be neglected, as both tissues contain much water. Within the dermis,
additional depot regions and metabolic sites may intervene in the progress
of the drug to a blood capillary, its partitioning into the capillary wall,
thence out into the blood, and its subsequent removal by the systemic circulation. Very little is known about equilibration in the subepidermal environ-

ment and the pharmacokinetic factors which operate there. Such knowledge would be particularly important for pro-drugs designed to operate in the dermis. A fraction of the diffusant may partition into the subcutaneous fat to form a further depot.

Although the aforementioned sequence is already too complex for a full theoretical analysis together with a practical investigation, the situation is further complicated. Such factors may be important as the nonhomogeneity of the various tissues; the presence of hair follicles, sweat glands, interstitial fluid, and lymphatics; and the division of cells in the basal layer, their transport through the stratum corneum, and their surface loss. In addition, drugs permeate the skin under dynamic conditions. Thus, the drug, the components of the vehicle, and the disease may progressively modify the skin barrier, as may the healing process. As components of the vehicle may diffuse into the skin, so physiological materials, including sweat, sebum, and cellular debris, may pass into the formulated product and change its physicochemical characteristics. Emulsions may invert or crack when rubbed into the skin, and volatile solvents may evaporate into the atmosphere.

To discuss, in a comprehensible fashion, such a complex of mutually dependent phenomena, it is necessary to simplify the organization of the material under the separate headings of Biological Factors and Physicochemical Factors. In general, we will look at each factor in turn, but we will bear in mind the dynamic nature of percutaneous absorption. It is relatively rare, in vivo, for a significant change in the magnitude of any one variable to have only a single effect on the flux of the drug.

General reviews, which are useful as an introduction to the biopharmaceutical concepts to be dealt with in this chapter, include those of Idson (1971, 1975), Katz (1973), Katz and Poulsen (1971, 1972), Poulsen (1972, 1973), T. Higuchi (1977), and Dugard (1977). Loomis (1980) reviews studies of the skin as a portal of entry for systemic effects in the context of cutaneous toxicity.

II. BIOLOGICAL FACTORS

A. Skin Age

The relation between a patient's age and the permeability of his or her skin to drugs has rarely been investigated. This neglect is perhaps not surprising when we consider the biological variability of samples of skin taken from one individual at the same time, together with intersubject differences. In recent years, most interest in skin age as it affects drug permeation has revolved around the use of potent topical steroids for the treatment of inflammatory dermatoses. Normal or inflamed skin sites in infants appear to be more permeable than comparable areas in adults, as judged by reports of cushingoid side effects consequent on topical steroid treatment (Malkinson and Gehlmann, 1977). However, in case reports which suggest that topical corticosteroids are more dangerous in children than in adults, hard evidence is often lacking (Fanconi, 1962; Benson and Pharoah, 1960). Three publications which deal with the kinetics of topical corticosteroid use and their side effects in children have implicated hydrocortisone used under occlusion and betamethasone valerate (Fienblatt et al., 1966; Feiwel et al., 1969; Munro, 1976). In these studies, plasma cortisol values fell dramatically.

However, Rasmussen (1978) applied 0.1% triamcinolone acetonide ointment four times a day for 6 weeks to children with severe atopic eczema. Plasma and urinary cortisol levels did not indicate any notable adrenal suppression. The author concludes that the use of a medium strength topical corticosteroid for this length of time probably poses no significant hazard from percutaneous absorption.

Although we lack sufficient detailed quantitative data, it is usually assumed that the skins of the fetus, the young, and the elderly are more permeable than adult tissue (Feldmann and Maibach, 1970; Feiwel, 1969; Vickers, 1966; Nachman and Esterly, 1971). However, Kligman (1978) classifies as maternal folklore such statements as that infants and children have more "tender" skin than adults. His studies have failed to show any differences at either end of the age spectrum. Rasmussen (1979), in a balanced treatment, reviewed percutaneous absorption in children, particularly for allergens and irritants, boric acid and borates, phenol, salicylic acid, mercury, hexachlorophene, lindane (gamma benzene hexachloride), and topical steroids.

B. Skin Condition

The skin is a tough barrier to penetration, but only if it is intact. Many agents can damage the tissue. Vesicants such as acids, alkalies, and mustard gas injure barrier cells and thereby promote penetration. Although cuts, abrasions, and dermatitis occur commonly, little fundamental information is available, as distinct from speculation, as to the extent to which the permeability of the skin alters under such stresses. It is possible that even a mild dermatitis may increase permeability by deranging epidermal function so that an abnormal stratum corneum grows.

A somewhat surprising result was obtained by Wickrema Sinha et al. (1978). They applied diflorasone diacetate cream to rats at depilated sites and at depilated sites which had been abraded to produce hyperemia. No marked differences in the excretion of the topical steroid were observed between rats with unabraded and with abraded skin. However, as the extent of percutaneous absorption (as measured by excretion) was almost 88%, any differences may well have been undetectable. In the monkey, a significant result was the prolonged retention of the steroid or its metabolites in the superficial cell layers of the epidermis of animals with abraded skin. The investigators concluded that such retention is related to the skin damage.

The in vitro percutaneous absorption of topically applied hydrocortisone increases in the experimental epidermal hyperproliferation of mice deficient in essential fatty acids (Solomon and Lowe, 1978). A similar increase occurs in abnormal hairless mouse epidermis produced by UV light irradiation, topical vitamin A acid, or topical 10% acetic acid in acetone (Solomon and Lowe, 1979). It is interesting to note that hydrocortisone penetration increases in spite of hyperkeratosis, parakeratosis, and acanthosis. Solomon and Lowe conclude that a combination of abnormal cell membrane phospholipids and abnormal stratum corneum increases skin permeability.

In heavy industry, workers' skins may lose their reactivity, or "harden," because of frequent contact with irritant chemicals. It remains to be elucidated whether a change in biochemical sensitivity or an alteration in the permeation properties of the skin causes this resistance to further damage.

In general, the entire complex of factors which determines penetration rates in damaged or diseased skin requires further study.

Cellophane tape stripping provides an experimental method for damaging skin. This treatment removes the stratum corneum, and the resultant evaporative water loss from the skin increases to a value similar to that from a free water surface. Stripping also enhances the absorption of almost any substance. Thus, up to 90% of the applied dose of radioactive hydrocortisone penetrates stripped skin (Malkinson, 1958) while the intact epidermis absorbs only 2% or less (Malkinson and Ferguson, 1955; Liddle, 1956). Five times as much radiolabeled strontium chloride permeates abraded rat skin compared with intact skin (Loeffler and Thomas, 1951). A wide variety of compounds, ranging from phenol to testosterone, demonstrates marked increases in penetrability (often 100-fold or more) after extensive barrier damage (Malkinson, 1958; Monash and Blank, 1958).

The evidence for permeability increases which may arise from UV, infrared (IR), and ionizing radiation, as well as mild thermal burns, was reviewed by Malkinson (1964), although some of the claims are unconfirmed. Absorption changes arising from trauma instigated by allergen contact need investigation.

Many solvents markedly alter the permeability of the skin barrier, often opening up the complex, dense structure of the stratum corneum (T. Higuchi, 1960; Blank and Gould, 1961a,b; Blank et al., 1964; Tregear, 1964; Stoughton and Fritsch, 1964; Sweeney et al., 1966). Other liquids change the skin's permeability relatively little (Dugard and Scott, 1978). A mixture of a nonpolar and a polar solvent such as chloroform and methanol removes the lipid fraction of the stratum corneum, forming artificial shunts in the membrane through which molecules pass more easily (Blank and Scheuplein, 1969). Hexane, acetone, and alcohol increase the permeability of the skin to water (Onken and Moyer, 1963) whereas ether does not affect surfactant and salicylate penetration (Blank and Gould, 1961a,b). Corrosive chemicals and protein denaturants, such as acids and alkalies, damage skin; and common industrial solvents, for example, phenols and anilines, are toxicological and dermatological hazards (Allenby et al., 1969; Malten et al., 1968; Conning and Hayes, 1970; Dutkiewicz and Piotrowski, 1962; Bettley, 1963).

A useful physical technique for assessing water permeability determines the electrical impedance of the skin. Some aliphatic acids, bases, and neutral compounds, including dimethylsulfoxide, dimethylformamide, and dimethylacetamide, markedly change the impedance of excised human skin. The corresponding increases in water permeability arise from a combination of mechanisms, including the relaxation of binding forces between skin elements, the dissolution of components, and the hydration and subsequent swelling of the skin to form additional channels for permeation (Allenby et al., 1969).

So far the discussion concerning the role of solvents in modifying skin permeability has concentrated on their incidental (usually damaging) effects. However, certain solvents such as dimethylsulfoxide (DMSO), dimethylacetamide (DMA), and dimethylformamide (DMF) may be employed in a more positive way to potentiate the absorption of drugs in clinical use. The topic of such sorption promoters, enhancers, or accelerants will be developed later (Sec. III.B.3).

Probably the most widespread cause of an alteration in skin condition is a disease. Injury to the tissue, with resultant inflammation, occurs more often in skin than in any other organ of the body. When sampling a dermatology text, the nondermatologist may be readily confused by the many often exotically named skin lesions listed. However, for our requirements it is sufficient to realize that the histopathological changes occurring in dermatitis are relatively few and simple. For general biopharmaceutical purposes we need only an elementary understanding of the gross changes which diseased skin undergoes. As they evolve, the signs of such dermatitis progress from swelling and acute erythema, to oozing and vesiculation, then to scaling and crusting, and finally to thickening and lichenification (Katz and Poulsen, 1971). Thus, we are mainly interested in visible damage. Is the skin inflamed, with loss of stratum corneum and altered keratinization? Then permeability increases. Is the organ thickened, as in ichthyosis or at the site of corns and calluses? Drug permeation should now decrease. However, it is still necessary to bear in mind that we do not have fundamental information as to the permeability of a scab to different chemicals.

In general, in diseases characterized by a defective stratum corneum, percutaneous absorption increases (Felsher and Rothman, 1945; Elliott and Odel, 1950; Scott, 1959; Malkinson and Rothman, 1963; Blank, 1964). Thus, testosterone and pyribenzamine penetrate psoriatic plaques more readily than at normal skin sites (Malkinson, 1964; Michelfelder and Peck, 1952). Drug concentrations in diseased skins can be higher than in normal skin sites adjacent to the lesion (Schaefer, 1979).

After injury or removal of the stratum corneum, within 3 days parakeratotic cells build a temporary barrier which persists until the regen-
erating epidermis can form normal keratinizing cells (Malkinson, 1958).
Usually, between 6 and 11 days after stripping, these parakeratotic cells
slough off. Complete regeneration of the stratum corneum, with its functional integrity entirely restored, requires approximately 2 weeks (Spruit
and Malten, 1965). However, even the first complete layer of new stratum
corneum cells formed over a healing layer can markedly reduce permeation (Monash, 1957; Monash and Blank, 1958; Matoltsy et al., 1962).

C. Regional Skin Sites

Few fundamental studies investigate how drug absorption varies with body
site. We may predict that variations in cutaneous permeability will depend
on the thickness of the stratum corneum, its nature, and—to a degree over-
emphasized in some publications—the density of skin appendages. Many
reports conflict, with variable epidermal cell counts and histochemistry
(Burch and Winsor, 1944; Witten et al., 1956; Dienhuber and Tregear,
1960; Bettley and Donoghue, 1960; Wurster and Dempski, 1961; Malkinson
and Rothman, 1961; Kedem and Katchalska, 1961; Smith et al., 1961;
Marzulli, 1962; Fredricksson, 1963; Blank and Scheuplein, 1964; Scheuplein,
1965; Vinson et al., 1965; McCreesh, 1965; Brown et al., 1967; Maibach
et al., 1971). Estimates of horny layer thickness (osmium tetroxide fixa-
tion) provide values of 8.9, 9.4, 10.9, and 12.9 μm for abdomen, back,
thigh, and flexor forearm, respectively. On average, 19 cells each 0.55 μm
thick give stratum corneum an overall thickness of 10.4 μm (Holbrook and
Odland, 1974).

Biological variability further complicates the situation in that the
absorption rate varies widely for a specific substance passing through
identical skin sites in different healthy volunteers. Extremes occur frequently in which flux rates for the most permeable regions in some individuals compare with rates for the least permeable sites in other subjects
(Marzulli, 1962). Further confusion arises when reports erroneously compare flux data derived from steady state experiments with transient data,
or they attempt to correlate an in vivo pharmacological response with an
in vitro diffusion analysis.

In particular, Scheuplein and Blank (1971) are concerned about the
error that may be made if we assume that skin from the palm and sole is
similar to that from other body sites (see also Scheuplein, 1978a). Although
plantar and palmar callus may be 400 to 600 μm thick compared with 10 to
20 μm thick from other regions (Rushmer et al., 1966), it is an inferior
barrier. Thus, the water flux and the permeability coefficient for plantar
skin are 10 times those for abdominal skin, yet the plantar diffusion coefficient is some 150 times that for abdominal skin. Thus, although plantar

skin is relatively weak, its very thickness imposes a protracted lag time for diffusion, which may give rise to erroneous concepts with respect to skin permeability. It is important to note that the two practical permeation measurements, the lag time and the steady state flux, yield estimates of h^2/D and D/h, respectively [see Chap. 2, Eqs. (2.9) and (2.10)]. Thus, lag times emphasize thickness differences at the expense of differences in diffusivity.

The inferior barrier nature of palmar and plantar callus is also indicated in the way in which weakly basic solutions, and even water, will eventually dissolve it (Kligman, 1964) and parathion will penetrate it (Maibach et al., 1971). These observations bring into question much of the earlier work on skin permeability, which attempted to make general observations from experiments performed on horny pads.

Regional variations in water permeability are not nearly as large as they would be if the stratum corneum were equal in thickness over all the body. As the thickness of the horny layer increases, so diffusivity increases so as to provide the skin with a relatively uniform steady state permeability.

Turning to materials other than water, we find that compounds such as salicylic acid, hydrogen sulfide gas, and lidocaine base penetrate the scrotum more readily than the abdomen (Smith et al., 1961). Scrotal and postauricular skin are the most permeable to tributyl phosphate (Marzulli, 1962). Feldmann and Maibach (1967), using radioactive hydrocortisone and analyzing its urine excretion, show that the scrotum absorbs the greatest total amount, with absorption decreasing in the following order: forehead, scalp, back, forearms, palms, and plantar surface of the foot arch. Normal vulvar skin (labia majora) absorbs hydrocortisone to a greater extent than does forearm skin (Britz et al., 1980).

Other workers attempt to assess regional variations in permeability by measuring a pharmacological response, e.g., the erythema reaction produced by vasodilators such as ethyl nicotinate or histamine (Cronin and Stoughton, 1962; Shelley and Melton, 1949). As indicated earlier, fundamental interpretation of such experiments is difficult because of the likelihood that transient and shunt diffusion trigger the physiological reaction.

Depending on the nature of the experiment and the permeant used, various investigators arrive at somewhat different rank orders for the permeability of skin sites. The most fundamental physicochemical work tentatively ranks the order of diffusivity for simple, small molecules in decreasing order as: plantar, palmar, and dorsum of hand, scrotal and postauricular, axillary and scalp, arm, leg, and trunk (Scheuplein and Blank, 1971).

Among the most interesting biopharmaceutical applications of such studies is the selection of a suitable regional site to use as a window for systemic therapy. Because of its relatively high permeability and its ease of access, the Transiderm, Transderm, or Transdermal Therapeutic System (TTS) employs the postauricular skin as the site of application to insert drugs percutaneously into the bloodstream (see Secs. III.B.2 and III.D.4; also Shaw et al., 1975, 1977; Michaels et al., 1975; Chandrasekaran et al., 1976, 1978a, b; Chandrasekaran and Shaw, 1977; Shaw and Chandrasekaran, 1978, 1981). Thus, Taskovitch and Shaw (1978) determined the transdermal flux of scopolamine in vitro in human skin of approximately constant stratum corneum thickness (20 to 28 μm). The order of permeability was postauricular skin, back, chest = stomach, forearm, thigh, with a 20-fold difference in flux between the postauricular skin and that of the thigh. These authors consider that the relatively high permeability of the skin behind the ear arises from a combination of morphological features. In this region, the squamous layers of the stratum corneum are thinner and less dense, there are more sweat glands and sebaceous glands per unit area, and the deep indentations of the dermal papillae into the epidermis bring many capillaries closer to the skin surface. This last factor increases the in vivo surface temperature of this area by some 4° to 6°C relative to thigh temperature. With a raised temperature, the percutaneous absorption of a drug increases (Shaw et al., 1980). In this context, Craig et al. (1977) showed that the percutaneous absorption of a cholinesterase inhibitor was a function of skin temperature.

Recently, Horhota and Fung (1978) investigated the percutaneous absorption of nitroglycerin through the shaved abdomen and back of the rat by measuring plasma concentrations after topical administration. Abdominal absorption was significant, whereas adhesive tape had to be used to strip the dorsal site before plasma concentrations of nitroglycerin could be detected. Photomicrographs of back and abdominal tissue sections from a rat showed marked differences in the epidermis at the two sites. The relative depth and number of layers of the stratum corneum on the back area were significantly greater than on the abdomen. These findings may have general relevance when it is realized that, for practical purposes, many screening studies on topical absorption utilize the back of the rat as the primary testing site (Gross et al., 1960; Bartek et al., 1972; Moore et al., 1976; Keen and Hurley, 1977). Site dependence for absorption of nitroglycerin has been reported in humans (Hansen, 1978), but not in the rhesus monkey (Noonan and Wester, 1980).

D. Skin Metabolism

When the pharmaceutical industry develops a new systemically active drug, a full biopharmaceutical investigation considers in detail the pharmacokinetics of the compound, including its absorption, distribution, metabolism, and excretion. However, in the past, for a topical drug, what happens to it after it penetrates the stratum corneum barrier has received much less attention than the fundamentals of the percutaneous process itself. In particular, this has been the situation with respect to the metabolism of drugs

by the skin. There are fertile fields for investigation in this area, with
respect to drugs in general and to the design and activation of pro-drugs in
particular (T. Higuchi, 1977, 1979; Yu, 1978; Fox et al., 1979; Yu et al.,
1979a, b). Hadgraft (1980) published a study on the theoretical aspects of
metabolism in the epidermis.

The major groups of chemicals which have been investigated to date
are the carcinogens and steroidal compounds. For the latter group, most
investigations concentrate on determining the chemical routes which lead
to the biosynthesis of naturally occurring hormones. Human skin may store
steroids and may be an important site for their metabolism and their biosynthesis. Inflammation, hirsutism, testicular feminization syndrome,
sebum production, and acne may all cause abnormalities in these functions
(Berliner, 1972).

Several investigators have studied androgen metabolism in whole human
skin and in plucked hair follicles (Wotiz et al., 1956; Wilson and Walker,
1969; Gomez and Hsia, 1968; Sansone and Reisner, 1971; Sansone-Bazzano
et al., 1972). Baseline data for the metabolism of testosterone, dehydro-
epiandrosterone, progesterone, and estradiol in skin and in sebaceous glands
were developed by Sansone-Bazzano et al. (1979), who also investigated,
in vitro, the effect of skin age.

The biotransformation of compounds absorbed by the skin usually
produces inactive metabolites, but sometimes metabolically active compounds form. For example, cortisone may convert to hydrocortisone in vitro
(Malkinson et al., 1959). Greaves (1971) and, in particular, Hsia and his
co-workers report that incubating hydrocortisone with slices of human skin
produces several different metabolites (Hsia et al., 1964, 1965; Hsia and
Hao, 1966, 1967). O'Neill and Carless (1980a,b) considered the influence
of the side chain on the hydrolysis of some hydrocortisone esters and how
such esters may also inhibit enzyme activity in skin. Little is known about
the biotransformation of highly potent fluorinated corticosteroids in the skin.
However, esterases in the skin of rats and guinea pigs rapidly hydrolyze
diflucortolone valerate, whereas in vitro tests with human skin reveal a
very slow degradation rate for this steroid (Tauber, 1976). In vitro metabolism of testosterone in human skin produces various derivatives, of which
5-α-dihydrotestosterone is the main one (Gomez and Hsia, 1968; Wilson
and Walker, 1969).

Berliner (1972) reviews the biotransformation of steroids by the skin
and provides further relevant references; Gomez and Frost (1972) do the
same for testosterone metabolism. Hsia (1980) provides a general outline
of the metabolism of steroids in human skin. Schaefer (1979) considers that
there is little skin metabolism of topically applied anti-inflammatory steroids
at therapeutic concentrations. Longcope (1980) concludes that normal skin
contributes to the overall metabolism of estrogens, but the tissue is not the
major site of metabolism despite its mass and blood flow. Kuttenn et al.
(1980) report results on androgen metabolism in normal and pathological
human skin.

Ando et al. (1977a,b) propose an in vitro model for determining the simultaneous transport and metabolism of the antiviral agent vidarabine. Leung and Ando (1979) assess the aqueous diffusion coefficient for the drug, the diffusion layer thickness, and the enzyme metabolic rate constant, using the rotating disk theory (Levich, 1962) with benzoic acid standardization (Prakongpan et al., 1976). Fox et al. (1979) present a general physical model for simultaneous diffusion and metabolism in biological membranes. This computational approach can model a wide variety of complex metabolic schemes, including nonuniform enzyme distributions and composite membranes with any number of layers. Further details relevant to vidarabine appear in the publications of Yu et al. (1980a,b,c).

Bickers (1980) has recently reviewed the role which the skin plays as a site of drug and chemical metabolism. He concludes that the skin actively metabolizes steroid hormones, chemical carcinogens, and drugs and that such metabolism may ultimately prove to be a critical determinant of therapeutic efficacy of topically applied drugs and of the carcinogenic responses in skin.

E. Circulatory Effects

Theoretically, changes in the peripheral circulation, or blood flow through the dermis, could affect percutaneous absorption. Thus, an increased blood flow could reduce the time for which a penetrant remains in the dermis and also raise the concentration gradient across the skin. For example, the penetration of tributyl phosphate in perfused dog skin preparations depends to some extent on the perfusate flow rate (Kjaersgaard, 1954). In vivo, the large area of the capillary bed should ensure the prompt removal of a diffusant and only if the blood flow drastically reduces would skin clearance have a measurable effect (Tregear, 1966). In other situations, the rate-limiting step in percutaneous absorption would remain located in the stratum corneum. Any effect of an increased blood flow, as in clinical erythema, would significantly influence only the absorption of rapidly penetrating molecules such as gases. Thus, when carbon dioxide induces vasodilation, radon is more readily absorbed (McClellan and Comstock, 1949). However, in clinically hyperemic skin, any consequent increase in absorption almost always arises from a disease process damaging the skin barrier (Vickers, 1966). Potent rubefacients such as nicotinic acid esters would also only have a significant effect after damaging the skin.

When one considers the opposite effect, vasoconstriction, the evidence is more clear-cut. It is possible that potent vasoconstricting agents such as topical steroids could reduce their own rate of clearance from the skin or the rate of a second drug administered either with the steroid or immediately after its application. Thus, topical application of 6-methylprednisolone to stripped skin sites slows the absorption of [^{14}C]testosterone applied sub-

sequently (Malkinson, 1958). Presumably, to detect any such effect, a potent
vasoconstrictor would be required or the stratum corneum would need to be
removed. When a weak vasoconstrictor such as hydrocortisone is applied
simultaneously with the testosterone, if it produces any effect at all it is to
increase the total amount of testosterone absorbed (Feldmann and Maibach,
1969).

Caution is required when interpreting results such as those just discussed. It is tempting to assume that, as potent steroids blanche the skin,
this "vasoconstriction" necessarily implies a decreased blood flow. (Not all
investigators are convinced that skin blanching arises from vasoconstriction.) From experimental measurements, blanching may or may not correlate with changes in blood flow. For example, one method for measuring
cutaneous blood flow determines the clearance rate of xenon-133 applied
either epicutaneously or by intracutaneous injection (Sejrsen, 1966, 1969,
1971). With fluandrenolide, the mean blood flow declines (Greeson et al.,
1973), but in other investigations anomalous dose-dependent effects arise.
Application of 0.1% betamethasone valerate in a cream base four times at
six hourly intervals reduces the blood flow in cutaneous tissue within 24 hr.
However, 0.1% hydrocortisone butyrate has no effect. Application of 0.5%
betamethasone valerate produces no difference compared with a placebo
cream, but 1.0% valerate increases the blood flow. Dosing with 0.1% hydrocortisone butyrate under plastic occlusion also increases cutaneous blood
flow. Kristenson and colleagues conclude that if the bioavailability of a
topical steroid is low, the blood flow may remain unaltered or my decrease;
but if the steroid is applied at high concentrations or under conditions which
promote percutaneous absorption (e.g., plastic occlusion), blood flow will
increase (Kristensen and Wadskov, 1977; Kristensen et al., 1978). These
authors do not explain the mechanism of this effect, but it may depend on
catecholamine depletion and/or interference with the intrinsic reactivity of
smooth muscle cells.

F. Species Differences

Mammalian skins from different species display wide differences in anatomy
in such characteristics as the thickness of the stratum corneum, the numbers
of sweat glands and hair follicles per unit surface area, and the condition of
the pelt. The behavior and distribution of the papillary blood supply (Montagna, 1963, 1967; Montagna and Ellis, 1961; Montagna and Yun, 1964) and
the sweating ability (Montagna, 1967) differ between humans and the common
laboratory animals. Such factors will obviously affect both the routes of
penetration and the resistance to penetration.

Frequently, laboratory animals such as rats, mice, and rabbits are
used to assess percutaneous absorption, but their skins have more hair
follicles than human skin and they lack sweat glands. To apply experimental

samples to such animals, often the hair must first be clipped and the skin shaved. It is often assumed that such shaving damages the stratum corneum and artificially increases penetration. Thus, when vasoconstrictors are applied to the shaved human forearm, the sites immediately blanche; a time delay intervenes for the unshaved limb. However, testosterone penetration through the shaved and unshaved forearm of the rhesus monkey shows no significant difference (Wester and Maibach, 1975a).

During experiments with nohuman subjects, precautions must be taken to prevent the animals from disturbing the topical sample or from ingesting it. Monkeys may be seated in a metabolism chair and their arms may be restrained with adhesive tape. Thus, the usual site of application, the ventral forearm, may be isolated from the fecal and urine collection area (Wester and Maibach, 1975a). Urinary catheters may also be used. Contamination can also be avoided by using special protective devices such as that employed with the pig (Bartek et al., 1972).

However, because experiments in humans are surrounded by so many restrictions, animals are often used instead despite their limitations. An additional complication is that subtle biochemical differences between human and animal skin may fundamentally alter the reactions between penetrants and the skin (Marzulli et al., 1969).

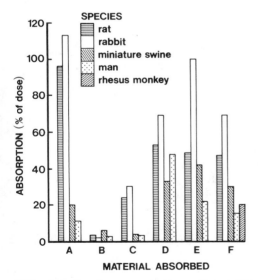

FIG. 4.2 In vivo percutaneous absorption of compounds in rat, rabbit, miniature swine, rhesus monkey, and man. Key: A = haloprogin, B = N-acetylcysteine, C = cortisone, D = caffeine, E = butter yellow, F = testosterone. (From Bartek et al., 1972; Feldmann and Maibach, 1969, 1970; Wester and Maibach, 1975a,b, 1977.)

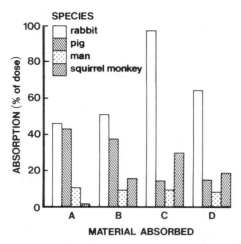

FIG. 4.3 In vivo percutaneous absorption of pesticides in rabbit, pig, squirrel monkey, and man. Key: A = DDT (monkey data not corrected by parenteral administration), B = Lindane, C = Parathion, D = Malathion. (Data from Bartek and La Budde, 1975; Feldmann and Maibach, 1974a.)

Wester and Maibach (1977), Wester et al. (1979), and Wester and Noonan (1980) recently correlated a number of publications in an attempt to obtain a perspective as to how percutaneous absorption in several animal models compares with penetration in humans. Basic clinical data were derived by applying radioactive material to the ventral forearm and by collecting the urine for analysis over 5 days. However, compounds may be excreted by routes other than the kidney or they may be stored in the body. To correct for such deviations, a parenteral tracer dose was given and the urine was similarly analyzed (Feldmann and Maibach, 1969, 1970, 1974a). The method does not allow for drug metabolism in the skin and it determines only total radioactivity. With obvious limitations, such data may be compared with results from other investigations in animals to determine approximate relationships. However, the accuracy of the analysis, which uses only a period of 5 days for urine collection, has been questioned (Franz, 1978).

The data in Fig. 4.2 compare clinical results with absorption studies in rats, rabbits, miniature swine, and rhesus monkeys. The topical antifungal agent Haloprogin penetrates well in the rat and rabbit but to a lesser degree in the pig and man, where results are similar. All species absorb little acetylcysteine. The rat and rabbit absorb about 25 to 30% of an applied cortisone dose, but little passes into the pig and man. Caffeine readily penetrates the epidermis of all four species. The banned food dye butter yellow passes particularly well through rabbit skin.

Wester and Maibach (1975a, b) compared percutaneous absorption in the rhesus monkey and in man. In both species, the order of increasing absorption is hydrocortisone, testosterone, and benzoic acid. For all species represented in Fig. 4.2, absorption of testosterone in the rhesus monkey is closest to that in man. For the guinea pig, absorption of hydrocortisone and benzoic acid is similar to man, but testosterone is absorbed to a greater extent (Andersen et al., 1980).

In summary, these results suggest that rabbit skin is the most permeable to topically applied compounds, with rat skin being second. However, while penetration through rabbit skin is rapid, the structures of the epidermis and its appendages do not appear to differ significantly from those of other animals which are more resistant to penetration (Steigleder, 1962; Wolff and Winkelmann, 1967; Winkelmann, 1969). The skins of miniature swine and rhesus monkeys behave somewhat similarly to that of man.

Figure 4.3 presents corresponding data for the percutaneous absorption of some pesticides in rabbit, pig, squirrel monkey, and man (Bartek and La Budde, 1975; Feldmann and Maibach, 1975). DDT [1,1,1-trichloro-2,2-bis(p-chlorophenyl)ethane] penetrates rabbit and pig well, man much less readily, and monkey only slightly; however, the monkey data are not corrected with parenteral control experiments. Lindane, parathion, and malathion readily penetrate the rabbit. Overall, in vivo percutaneous absorption of pesticides in the rabbit is much greater than in man, whereas the skins of the pig and the squirrel monkey behave somewhat similarly to that of man.

There is evidence that porcine skin shares some histochemical, anatomic, and penetration features with human skin (Montagna and Yun, 1964; Forbes, 1969; Winter and Wilson, 1976; Ayres and Hooper, 1978; Meyer et al., 1978; Meyer and Neurand, 1976).

The skin of the rhesus monkey functions like human skin for compounds such as testosterone, hydrocortisone, and benzoic acid in respect of both the total amount absorbed and how this relates to the applied dose. Thus,

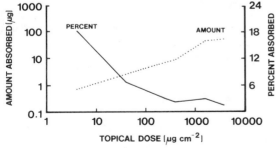

FIG. 4.4 Percutaneous absorption of topical doses of testosterone in the rhesus monkey; effect of increasing applied dose. (From Wester and Maibach, 1976.)

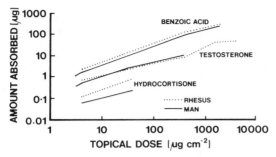

FIG. 4.5 Comparison between percutaneous absorption in man and in rhesus monkey: relationship between topical dose and amount absorbed for benzoic acid, testosterone, and hydrocortisone. (From Wester and Maibach, 1976.)

the efficiency of absorption, as judged both by the percentage of the dose absorbed as well as the total amount absorbed, varies with the dose applied. Figures 4.4 and 4.5 show these relationships.

Recently, the percutaneous absorption and disposition of a new topical corticosteroid, diflorasone diacetate, were studied in the rat, cynomolgus monkey, and man after a single cutaneous applications of a 0.05% steroid steroid cream (Wickrema Sinha et al., 1978). The site of application for the animals was the depilated back; the depilated ventral forearm was used for human studies. The extent of percutaneous absorption (as measured by urinary and fecal excretion) was high for the rat and the monkey, being about 90% and 50% of the net administered dose, respectively. However, only approximately 1% of the net dose was excreted in man. Wickrema Sinha and co-workers attribute the difference to anatomic variations in skin structure in particular to the greater density of hair follicles in the animals; they conclude that neither the monkey nor the rat is a suitable animal model for comparison with man, at least for this steroid. However, urinary excretion is the major route of elimination of this steroid and its metabolites in man, as it is in the monkey. In this respect, therefore, the monkey does resemble man. In the rat, fecal (bilary) excretion is more important.

Benzoic acid, progesterone, and testosterone penetrate less readily into the skin of the Mexican hairless dog than into human skin (Hunziker et al., 1978). Thus, this animal does not provide a good model for human skin.

An unresolved problem is to select an animal species which provides close correlation with the newborn human infant. Skin permeability in the newborn infant is of particular concern because of the cases of fatal poisoning which have occurred from, for example, topical application of hexachlorophene (see Tyrala et al., 1977; for a review, see Marzulli and Maibach, 1975), phenol (Brown, 1970), pentachlorophenol (Armstrong et al.,

TABLE 4.1 In Vitro Permeability Rankings for Different Species, Listed
in Decreasing Order of Permeability

Marzulli et al. (1969)	McCreesh (1965)	Tregear (1966)
1. Mouse	1. Rabbit	1. Rabbit
2. Guinea Pig	2. Rat	2. Rat
3. Goat	3. Guinea Pig	3. Guinea Pig
4. Rabbit	4. Cat	4. Man
5. Horse	5. Goat	
6. Cat	6. Monkey	
7. Dog	7. Dog	
8. Monkey	8. Pig	
9. Weanling Pig		
10. Man		
11. Chimpanzee		

Source: Wester and Maibach (1977).

1969), and Castellani's solution (Lundell and Nordman, 1973). For a recent
review of percutaneous absorption in children, see Rasmussen (1979). Because of ethical and technical difficulties, we cannot directly compare topical
absorption in the human infant with selected animal species. However, it
seems reasonable to make at least preliminary extrapolations from studies
in the newborn rhesus monkey to human neonates (Wester et al., 1977).

Turning from the in vivo to the in vitro situation, several publications
present data which rank skin permeability in different species (Table 4.1).
Although these studies use different compounds and different anatomic sites
for skin samples, in general it appears that the skins of laboratory animals
such as guinea pig, rat, and rabbit are more permeable than human skin.
Skin from the monkey and the pig is closest to that of man. This general
ranking correlates with the in vivo data discussed previously. Dugard (1977)
considers that rat and man have similar skin permeability properties to
small polar molecules such as water; the normal transepidermal water loss
is also similar for these species (see Prottey, 1976).

As part of their work on a transdermal therapeutic device, Campbell
et al. (1976) investigated the in vitro permeability of scopolamine through
human, rat, and rabbit skin. The results indicate that human skin is the
least permeable and that the relative order of rabbit and rat skin permea-

bilities depends both on the method used to remove the hair and the location of the skin (side or back).

In some investigations, mouse skin proves to be the most permeable, much more so than human skin (Marzulli et al., 1969). However, Stoughton (1975) reports that, in vitro, human and hairless mouse skin behave similarly toward some steroids, tolnaftate, 5-fluorouracil, and thiabendazole (Cohen and Stoughton, 1974). Durrheim et al. (1980) reach the same conclusion with respect to the n-alkanols.

From work designed to investigate the effect of surfactants on the percutaneous absorption of naproxen in vitro, Chowhan and Pritchard (1978) conclude that rabbit and rat skin are not comparable with human skin. They also emphasize that the rat is not a good in vivo model for man (Chowhan et al., 1978).

Other investigations include work which indicates that intact guinea pig skin provides results which are similar to those of human skin (Arita et al., 1970). Topical steroid absorption was studied in pigs (Desgroseilliers et al., 1969; Ayres and Hooper, 1978), and sodium salicylate was investigated in rabbits (Stolar et al., 1960a,b). Sweeney et al. (1966) used hairless mice to investigate the effect of DMSO on water permeation. Allergenic chemicals can be screened in guinea pigs (Magnusson, 1975; Magnusson and Kligman, 1970; Maguire, 1973). Lansdown (1978) has reviewed the role of animal models for the study of skin irritants.

We may summarize the comparative studies of skin penetration in vivo and conclude that in general the skins of the monkey and the pig are most like that of man. The Guidelines for Preclinical and Clinical Testing of New Medicinal Products (1977), published by the Association of the British Pharmaceutical Industry, recommend the use of piglets on the basis that their skin is similar in many ways to human skin. Rabbit and rat skins are highly permeable, and the skin of the Mexican hairless dog has characteristics different from those of man. In vitro, the skins of rabbit, rat, and guinea pig are more permeable than human skin. Again, the permeability of pig and monkey skins approximates to that of man.

We know little about the regional differences in permeability within an animal species, even though important differences probably exist as they do in man. Nor do we know if a specific anatomic site in an animal approximates to the same site in man, or even to another region in human skin. However, we do know that the absorption of testosterone in the rhesus monkey depends on the site of application (Wester et al., 1980), as does nitroglycerin absorption in the rat (Horhota and Fung, 1978).

It is worth mentioning that there is a diversity of skin types among the races of man; integumental differences are probably greater than for any other body organ (Kligman, 1978). However, we know almost nothing about physiological differences and vulnerability to irritation and percutaneous absorption between the races. We do know that black skin is hardier and more resistant to toxic chemicals, partly because it has greater density and more cell layers than Caucasian skin (Weigand et al., 1974). Fair-skinned people of Celtic ancestry (Irish, Welsh, or Scottish) sunburn easily, and their skins are hyperirritable to a variety of toxic chemicals such as croton oil, kerosene, alkalies, and sodium lauryl sulfate, compared with dark-complexioned Caucasoids from the Mediterranean region (Frosch and Kligman, 1977). The frequency of contact dermatitis in automobile factory workers is much higher in fair-skinned people (Newhouse, 1964).

Recently, Weigand et al. (1980) compared the stratum corneum from Negroes and Caucasians with respect to the ease of tape stripping, number of cell layers, buoyant density, and permeability to water. Their findings supported the view that Negro stratum corneum is a more effective barrier, and this may explain the relative resistance of Negro skin to chemical irritation.

III. PHYSICOCHEMICAL FACTORS

A. Factor Interactions

The principal physicochemical factors which control the passive diffusion of a solute from a vehicle into the skin arise from the molecular properties of the diffusant, the vehicle, and the skin. The fundamental properties of these three materials and how they interact determine to a large extent the penetration rate of a drug into the skin. If we follow the excellent treatment of Katz and Poulsen (1971), we can identify three possible interactions, each composed of two factors, i.e., drug-skin, vehicle-skin, drug-vehicle, and one three-factor interaction, i.e., drug-vehicle-skin. The following discussion will therefore be based on this useful artificial division of the subject matter. We will examine how these interactions may influence the rate and extent of percutaneous absorption and thus how they may affect the degree and duration of a pharmacological response. However, we will not consider specifically the pharmacokinetics or pharmacodynamics of the drug interaction at a receptor site. Standard pharmacological textbooks and monographs present information on this important topic.

B. Drug-Skin Interactions

1. Skin hydration

When water saturates the skin, the tissue softens, swells, and wrinkles and its permeability dramatically increases. Thus, scientists show much interest in the hydration state of the stratum corneum, and several groups of workers have measured water sorption isotherms (Blank, 1952, 1953; Fox et al., 1962; Singer and Vinson, 1966; Scheuplein, 1966; Middleton, 1968; Anderson et al., 1973; El-Shimi et al., 1975; Spencer et al., 1975;

Hey et al., 1978). The associated phenomenon of transepidermal water loss
is also important. Idson (1978a) has reviewed the methods available for
measuring this loss in vivo and the role of hydration in promoting percutaneous absorption (Idson, 1978b).

It is possible that some drugs which can rapidly penetrate the skin to
yield tissue concentrations that are high enough to exert an osmotic effect
may increase skin hydration. A compound which efficiently hydrates the
skin could significantly improve the treatment of dry, scaly dermatoses.
The search for such a skin "moisturizer" has been an important project in
the cosmetic industry for many years. The term most widely used by investigators to describe this elusive material is natural moisturizing factor
(NMF), introduced in 1959 (Jacobi, 1959, 1972; Pugh, 1976).

Middleton (1968) showed that after extraction with water, the water-
binding capacity of stratum corneum at 90% relative humidity is 38-39 mg
per 100 mg dry weight. The value is the same when the tissue is extracted
by ether following the water extraction. However, if the procedure is re-
versed (extract with ether, then with water) the water-binding capacity falls
to 28 mg per 100 mg. The data of Fox et al. (1962) confirm this effect. Extraction of hairless mouse skin with a range of solvents removes the lipids
and increases the rate of diffusion of water. Such lipids would normally
impede the access of water to hygroscopic materials in the skin (Sweeney
and Downing, 1970). Jacobi (1958) showed that skin becomes water repellent
after successive extractions first with ether, then with water. While
untreated skin holds from 30 to 70 percent of water, after extraction it no
longer holds water when placed in an environment of low relative humidity
(Blank, 1953). Soaking the skin in soap or synthetic detergent solutions
also reduces the water-holding capacity of the skin (Blank and Shapiro,
1955).

Recent studies on water sorption by human callus have employed
vacuum microbalance, x-ray powder diffraction, and nuclear magnetic
resonance (NMR) relaxation methods (Hey et al., 1978). The results are
consistent with a model in which the water-binding properties of callus
depend on the presence of water-soluble components. These allow a monolayer of water to form at low relative vapor pressure followed by physical
multilayer formation. Wurster (1978) has also considered the uptake of
water (as well as acetate esters) from the vapor state into human callus.

Investigations such as the examples just cited suggest that some form
of humectant normally resides in the skin, protected by a lipid component
which is soluble in suitable solvents. This humectant, now usually identified
as NMF, can be the material extractable by water from stratum corneum
after liberation by solvent treatment. The term is also used to identify
synthetically produced substitutes which are claimed to produce the same
effect as the natural material.

The water-soluble constituents of stratum corneum have been investigated by many workers, and Schneider and Schuleit (1951) have reviewed

several publications. Szakall (1955, 1957) showed that stratum corneum contains 11% lipids and 30% water-soluble NMF and that the NMF content drops in psoriatic skin and in sunburned skin. He attributes the NMF to products of disintegrated cell nuclei, whereas Matolsty and Blank (1955) consider whether the material is a precursor of keratin or a result of keratin formation. Spier and Pascher (1955a,b, 1956, 1957) analyzed NMF as 40% free fatty acids, 12% pyrrolidone carboxylic acid, 7% urea, 5% sodium, 1.5% calcium, 4% potassium, and 12% lactate. Blank and Shapiro (1955) found a relatively constant concentration of amino acids in detergent-extracted material, and Flesch and his co-workers discovered a high content of mucopolysaccharide in NMF (Flesch and Esoda, 1960, 1963; Flesch et al., 1961, 1962). Singer and Vinson (1966) prepared stratum corneum extracts of low-molecular-weight, water-soluble substances which avidly absorb water; they considered these materials to be primarily responsible for water binding in stratum corneum cells. According to Curri (1967), the NMF may be a mucoprotein complex or a lipomucopolysaccharide complex.

Laden and Spitzer (1967) identified the main humectant in the water-soluble extract from skin as sodium pyrrolidone carboxylate. They patented the use of the salt, showing that it is a more powerful humectant than glycerol and that the free acid has no humectant properties. Measurements on scraping from the hand illustrated that the pyrrolidone carboxylic acid content relates linearly to the moisture binding capacity. Idson (1969a,b), Pugh (1976), and Tartarini et al. (1976) have discussed sodium pyrrolidone carboxylate and sodium lactate in their roles as major humectants in NMF.

Middleton and Roberts (1978) found that a cream containing 5% sodium pyrrolidone carboxylate increased by some 13% the water-holding capacity of the isolated stratum corneum of the footpads of guinea pigs. In a consumer trial which assessed skin dryness and flakiness, this cream was more effective than the control product and was as effective as a marketed cream (name unspecified) which contains urea.

Hydration of the stratum corneum facilitates the penetration of most materials through the skin, including corticosteroids (Scheuplein, 1978a). Woodford and Barry (1977a), in a limited experiment, tried to increase skin hydration by applying sodium pyrrolidone carboxylate. They then determined the effect of the moisturizer on the skin penetration of a range of topical steroids, as assessed by the skin blanching test. However, they obtained a negative correlation, which provisionally suggests that the NMF retards the percutaneous absorption of the steroids. However, the effect may have been due to the NMF increasing the solubilities of the steroids in the vehicles used to apply the steroids to the skin. The NMF could also have reduced the thermodynamic activities of the steroids in the vehicle by complexation. In addition, the moisturizer may have altered the diffusional properties of the corticosteroid molecules in the skin (e.g., by an effect on skin structure, by binding of water, or by complex formation with the steroids). Such factors would reduce steroid flux through the skin.

It appears that hydration does not affect the permeation of small, highly polar nonelectrolytes (water, methanol, and ethanol), at least through hairless mouse skin (Behl et al., 1980). For the more hydrophobic alcohols, i.e., butanol and hexanol, the permeability coefficients for this tissue double during the first 10 hr of immersion in water. In our laboratories we have shown that hydration, promoted by occlusion, has little effect on the permeation of mannitol, ibuprofen, and flurbiprofen through human cadaver skin (unpublished data).

Jacobi (1972) claims that effective moisturizers should be nonhygroscopic. Rieger and Deem (1974) show that humectants in the skin increase the transepidermal water loss in vitro, which may be undesirable in vivo. Jacobi (1959) analyzed the components in NMF and patented a condensation product of a N-glycoside as a nonhygroscopic moisturizer. Stankoff (1962) reviews some of the work which led to the development of this synthetic NMF.

Padberg (1967, 1972) showed that a fraction of sugars which contributes to water retention by NMF is chemically bound to protein in the stratum corneum. He prepared a sugar complex with a high moisture-retaining capacity that shavings of stratum corneum take up. In a clinical trial, the complex had a positive effect on skin roughness (Padberg, 1969).

Cooperman (1972) showed that hydrolized proteins, which are highly substantive, increase the ability of callus to absorb and to retain moisture, even after prolonged extractions with water.

Pugh (1976) has concluded from these investigations that the effect of NMF on human skin arises from a combination of the humectancy of the sodium salt of pyrrolidone carboxylic acid and of sodium or calcium lactate, combined with the water-retaining properties of some sugar-protein complex.

The esters of pyrrolidone carboxylic acid (of chain length 8 to 30, either branched or straight chain) have also been claimed to increase skin moisture (German Patents 2,102,171, 2,102,172, 2,102,173, 2,542,794). A recent patent (Di Giulio, 1977) promotes the use of 2-pyrrolidone for the same purpose when formulated in an oil-in-water emulsion.

Wilkinson (1973) provides further information and references on NMF.

Turning to other materials, urea has attracted interest because of its ability to moisturize the skin and to act as a mild keratolytic, although the molecular mechanism of action is unknown. Both these effects should promote skin penetration, and therefore some topical anti-inflammatory steroid preparations employ urea.

Several reports suggest that a commercial cream containing 10% urea (Calmurid) is valuable in the management of ichthyosis. This disease is characterized by very rough skin which presents a dry, cracked appearance resembling fish scales (Steward et al., 1969; Rosen, 1970; Ashton et al., 1970; Pope et al., 1972). For example, in a double-blind trial with 14 patients with ichthyosis, Calmurid Cream improved the clinical condition. It increased the water-holding capacity of the stratum corneum by 100%, and

the cream had little effect on the epidermal water barrier as determined by
the transepidermal water loss (Grice et al., 1973). However, this cream
was reported to be no more effective than Aqueous Cream B.P. in the treatment of hyperkeratosis (General Practitioner Research Group, 1973).

Swanbeck (1968) showed that this 10% urea cream increases the uptake
of water by the horny layer and by scales of ichthyotic and psoriatic patients.
Feldmann and Maibach (1974b) applied 1% [^{14}C]hydrocortisone acetate in a
cream vehicle with and without 10% urea to the ventral forearm of five adult
male volunteers in a crossover experiment. Using the urinary recovery of
carbon-14 as an index of penetration, these investigators conclude that the
urea increases steroid penetration approximately twofold. Parallel work
with double-blind controlled clinical bioassays demonstrates increased
efficacy of a topical corticosteroid in the presence of urea (Swanbeck, 1968;
Hindson, 1971; Roth and Gellin, 1973). Thus, the results of Almeyda and
Fry (1973) show that in the treatment of atopic eczema, 1% hydrocortisone
in a 10% urea cream base (Calmurid HC) is as effective as a 0.1% betamethasone 17-valerate cream, a relatively potent fluorinated preparation
(Floden et al., 1971; Hersle and Gisslen, 1972; Laurberg, 1975).

One of the problems with such urea cream vehicles is the acidity of
the cream (pH 3), which may sting when applied to excoriated skin. To
counteract this irritant effect, a new delivery system has been developed.
In this, an insoluble matrix consisting largely of maize starch loosely binds
a hypertonic solution of urea. The urea is stable in this form and readily
diffuses into the skin. The powder matrix is evenly dispersed at skin pH in
a nonaqueous medium in which hydrocortisone is freely suspended. This
preparation, Alphaderm, readily hydrates the skin (Ayres, 1977). It performs well clinically compared with fluorinated steroid preparations, and
it is claimed to be superior to the acidic urea/hydrocortisone cream Calmurid HC (Almeyda and Burt, 1974; Jacoby and Gilkes, 1974; Khan, 1978;
Marion-Landais and Krum, 1979).

From in vivo experiments in the pig, Ayres and Hooper (1978) claim
that Alphaderm promotes the penetration of hydrocortisone into the skin.
However, their methodology has been criticized, as it adds minute quantities of radiolabeled hydrocortisone in solution to formulations which already
incorporate unlabeled hydrocortisone in a variety of physicochemical form
dispersed in different environments. It is incorrect to compare different
formulations for their effectiveness by multiplying the percentage of radioactive hydrocortisone absorbed into the skin by the total amount of hydrocortisone originally present in the preparations, without waiting for radiolabeled steroid to equilibrate with nonradioactive steroid (Whitefield, 1979;
Orr et al., 1979).

When employing urea to modify the hydration state of the horny layer,
the carbamide must be allowed sufficient time to act. Thus, Barry and
Woodford (1976) assessed the vasoconstrictor activity and bioavailability of
hydrocortisone in six commercial cream formulations. They used a single

application technique in which the creams were applied for only 6 hr under occlusion. Results for the two preparations which contained urea—Calmurid HC and Alphaderm—suggested that under such conditions the urea did not preferentially promote the skin penetration of hydrocortisone. Two possible reasons for this result were the short application time and the possible swamping effect of occlusion which would rapidly saturate all stratum corneum sites with water. In a subsequent trial which employed a nonoccluded, multiple dosage regimen over 5 days, the activity and bioavailability of the hydrocortisone in Alphaderm were much improved (Barry and Woodford, 1977). This difference presumably arose because the extended time scale allowed the urea to exert its moisturizing and keratolytic effects in the skin so as to promote steroid penetration.

More recently, a delivery system of urea and starch (Psoradrate) has been used to promote dithranol penetration, although the stability of the dithranol in the formulation is questioned (Hooper, 1979; Thorne, 1979; Yarrow, 1979).

Evaluations and discussions on the use of urea have been published (Anonymous, 1971, 1973).

It has been suggested that steroids such as pregnenolone and estrogens benefit aging skin by hydrating it. Thus, pregnenolone acetate reduces the degree of wrinkling in older skin (Sternberg et al., 1961). It would be logical to investigate the role of aldosterone in the hydration of skin because of its influence on water and ion transport.

2. Drug-skin binding

In many of the investigations devoted to various aspects of percutaneous absorption, the investigators pay little attention to the binding of the drug to tissue components, as distinct from the simple passage of a material through the various skin membranes. However, to reconcile the steady state diffusivity of a drug permeating skin with the non-steady-state value calculated from transient measurements, it may be necessary to allow for skin binding. Thus, for scopolamine penetrating human skin, a dual sorption model may be used (Chandrasekaran et al., 1976, 1978a, 1980; Chandrasekaran and Shaw, 1978). This model includes molecules which bind to skin sites and which are therefore immobile, together with mobile, freely diffusing species. The mathematical analysis was used to optimize a Transdermal Therapeutic System (TTS), particularly with regard to the magnitude of the priming dose of drug. This priming dose serves to saturate immobilization sites for scopolamine within the stratum corneum. Then a steady state in the urinary excretion rate of the drug can be rapidly reached in vivo (see Sec. III.D.4).

It is logical to assume that the high activation energies observed for the transport process of penetrants in general arise from the binding of the penetrant to the stratum corneum membrane. It is therefore theoretically useful to determine the heat of adsorption for the sorption of the diffusant on the membrane, and also to determine its two components—the heat of activation for adsorption and the heat of activation for desorption. Examples of this approach are found in Wurster's (1972) study of the desorption of diethylphosphite from keratin powder in n-heptane and in Wurster's (1978) work with sarin adsorbed onto p-dioxane-conditioned callus. If a penetrant shows a high activation energy for transport and the membrane strongly adsorbs it, then much energy will be required to disrupt the penetrant-membrane bonds. A large heat of activation for desorption would be measured for this interaction. Any influence which decreases the heat of activation for desorption, thus aiding desorption, helps the transport process through the skin. One practical application for this information is to use simple adsorption and desorption experiments to select membrane-conditioning agents (accelerants, penetration enhancers, or promoters) on the basis of their effect in decreasing the heat of activation for desorption (see Wurster, 1978). Such work on sarin transport across excised human skin has been reported by Wurster et al. (1979) and Matheson et al. (1979, 1980).

Most compounds which the skin absorbs must be bound in part to skin proteins or even, at inflamed sites, to serum albumin which has diffused into the dermis through damaged blood vessel walls (Goldstein et al., 1969; Gabourel, 1972; Weber, 1972). In the absence of data specific to skin we have to proceed by analogy from plasma protein-drug interactions, which have been extensively studied (Goldstein, 1949; Goldstein et al., 1969; Settle et al., 1971; Chignell, 1971; Keen, 1971; Solomon, 1971; Gabourel, 1972). Presumably, skin-bound compounds are as inactive as plasma-protein-bound drugs in the general circulation. They are also protected from biotransformation, and their diffusion out of the skin into the lumen of a blood vessel is hindered. Since binding is reversible, the drug-protein complex provides a local reservoir, releasing drug to replace the free species as the general circulation removes it. Both the specific proteins which bind compounds and the extent of such binding are undetermined, although keratin-drug binding will obviously be important in the epidermis.

Little is known about the effect on the binding of a drug and its pharmacological activity when we administer, locally or systemically, a second compound with high protein affinity which may dislodge the first drug. We understand still less about the effects which dermatological diseases may have on the amount or binding properties of tissue proteins (Malkinson and Gehlmann, 1977). Age factors may influence protein bindings—as has been noted for serum albumin, which binds less in neonates and the elderly (Krasner et al., 1973; Hooper et al., 1974). The usual physicochemical variables such as temperature, pH, pK, and ionic strength will also affect the number of protein binding sites and their dissociation constants (Lunde et al., 1970; Sellers and Koch-Weser, 1974).

Turning to a few specific examples of drug-skin binding, Wurster and Dempski (1960) showed that powdered human callus tissue selectively adsorbs some unsaturated and 2-hydroxy fatty acids. Although we constantly apply surfactants, including soaps, to the skin, even to an irritant level, few data exist in the literature concerning the sorption of surfactants by human skin or hair. Exceptions include studies dealing with hair sorption of low concentrations (less than 1%) of long-chain quaternary ammonium halides (Scott et al., 1969; Finkelstein and Laden, 1971) and a brief study of sodium acyl sarcosinates, with concentrations up to 5% (Nelson and Stewart, 1956). For skin, Harrold and Pethica (1958) and Blank and Gould (1959) worked with anionics applied for long periods of time (18 to 24 hr) at low concentrations. Garrett (1965) studied the sorption of surfactants by hide powder. In a study designed to assess the uptake of sodium lauryl sulfate by the keratinous substances in human hair and neonatal rat stratum corneum, Faucher and Goddard (1978a) employed shorter periods of application (up to 8 hr) and higher concentrations of surfactant (up to 15%). These times and concentrations correspond in some degree to normal-use conditions. They conclude that the uptake of anionic surfactants by hair and by stratum corneum is appreciable. With sodium lauryl sulfate, the uptake increases markedly with concentration, even above the CMC. The uptake also increases in the presence of salt but decreases when nonionic surfactant is present. Lauryl ether sulfates are sorbed to a lesser extent than sodium lauryl sulfate and their uptake decreases with ethylene oxide content. The same authors showed that a cationic cellulose polymer (which itself strongly sorbs to stratum corneum) has no effect on the sorption of sodium lauryl sulfate. Therefore, it does not block the adsorption sites, although the polymer does reduce the amount of surfactant passing through the membrane (Faucher and Goddard, 1978b).

Breuer (1979) reviewed the interaction between surfactants and keratinous tissues in general. He concluded that the extent of the binding depends on the nature of the head group and the length of the hydrophobic tail of the detergent. Some detergents can penetrate both the amorphous region of the keratin and the crystalline microfibrils so as to change their structures and to affect their tensile properties.

Shaw et al. (1975) pretreated stratum corneum in vitro with 0.1 M aqueous solution of sodium lauryl sulfate; the surfactant reduced the binding of scopolamine and enhanced its permeation rate. In vivo, such pretreatment alters the pattern of urinary excretion of scopolamine when a TTS is applied to the skin surface (see Sec. III.D.4).

The effect of adsorbed sodium dodecyl sulfate and dodecyl trimethyl-ammonium bromide on the uptake of water by callus was determined by Hey et al. (1978). The anionic surfactant increases the monolayer uptake of water, whereas the quaternary ammonium compound has no effect.

In developing sunscreens, the skin substantivity of candidate molecules, i.e., their ability to adhere to or combine with keratin in the stratum corneum, is important (Lorenzetti et al., 1975). The affinity of sunscreens for human skin in vivo has been investigated (Willis and Kligman, 1970; Cumpelik, 1976), as has binding to animal skin in vitro (Hoppe, 1973). The interactions of four p-aminobenzoates (methyl, ethyl, n-propyl, and isopropyl) with human skin and animal wool were investigated by Bottari et al. (1978). For all compounds, they obtained linear absorption isotherms. Such esters are widely used as effective and safe sunscreens (Markland, 1976).

The interactions between a drug and the skin can be expected to range from weak physical attractions of the van der Waals type to strong chemical bonding. Materials which form the stronger type of bond with skin or hair may resist dislodgement when rinsed with water; i.e., these compounds may have substantive properties. Such properties are desirable for hair-grooming or -conditioning aids. Idson (1967) has reviewed the substantive properties of many topical antibacterial agents.

The most important clinical examples to date which involve drug-stratum corneum binding arise in the so-called reservoir effect of topical steroids and, to a lesser extent, antibiotics. This phenomenon is dealt with in Chap. 3, Sec. III.

A specific type of binding, namely, a drug-melanin interaction, can occur in skin, although once again the subsequent pharmacological effects are unclear. Initial clinical interest in this topic arose from cases of loss of vision and pigmentary retinopathy after the administration of phenothiazine drugs (Kinross-Wright, 1956; May et al., 1960; Weekley et al., 1960). Subsequently it was shown that phenothiazines such as chlorpromazine, as well as the antimalarial chloroquine, concentrate in melanin-containing tissues such as the pigmented structures of the eye (for a review of this topic, see Blois, 1972). It became apparent that the binding of such compounds to melanin granules is fairly specific, largely physical, and apparently reversible. As far as skin therapy is concerned, one obvious specific application of such binding would be to selectively concentrate an anti-cancer agent in the pigmented metastases of malignant melanomas. To further this study, Blois (1972; also Blois and Taskovitch, 1969) investigated screening techniques for melanin binding that use melanin and a number of other biopolymers. Although in vivo and in vitro experiments demonstrated that melanin binds a number of compounds, no fundamental information as to the mechanism of binding was obtained. However, clinical evidence of the production of retinopathies suggests that a drug bound in large quantities to eye pigment may act as a depot which slowly releases drug over an extended time period. This phenomenon could have a similar significance in the treatment of skin melanomas as does the steroid reservoir in the treatment of inflammatory skin diseases.

C. Vehicle-Skin Interactions

The skin interacts dynamically with the environment, and thus the epidermal microenvironment changes throughout a normal day's activity. When we apply pharmaceutical vehicles to the skin such as solutions, lotions, creams, ointments, gels, powders, and aerosols, these materials may well superimpose further changes on the physical state of the integument and they may affect its permeability. If the applied vehicle does modify the skin permeability, its mechanism of action will probably be a solvent action on the stratum corneum, a hydration effect, or an effect on the skin temperature. Often, more than one process operates at the same time. In this section we will consider each of these effects separately.

1. Vehicle effects on skin hydration

In Sec. III. B. 1, we saw that the water-binding properties of the horny layer depend on the presence of the so-called natural moisturizing factor (NMF). This material is necessary to maintain the water content of the stratum corneum above about 20%, when the tissue is soft and pliable (Blank, 1952, 1953). The skin chaps if the hydration falls below this critical level. The condition can only be remedied by restoring the water content of the skin.

An almost invariable side effect to a raised hydration level is an increase in the permeation rate of a skin penetrant. Thus, occlusive vehicles such as fats and oils reduce water loss to the atmosphere, increase the moisture content of the skin, and promote drug penetration.

A topical vehicle may either increase or decrease the moisture content of the stratum corneum. Thus, oily materials such as lanolin, isopropyl myristate, and the paraffins efficiently retard moisture loss from the skin. Thus, they are good moisturizers, although they are not cosmetically elegant (Powers and Fox, 1959; Spruitt, 1961; Jolly and Sloughfy, 1975). One way of increasing acceptability and patient compliance is to formulate a moisture retardant as a bath additive. Thus, Oilatum Emollient (Stiefel) contains acetylated wool alcohols (as a dispersant) and liquid paraffin. The patient soaks in a bath containing the additive and hydrates his stratum corneum. Upon leaving the water, a thin layer of liquid paraffin deposits on the skin to retard reflex drying.

Commercial products are often promoted to the consumer as skin softeners, with the presumption that these preparations increase the moisture content of the skin. Such formulations often contain humectants such as glycerol and emulsifiers which actually withdraw moisture from the skin. One such product increases water loss by as much as 56% (Powers and Fox, 1959).

As a general principle, we expect water-in-oil emulsions to be less occlusive than lipid materials but more occlusive than oil-in-water emulsions. This is because in a water-in-oil emulsion the continuous oil phase retards water diffusion. Results from in vitro experiments with a water-impervious polymer film, petrolatum, an isopropyl myristate gel, and three oil-in-water creams indicate that the first three preparations are approximately equal in their resistances to moisture loss. The commercial creams are relatively permeable to water (Dempski et al., 1965).

Dramatic examples of the importance of hydration in promoting the penetration of drugs through the skin can be found in investigations which employ occlusive plastic films in topical steroid treatment. Without exception, the prevention of water loss from the stratum corneum and the subsequent increased water content in the skin apparently enhances the penetration of the steroid (Scholtz, 1961; Sulzberger and Witten, 1961; McKenzie and Stoughton, 1962; Vickers, 1963; Hall-Smith, 1962; Witten et al., 1963; Stoughton, 1972). The penetration of corticosteroids may increase 100-fold under occlusion (a factor possibly exaggerated by the assessment method), and this increase may cause side effects because of too much drug absorption. Just as occlusion enhances the reservoir effect in the stratum corneum (see Chap. 3, Sec. III), it also promotes steroid penetration as judged by the vasoconstrictor test (Stoughton, 1972; Woodford and Barry, 1974, 1977a,b; Barry and Woodford, 1974, 1975, 1976, 1977, 1978; Barry, 1976).

Penetration of steroids and naphazoline nitrate increases when the humidity over the skin increases or the tissue is soaked in water (Fritsch and Stoughton, 1963; Stoughton, 1964, 1972). Thus, for triamcinolone acetonide, fluocinolone acetonide, and hydrocortisone, the percentage of steroid penetrating the skin increases 10-fold when the relative humidity rises from 50 to 100%.

Glycerol and the lower glycols, such as propylene glycol and polyethylene glycol, are distinctly hygroscopic. They withdrew water from the skin, especially when present in high concentrations in gels.

Powders, either formulated as dusting powders or as lotions, provide a large surface area for evaporation and they can thus function as drying agents.

Table 4.2 provides a brief summary of the effects which common dermatological bases (without active ingredients) may exert on skin hydration and skin permeability.

In theory, the pH of a topical vehicle could modify skin keratin (isoelectric point 3.7 to 4.5) and thereby alter skin hydration. However, from studies on neonatal rat skin (Singer and Vinson, 1966), hairless mouse skin (Matoltsy et al., 1968), and human fingernails and skin (Memschel, 1925), it appears that between pH 1 and 10 the tissue neither swells nor hydrates markedly. Above pH 10, water diffusion rates increase and water-binding capacities decrease as the buffer extracts water-binding materials and dissolves the keratin. Thus, under normal physiological conditions, within the pH range tolerated without skin irritation and obvious damage, the vehicle pH has little effect on hydration.

Wurster and Kramer (1961) provided an interesting example of how the in vivo hydration state of normal skin affects its permeability. These investigators fitted two-compartment absorption cells containing either a desiccant or water together with salicylates to the forearms of volunteers. Thus, they could monitor the in vivo percutaneous absorption rates of the salicylate series, ethyl, methyl, and ethylene glycol under hydrous and "anhydrous"

TABLE 4.2 Theoretically Expected Effects of Common Vehicles on Skin
Hydration and Skin Permeability—in Approximate Order of Decreasing
Hydration Effect

Vehicle	Examples/ constituents	Effect on skin hydration	Effect on skin permeability
1. Occlusive Dressing	Saran Wrap Melinex Film, unperforated water-proof plaster	Prevents water loss; full hydration	Marked increase
2. Lipophilic	Paraffins, oils, fats, waxes, fatty acids, alcohols, esters, silicones	Prevents water loss; may produce full hydration	Marked increase
3. Absorption base	Anhydrous lipid material plus water/ oil emulsifiers	Prevents water loss; marked hydration	Marked increase
4. Emulsifying base	Anhydrous lipid material plus oil/ water emulsifiers	Prevents water loss; marked hydration	Marked increase
5. Water/oil emulsion	Oily creams	Retards water loss; raised hydration	Increase
6. Oil/water emulsion	Aqueous creams	May donate water; slight hydration increase	Slight increase?
7. Humectant	Water-soluble bases, glycerol, glycols	May withdraw water; decreased hydration	Can decrease or act as penetration enhancer
8. Powder	Clays, organics, inorganics, "shake" lotions	Aid water evaporation; decreased excess hydration	Little effect on stratum corneum

conditions by monitoring total salicylate excretion in the urine. For all
three compounds, the absorption rate increased under hydrating conditions.
The more water soluble the compound and the lower its partition coefficient
into the skin (as assessed by the olive oil-water partition coefficient), the
greater was the effect of hydration. Table 4.3 provides relevant data. Figure 4.6 illustrates results obtained for glycol salicylate.

Wurster and Munies (1965) extended the work to measure the excretion
rate of methyl ethyl ketone in expired air. Hydrated skin provided a transient
large increase in penetration compared with dehydrated or normal skin.
This sharp increase probably arose because partial dehydration of the
stratum corneum dramatically altered the barrier property of the skin. After
about 2 hr, transient effects disappeared and the excretion rate (and therefore, presumably, the absorption rate) for hydrated skin was about double
that for nonhydrated skin.

TABLE 4.3 Effect of Hydration on the In Vivo Penetration of Salicylate
Esters Through Human Skin

	Ethyl salicylate	Methyl salicylate	Glycol salicylate
Relative excretion rate[a]	2.0	3.2	9.0
Water solubility (%)	0.03	0.08	1.27
Partition coefficient[b]	1170	343	7.7
Relative partition coefficient[c]	152	45	1

[a]Relative excretion rate = $\dfrac{\text{hydrous system rate calculated as ester}}{\text{anhydrous system rate calculated as ester}}$.

[b]Partition coefficient = $\dfrac{\text{concentration in olive oil at equilibrium}}{\text{concentration in water at equilibrium}}$.

[c]Relative partition coefficient = $\dfrac{\text{partition coefficient of ester}}{\text{partition coefficient of glycol salicylate}}$.

Source: Wurster and Kramer, 1961.

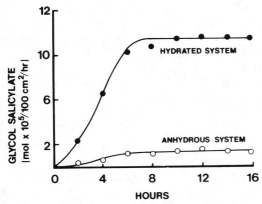

FIG. 4.6 Influence of hydration on the percutaneous absorption of glycol
salicylate, as determined by the urine excretion rate. (From Wurster and
Kramer, 1961.)

The vapor state transport of n-propyl and n-amyl acetates increases in hydrated stratum corneum (Amin, 1967). Sarin (isopropoxymethylphos phonofluoridate) passes more readily across hydrated callus than across dehydrated material (Ostrenga, 1967).

The previous four examples of hydration effects were reviewed by Wurster (1978).

Hydration of the epidermis increases the percutaneous absorption of nicotinic acid (Cronin and Stoughton, 1962), salicylic acid (Malkinson, 1964), and aspirin (Fritsch and Stoughton, 1963; Stoughton and Fritsch, 1964).

Many more examples in the literature deal with the effect which hydration can have on the flux of a drug through the skin. However, we should be cautious when interpreting in vitro experiments which use excised skin to gain an insight into the clinical use of drugs. In the in vitro test, investigators often maintain the skin sample between an essentially aqueous sink and an aqueous or occlusive donor phase. The practical advantage of this design is that the controlled environmental conditions allow us to make a more or less rigorous analysis under Fickian, steady state conditions. However, the skin hydrates extensively to a nonphysiological level. The aqueous condition of the stratum corneum then correlates only with the therapeutic treatment of rigorous occlusion or with the state of a body which has been immersed in water for some hours. The level of hydration is much higher than that in the more usual clinical condition.

Because of such considerations, an alternative in vitro method has been developed (Foreman et al., 1977). The skin sample has the dermal side in contact with a normal aqueous receptor solution; the epidermal surface is open to the ambient atmosphere (the relative humidity of which should be controlled). The investigators apply the diffusant to the stratum corneum as a thin surface film. Such an arrangement approximates to many nonoccluded dermatological treatments. Data may be analyzed by an elementary Monte Carlo simulation. Rather surprisingly, Foreman et al. (1978) report that, using this method, the diffusion parameters for nandrolone penetrating human skin are similar under occluded and nonoccluded conditions. A similar experimental approach is the "finite dose" technique of Franz (1978).

2. Effect of temperature

The stratum corneum is an excellent barrier to the permeation of molecules through the skin, as penetration depends on the translational movement of such molecules. However, the tissue is a poor heat insulator as heat can flow by contact between molecules and the membrane is very thin (Tregear, 1966). Thus, a sharp temperature gradient develops across the horny layer from the epidermal body temperature to the temperature of the nearly stagnant air layer at the free surface. The stratum corneum under normal conditions in temperate climates operates therefore between about 30 ° and 37 °C.

Clinically, skin temperature increases under occlusive dressings or in diseased states. Under occlusion, sweat cannot evaporate nor can heat radiate as readily and the surface temperature may rise by a few degrees. However, any consequent increased permeability is small compared with the more dramatic effect which the resultant increased hydration causes (see Sec. III.C.1). In diseased skin, other effects such as the disruption of the horny layer are much more important than an elevated temperature in promoting penetration.

Cooling lotions are even less important for their temperature effect on skin penetration. A solvent with a low boiling point cools the skin as it evaporates, but the change is transitory. The skin returns to its normal temperature within a period negligible compared with the time scale of diffusion.

The stratum corneum resists heat damage, tolerating temperatures as high as 60 °C for several hours without serious alteration to its barrier properties (Blank and Scheuplein, 1964). However, when heated above 65 °C or when incubated in aqueous media below pH 3 or above pH 9 the horny layer suffers irreversible structural changes (Allenby et al., 1969).

The usual method for studying the effect of temperature on the diffusion of molecules through the skin in vitro determines the activation energy for diffusion or for permeation (see Chap. 2, Secs. I.B.7, II.A.2, and II.B.1).

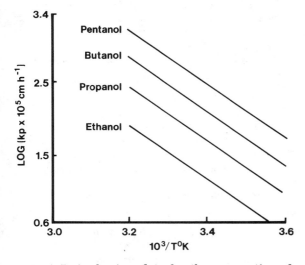

FIG. 4.7 Arrhenius plots for the permeation of polar alcohols through epidermis. (From Scheuplein and Blank, 1971.)

We can construct Arrhenius-type plots which illustrate the effect of temperature on the transport of alcohols across the epidermis (Blank and Scheuplein, 1964; Blank et al., 1967; Scheuplein and Blank, 1971). Figure 4.7 illustrates such graphs for the polar alcohols ethanol to pentanol. Good straight lines yield an average activation energy of 16.5 kcal mol^{-1} (see Table 3.2). For the lipid-soluble alcohols (hexanol, heptanol, and octanol) the Arrhenius plots are nonlinear. Below 25 °C the average value of their activation energy is about 17.0 kcal mol^{-1}. This decreases to 8-10 kcal mol^{-1} at temperatures above 25-30 °C. The suggested reason for this is that the lipid-soluble alcohols appear to penetrate via a lipoidal pathway within the stratum corneum. With temperature rise, the lipid may partially melt to become less viscous and thus the activation energy for diffusion of the alcohols falls. Durrheim et al. (1980) recently produced similar results for alcohol permeation in hairless mouse skin.

The effect of temperature on the penetration of other materials such as aspirin and aniline has been determined also. In the experiment referred to in respect of skin hydration (Sec. III.C.1), hydration increases the penetration rate of aspirin. In addition, in vitro a 30 °C temperature rise (from 10° to 40 °C) increases penetration 8 times at 88% relative humidity and 15 times at 50% relative humidity (Frisch and Stoughton, 1963). In vivo Piotrowski (1957) showed that the penetration rate for aniline in humans increases fourfold when the temperature rises from 29.8° to 35.0 °C.

From the practical aspect we can conclude that the penetration rate of a material through human skin can change by an order of magnitude if we expose our bodies to a large temperature change, e.g., if a person leaves a sauna to travel in very cold weather. Thus, the temperature coefficient for a 10° temperature change (Q_{10}) ranges between 1.4 and 3.0 for several substances (Tregear, 1966; Scheuplein, 1978a). In normal situations, of course, for most of the body adequate clothing would prevent such a wide fluctuation in penetration rates.

3. Penetration enhancers

For many years, clinical investigators and chemical warfare experts have suggested that substances must exist which could temporarily diminish the impermeability of the skin. Such materials, if they are safe and nontoxic, could be used in dermatology to enhance the penetration rate of drugs and even to treat patients systemically by the dermal route. Katz and Poulsen (1971) define a spectrum of properties which such a material should ideally possess. An expanded list of desirable attributes is as follows:

1. The material should be pharmacologically inert and it should possess no action of itself at receptor sites in the skin or in the body generally. In fact, the most widely studied penetration enhancer, dimethyl sulfoxide, is clinically active in many disease states.
2. The material should not be toxic, irritating, or allergenic.

3. On application, the onset of penetration-enhancing action should be immediate; the duration of the effect should be predictable and should be suitable.
4. When the material is removed from the skin, the tissue should immediately and fully recover its normal barrier property.
5. The barrier function of the skin should reduce in one direction only, so as to promote penetration into the skin. Body fluids, electrolytes or other endogenous materials should not be lost to the atmosphere.
6. The enhancer should be chemically and physically compatible with a wide range of drugs and pharmaceutical adjuvants.
7. The substance should be an excellent solvent for drugs.
8. The material should spread well on the skin and it should possess a suitable skin "feel."
9. The chemical should formulate into lotions, suspensions, ointments, creams, gels, aerosols, and skin adhesives.
10. It should be inexpensive, odorless, tasteless, and colorless so as to be cosmetically acceptable.

It is unlikely than any single material would possess such a formidable array of desirable properties. However, some substances do possess several of these attributes, and they have been investigated clinically or in the laboratory. Such materials appear to increase skin permeability by reducing the diffusional resistance of the stratum corneum, by reversibly damaging it, or by altering its physicochemical nature. In extreme situations (with materials which are too drastic in their effects to be used clinically) the reduction in skin resistance is large and is easily measured. For example, after a mixture of chloroform and methanol removes lipids from epidermal membranes, the activation energy for diffusion of water through the epidermis falls from the normal value of approximately 15 kcal mol^{-1} (Scheu (Scheuplein, 1965) to around 6.0 or 6.5 kcal mol^{-1} (Blank et al., 1967). Similarly, in a delipidized epidermis the activation energies for diffusion of propanol and heptanol fall. For clinical use, one would look for a less drastic change, possibly involving a simple reduction in the extent of hydrogen bonding in the skin.

We refer to materials which promote the topical penetration of drugs as accelerants (Allenby et al., 1969b), sorption promoters (Ritschel, 1969), or penetration enhancers. We will limit the use of these terms to materials which significantly enhance drug penetration through the epidermis but which do not severely irritate or damage the skin. The definition also implies that the mode of action is by a reversible change in the specific barrier properties of the skin. We can often increase the flux rate of a drug through the skin in other ways. For example, we can optimize the thermodynamic activity of a penetrant in a vehicle by using a cosolvent, or we can increase the partition coefficient of the drug and thus promote its release from the vehicle into the skin. When a material acts in such ways, we will not consider it as functioning as a penetration enhancer as just defined. In practice, it is often difficult to isolate the effect of an agent on a single parameter in the overall process of percutaneous absorption. Many of the experiments which are quoted in the literature as examples of the penetration enhancer effect can be attributed, at least in part, to an action other than a simple reduction in barrier permeability.

In the clinical literature particularly, some authors imply that a mechanism exists whereby a solvent can actually transport a dissolved drug from a vehicle into and through the skin. Such a mass transport mechanism, in which solvent and drug remain together throughout the percutaneous absorption process, is highly unlikely, as it does not correlate with what we know about the structure and physicochemical properties of normal stratum corneum. For dissolved drug to sweep through the skin in this manner would imply that the horny layer is a porous membrane with channels large enough to allow mass flow of solvent. For intact skin this is not so, and materials applied to the epidermis diffuse independently. Penetration enhancers operate by conditioning the stratum corneum so as to promote drug diffusion.

a. Dimethyl sulfoxide Dimethyl sulfoxide (DMSO) is the lowest member of a group of compounds with the general formula RSOR (Fig. 4.8). It is a nearly odorless, water-white, dipolar, aprotic solvent which is completely miscible with water and with common organic solvents. A 2.16% solution is isosmotic with serum. DMSO is hygroscopic and it mixes exothermically with water to produce considerable heat. It is a powerful solvent which dissolves most aromatic and unsaturated hydrocarbons, many inorganic salts, organosulfur compounds and organic nitrogen compounds.

Therapeutic applications of DMSO date from the mid-1960s. When it was discovered that DMSO easily penetrates the bark of trees, medically orientated studies started at the University of Oregon in cooperation with the Crown Zellerbach Corporation. In the United States, Syntex, Squibb, Merck Sharp & Dohme, Schering, Geigy, and American Home Products began clinical studies. In 1964, Jacob et al. published their program for a pharmacotherapeutic investigation into the possibilities of using DMSO as a resorption agent (vehicle), bacteriostatic, local analgesic, anti-inflammatory agent, diuretic, tranquilizer, and synergen.

In Germany, a symposium was published which included 18 papers that evaluated the results of clinical investigations (Laudahn and Schlosshaur, 1965).

DMSO then became widely used until the Huntingdon Research Centre in the United Kingdom issued an alarming report that DMSO can change the refractive index of the lens in the eyes of rabbits, pigs, and dogs. In the United States, the Food and Drug Administration (FDA) then prohibited the use of DMSO in humans despite the fact that the Huntingdon results contradicted earlier conclusions as to the safety of DMSO.

An intensive investigation of the toxicity of DMSO then began (Laudahn and Gertich, 1966; Jacob and Wood, 1967). It was found that nobody had

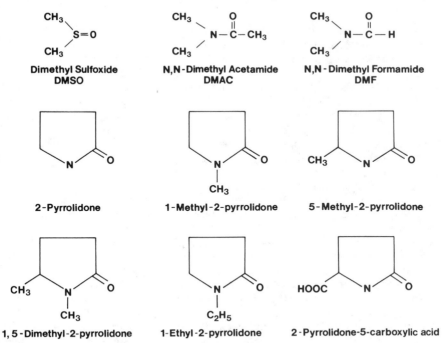

FIG. 4.8 Some penetration enhancers.

observed a single case of damage by DMSO to human eyes. An extensive toxicological study of DMSO was conducted at 3 to 30 times the usual treatment dose in humans for 3 months. Brobyn (1975) concluded that DMSO is a very safe compound for human administration. In particular, the lens changes which take place in certain other mammals do not occur in humans under this prolonged, intensive treatment regime.

However, DMSO does exhibit some undesirable effects on topical application. Sulzberger et al. (1967) applied a single drop of 100% DMSO to the backs of human volunteers and they produced follicular papules within 5 to 15 min and a wheal within 30 min. Concentrations as low as 10% DMSO can produce erythema (Brown, 1967). The neck, face, and axillae are more sensitive to topical application of DMSO than the back or extremities. In the majority of patients, cutaneous reactions usually subside after 7 to 10 days, when patients become tolerant to the compound (Scherbel et al., 1967). Zuckner et al. (1967) claim that DMSO always causes a burning sensation in the skin, which is usually accompanied by a rash, peeling, scaling, pruritis, redness, and occasional vesiculation of the tissue. Steinberg (1967) and Arno et al. (1967) also observed erythema and burning when they applied DMSO to their patients. However, when Goldman et al. (1967) treated 1,300 patients and Ayres and Mihan (1967) dealt with 174 patients, both teams considered that local irritation did not pose a significant problem. The wealing response of human skin to DMSO has been quantified by Frosch et al. (1980).

The initial local irritation which DMSO produces diminishes with continued application. The histamine liberated in skin exposed to DMSO provokes the primary irritant or allergic contact-like effects. Occlusive wraps accentuate the irritant effects of DMSO. Erythema and urticaria become constant features and in some patients an erythematous papulovesicular response occurs. However, even this injury reverses and the skin recovers with no permanent damage done (Kligman, 1965a).

Possibly a more inconvenient side effect is the foul breath and taste (oyster- or garlic-like) which DMSO application produces in the patient. This is due to the excretion of the metabolite dimethyl sulfide (Di Stefano and Borgstedt, 1964; Borgstedt and Di Stefano, 1967; Berger and Hauthal, 1976). These oral complications may hinder treatment because of problems with patient compliance. The smell makes it difficult to perform double-blind clinical trials, as it soon becomes only too obvious which patients have received the DMSO-containing product!

In the United States, official permission for the experimental clinical use of DMSO was granted toward the end of 1966. The FDA allowed clinical studies on a larger scale in September 1968. DMSO preparations have been available in West Germany since June 1967. The number of European products which contain DMSO is slowly increasing.

DMSO is probably the most widely publicized medicinal agent since penicillin (Katz and Poulsen, 1971). To quote Leake (1975), "rarely has a new drug come so quickly to the judgement of the members of the health professions with so much verifiable data from so many parts of the world, both experimentally and clinically, as to safety and efficacy." It is impracticable to attempt to deal in this section with all this material. Of necessity, we must be selective and mention only those publications which are directly relevant to the biopharmaceutics of topical dermatologicals. For further study for the interested reader, some of the most informative publications on DMSO are Kligman (1965b), Jacob and Rosenbaum (1967), Leake (1966), Laudahn and Gertich (1966), Schumacher (1967), Jacob et al. (1971), Jacob and Herschler (1975), Martin and Hauthal (1976), and the National Academy of Sciences Report (1973). In particular, Beger and Hauthal (1976) deal with the role of DMSO in medicine and pharmacology, with 421 references and an appendix listing reviews and general literature.

Soon after the introduction of DMSO into medicine, patents were registered to protect the compositions and applications of combinations of active substances with DMSO (Crown Zellerbach Corp. 1964; Olin Mathieson Chemical Corporation, 1965a,b; Imperial Chemical Industries Ltd., 1964a,b,c; Smith, Kline & French Laboratories, 1965; Société Pluripharm, 1964; Schering A.G., 1965; Laboratoires Laroche Navarron, 1965a,b).

In many in vivo and in vitro experiments, DMSO enhances the skin penetration of water (Sweeney et al., 1966; Baker, 1968; Scheuplein and Ross, 1970; Astley and Levine, 1975) and a wide range of drugs. These drugs include hexopyrronium bromide, naphazoline, fluocinolone acetonide, and hydrocortisone (Stoughton and Frisch, 1964), dyes (Jacob et al., 1964; Kligman, 1965a,b; Fabianek and Herp, 1966; Sulzberger et al., 1967), organic phosphates (Allenby et al., 1969b; Allenby et al., 1969a), alkyl sulfates (Embery and Dugard, 1969; Dugard and Embery, 1969), local anesthetics (Brechner et al., 1967; Sams et al., 1966), narcotics (Jacob, 1965; Collon and Winek, 1968), antimetabolites (Davis, 1966), antibiotics (Kamiya et al., 1966; Kligman, 1965b; Vickers, 1969), antiperspirants (Dobson et al., 1970), antibacterials (Stringer and Engel, 1966), salicylic acid (Kligman, 1965b; Stelzer et al., 1968), tubocurarine hydrochloride, amphetamine sulfate, and barbiturates (Horita and Weber, 1964), picric acid (Elfbaum and Laden, 1968a,b,c), fluocinolne acetonide, triamcinolone acetonide, and hydrocortisone (Stoughton, 1965a), griseofulvin and hydrocortisone (Munro and Stoughton, 1965), hydrocortisone (Maibach and Feldmann, 1967; Stoughton, 1965b; Vickers, 1963), triamcinolone acetonide (Vickers, 1963; Groel, 1968), fluocinolone acetonide (Brode, 1968; Stoughton, 1965b; Coldman et al., 1971), hydrocortisone sodium succinate (Cramer and Cates, 1974), iodone, cortisone, and penicillin (Jacob, 1965), cortisone acetate and estradiol (Djan and Grunberg, 1967; Highman and Altland, 1969), estradiol benzoate (Smith and Allison, 1967), testosterone and its esters (Malkinson, 1958; Feldmann and Maibach, 1966; Maibach and Feldmann, 1967), fluorouracil (Kitzmiller, 1967; Stjernvall, 1969), iodine (Sears et al., 1956), hexachlorophene (Stoughton, 1966), physostigmine and phenylbutazone (Hausler and Jahn, 1966; Pontio and Karki, 1965; Wepierre et al., 1966), quaternary ammonium compounds (Rosen et al., 1965), quaternary oximes (McDermot et al., 1965), p-aminohippuric acid (Giorgi and Segre, 1966), sugars (Braudé and Monroe, 1965; Csaky and Ho, 1966), colchicine (Siddiq and Majid, 1969), and scopolamine (Chandresekaran et al., 1977).

A few authors deny that DMSO increases skin absorption (Caccialanza and Finzi, 1966; Vogel et al., 1967).

DMSO enables low molecular weight substances to penetrate quickly into the deep layers of the skin and from there into neighboring structures and into the blood stream. However, the sulfoxide does not abolish the skin barrier nor does it allow the percutaneous absorption of macromolecules. Substances with molecular weights of 3,000 or more cannot be transported appreciably into the stratum corneum (Ritschel, 1969). Thus attempts to use DMSO to administer polypeptides such as corticotropin* and vasopressin, as well as allergens from house dust, dog hair, timothy pollen, and castor bean, have been unsuccessful (Kastin et al., 1966; Sulzberger et al., 1967; Perlman and Wolfe, 1966).

---

*Also called adrenocorticotropin or ACTH.

Human and animal skin is highly permeable to DMSO. Radiolabeled DMSO applied cutaneously to humans can be detected in the bloodstream within 5 min (Kolb et al., 1967). The radioactivity reaches a maximum plateau within 4 to 6 hr. Whole-body radioautograms of rats treated topically with DMSO reveal intense contamination of all bones within 1 hr; the radioactivity does not accumulate in the brain, spinal chord, vertebral disks, fatty tissues, or the adrenals of these animals 24 hr after topical application.

In experimental animals and man, more than 50% of the DMSO applied cutaneously appears in the urine within 6 to 8 hr. Only about 3% is recovered in human breath (Cortese, 1971; Hucker et al., 1967).

Allenby et al. (1969b) report a permeability coefficient of 300 $\times$ 10^{-8} mmin^{-1} for 100% DMSO penetrating excised stratum corneum. This value is much greater than the comparable one for water: 45 $\times$ 10^{-8} mmin^{-1} (Tregear, 1966).

We still do not possess an absolutely clear concept of the mechanism by which DMSO enhances the migration rate of drugs through the skin. The capability of the sulfoxide at moderate concentrations to penetrate tissues without damaging them significantly probably relates to its relatively polar nature, its small, compact structure, and its capacity to accept hydrogen bonds. This combination of properties allows DMSO to associate with water, proteins, carbohydrates, nucleic acid, ionic substances, and other constituents of biological tissue. The ability of the aprotic solvent to replace some of the water molecules associated with cellular constituents or to affect the structure of biological water is of fundamental importance (Szmant, 1975).

DMSO appears to stabilize ice-like water clusters and it may therefore displace the equilibrium in a tissue from less structured to more highly structured water. Since the activity of water in general is not necessarily the same in different states, DMSO may indirectly affect biological systems by the changes it causes in liquid structure. The solvent may thus alter the conformation and the association of proteins and other molecules (Rammler and Zaffaroni, 1967; Henderson et al., 1975). Elfbaum and Laden (1968b) report that DMSO unfolds or expands protein chains in hair keratin, bovine serum albumin, and β-lactoglobulin.

Another possible mode of action for DMSO at high concentrations could be its ability to damage skin or to produce gross structural changes in the skin. The high osmotic activity of DMSO may distort the laminated structure of the stratum corneum, swell it, and induce channels to form within the matrix. Such channels would promote the passage of various compounds (Elfbaum and Laden, 1968c; Morain et al., 1966; Dugard and Embery, 1969; Chandrasekaran et al., 1977; Chandrasekaran and Shaw, 1978; Creasey et al., 1978). In addition, the stratum corneum may hold relatively large amounts of DMSO. The solvent may in effect become the membrane phase. Since most drugs are much more soluble in DMSO than in water, the high concentrations of drugs attained within the stratum corneum would further promote percutaneous absorption (Katz and Poulsen, 1971).

However, Kligman (1965b) exposed stratum corneum to 90% and 100% DMSO for 20 days at 37 °C and found that the tissue's integrity did not change. He concluded that this treatment does not affect the intercellular cement which holds the horny layer cells together. In contrast, Montes et al. (1967) and Skog and Wahlberg (1967) applied DMSO to stratum corneum and produced microscopic and submicroscopic changes. Canals of edema formed extending from the surface down to the dermis. Soaking epidermal specimens in DMSO extracts cholesterol, phospholipid, and lipoprotein (Allenby et al., 1969b; Mustakallio et al., 1967; Creasey et al., 1978). These experiments support the contention that DMSO operates by direct insult to the stratum corneum.

DMSO interacts exothermically with water in the skin and the temperature of horny layer may rise slightly. However, the effect is transient and it is not sufficient of itself to significantly increase the penetration rate of a compound administered at the same time.

DMSO shows an unusual concentration dependence connected with its penetration enhancing properties. Below about 50% DMSO in water, the penetration rate for many compounds is little higher than that from water. Depending on the particular experiment, the drug penetration rate rises exponentially as the DMSO concentration increases above 60-70% (Sweeney et al., 1966; Allenby et al., 1969b; Elfbaum and Laden, 1968b; Dugard and Embery, 1969; Embery and Dugard, 1969; Chandrasekaran et al., 1977). DMSO forms a stable 2:1 water hydrate (67% v/v DMSO) and this may explain its dehydrating and penetration enhancing effect at high concentrations (Scheuplein and Ross, 1970; Scheuplein, 1978a).

Chandrasekaran and Shaw (1978) have shown that the effects of dimethyl sulfoxide on skin permeability are consistent with their sorption-diffusion model for membrane transport (see Secs. III.B.2 and III.D.4), provided that we allow for changes in penetrant activity with changes in solvent composition. The marked distortion and intercellular delamination of the stratum corneum, which they claim accompanies the osmotic shock due to the sulfoxide, must also be considered.

Some dermatologists consider that the use of idoxuridine in dimethyl sulfoxide constitutes a major advance in therapy for the treatment of herpes simplex and herpes zoster (MacCallum and Juel-Jensen, 1966; Dawber, 1972, 1974; Watson, 1973; Juel-Jensen and MacCallum, 1974; Simpson, 1975; for further references and reviews, see Martindale: The Extra Pharmacopoeia, edited by Wade and Reynolds, 1977).

b. Dimethylacetamide and dimethylformamide N,N-Dimethylacetamide (DMAC) and N,N-dimethylformamide (DMF) are two organic solvents that promote permeability changes in the skin which appear to be very similar to those produced by DMSO. However, DMSO has overshadowed both compounds and neither has been as extensively studied.

DMSO, DMAC, and DMF were better than ethanol, benzene, and a cream for promoting the in vitro penetration of griseofulvin and hydrocortisone. DMAC and DMF were not as active as DMSO (Munro and Stoughton,

1965; Munro, 1969). Stoughton (1966) found that DMAC established and maintained an effective concentration of hexachlorophene in the stratum corneum.

DMSO, DMF, and DMAC increase transepidermal water loss when applied to human skin, in the order of rank as written. All three compounds can thus profoundly alter the resistance of the horny layer. The barrier function restores to normal within about 6 hr when DMF and DMAC are used, and slightly longer for DMSO (Baker, 1968).

Patients tolerate topical application of DMAC and DMF better than they do DMSO, and neither compound produces the foul mouth odor and taste which is so characteristic of the sulfoxide. Stoughton (1969) has a patent covering the use of DMAC and other lower alkyl amides for enhancing percutaneous absorption.

Spiegel and Noseworthy (1963, 1966) discuss aspects of DMAC.

c. Alkyl sulfoxides, phosphine oxides, and sugar esters The Proctor & Gamble Co. (1976) have several patents which claim to enhance the penetration through the skin of pharmacologically active agents. The formulations use alkyl sulfoxides or a sugar ester combined with a sulfoxide or a phosphine oxide. A number of compounds are listed, with typical examples being sucrose monooleate (sugar ester), decyl methyl sulfoxide (alkyl sulfoxide), and dodecyl dimethyl phosphine oxide (phosphine oxide). Typical pharmacologically active agents include antimicrobials, steroids, sunscreens, and antiperspirants.

Wechsler et al. (1978) and McKinivan (1979) present clinical evidence that topical tetracycline hydrochloride in an ethanol-water solution with n-decyl methyl sulfoxide as a penetration enhancer is effective in the treatment of acne when applied over a prolonged period of time, even though the concentration of sulfoxide in the marketed product (Topicycline) is only 0.125%. Presumably, the sulfoxide acts here as a surfactant, complementing the sucrose esters which are also present.

Trimethyl phosphine oxide promotes the absorption of a polar steroid (hydrocortisone sodium succinate) through rat skin; it has little effect on the penetration rate of the lipid-soluble steroid cortisone acetate (Cramer and Cates, 1974).

Sekura and Scala (1972) investigated a homologous series of alkyl methyl sulfoxides from DMSO to C_{14}-MSO for their penetrability and their ability to affect the skin's permeability to other materials. Penetration rates through rabbit and guinea pig skin were a function of the alkyl chain length with a maximum at 10 carbon atoms. All sulfoxides increased the permeability of the skin for sodium nicotinate and thiourea.

d. Pyrrolidones The pyrrolidones can be used with a variety of compounds to promote penetration and to establish a reservoir of drug in the stratum corneum and in the nails. Thus, Stoughton (1976a) reports that if griseofulvin is presented in a vehicle containing 2-pyrrolidone or an

N-lower alkyl 2-pyrrolidone the formulation produces a high degree of epidermal retention (see also Resh and Stoughton, 1976).

A second patent achieves this result by combining 2-pyrrolidone with N-methyl 2-pyrrolidone in ratios ranging between about 1:4 and 4:1 (Stoughton, 1977). 2-Pyrrolidone and N-lower alkyl 2-pyrrolidones also promote topical absorption of antibiotics of the lincomycin family in the treatment of acne (Stoughton, 1976b). The same compounds promote the penetration of theophylline from formulations designed as anti-inflammatory treatments (Schroer, 1976). Pfizer Inc. (1976) uses 2-pyrrolidone to formulate high-potency oxytetracycline solutions for topical use. However, it appears that under idealized in vitro conditions, 2-pyrrolidone is not a strong penetration enhancer for alcohols (C_1-C_8), at least as judged by its effect on partition coefficient and steady state flux, using the same solvent in donor and receptor compartments (Southwell et al., 1980). 2-Pyrrolidone enhances caffeine penetration in the finite dose technique (Southwell and Barry, 1981).

e. Azocycloalkan-2-ones Nelson Research & Development Co. (1976) suggest the use of substituted azocycloalkan-2-one penetrants in topical compositions—especially for antibacterials, antifungals, steroids, iododeoxyuridine, and 5-fluorouracil.

f. Tetrahydrofurfuryl alcohol Tetrahydrofurfuryl alcohol (THFA), a liquid which moderately irritates the skin and mucous membranes, can enhance the percutaneous absorption of drugs. Sarkany et al. (1965) conclude that, as judged by vasoconstrictor assays, THFA and DMA promote the skin penetration of hydrocortisone. Barrett et al. (1965) and Reid and Brookes (1968) also report that THFA increases the permeation of corticosteroids. Brode (1968) showed that THFA aids the percutaneous absorption of fluocinolone through rat skin.

g. Propylene glycol and ethanol The evidence for the effect of solvents such as propylene glycol and ethanol in promoting skin penetration is conflicting (Mackee et al., 1945; Poulsen et al., 1968; Busse et al., 1969; Feldmann and Maibach, 1966; Christie and Moore-Robinson, 1970; Sarkany et al., 1965; Caldwell et al., 1968; Tissot and Osmundsen, 1966; Brode, 1968; Dillaha et al., 1966; Barrett et al., 1965; Portnoy, 1965).

In many instances, the liquids function simply as cosolvents to produce saturated or nearly saturated solutions of the active ingredient and thereby they maximize the thermodynamic activity of the penetrant. This optimization procedure increases percutaneous absorption even if the stratum corneum remains unaffected. A true penetration-enhancing effect, as defined at the beginning of this section, would probably only be apparent at high concentrations of the solvent. Even then, the effect would be much less than with materials such as DMSO, DMAC, and DMF.

Higher glycols (e.g., polyethylene glycols—PEG 300 and 400) do not penetrate stratum corneum significantly and may form hydrogen bonds with

penetrants, thus reducing the compound's thermodynamic activity and penetration rate (T. Higuchi, 1980; T. Higuchi et al., 1969; Creasey et al.,
1978).

h. Surfactants The role which surfactants can play in altering the
effective concentration (the thermodynamic activity and chemical potential)
of a diffusing species has been considered in Chap. 2, Sec. III.C.3)

Topical creams contain surfactants as emulsifying agents, but in the
concentrations used they probably have little effect on skin permeability.
However, when we apply even dilute solutions of ionic surfactants to the
skin, they may alter the physical state of water in the skin in such a way
as to promote the passage of charged hydrophilic substances. The surfactants may also affect the permeability of the skin to water (Sprott, 1965;
Mezei and Ryan, 1972; Dugard and Scheuplein, 1973).

The effect of surfactants and soap on the loss of water from the skin
has been studied (Bettley and Donoghue, 1960; Bettley, 1961, 1963, 1965;
Isherwood, 1963), and the part played by surfactants in percutaneous absorption has been reviewed (Barr, 1962; Sprott, 1965; Minato et al., 1967;
Scala et al., 1968; Ritschel, 1969; Scheuplein, 1978a). Blank and Gould
(1961a) reviewed the possible complex ways by which the skin may restrict
the migration of synthetic anionic surfactants. However, anionic surfactants
can irritate the skin, which suggests that a material such as sodium lauryl
sulfate can penetrate through the stratum corneum to reach the viable
epidermis (Bettley, 1965).

As for materials in general, the stratum corneum is an effective barrier
to the percutaneous absorption of soap and other surfactants (Scala et al.,
1968; Blank, 1965; Blank and Gould, 1959, 1961a,b; Blank et al., 1964;
Embery and Dugard, 1969; Dugard and Embery, 1969). However, measurable amounts of surfactants do penetrate the skin, with the usual order of
decreasing penetration being anionics, cationics, and nonionics (Wahlberg,
1968; Bettley, 1965).

Among anionic surfactants, the laurate ion penetrates best and has the
greatest effect on the permeation of other solutes. Sodium salts of fatty
acids with alkyl chains of 10 carbon atoms or less penetrate significantly,
and fatty acids with longer chains provide modest flux rates (Bettley, 1961,
1963, 1965; Sprott, 1965; Blank and Gould, 1959, 1961a; Chowhan and
Pritchard, 1978). Potassium methyl sulfate and potassium butyl sulfate
migrate across intact skin, with the methyl ester providing the greater
flux rate (Dugard and Embery, 1969). Alkyl sulfates, sulfonated fatty acids,
and carboxylic acid esters of isethionic acid penetrate rat stratum corneum
(Faucher and Goddard, 1978c; Sprott, 1965). Alcohol sulfates and ether
sulfates penetrate rat skin less readily than do alcohol ethoxylates (Black
and Howes, 1979).

Anionic surfactants bind strongly to skin proteins and the stratum corneum swells grossly. This swelling arises as the surfactant binds coopera-
tively to the protein and uncoils the filaments in a reversible conformational
change (Scheuplein and Ross, 1970; Putterman et al., 1977).

The penetration of fatty acid soaps varies inversely with pH from pH 6.0 to 10.8. Above pH 10.8, the alkalinity itself overshadows the effect of pH change on ionic equilibria in the soaps (Sprott, 1965; Blank and Gould, 1959, 1961a). Bettley (1965) found no correlation of permeation with pH. It is possible that as surfactants permeate through the stratum corneum, they progressively alter the nature of the barrier and promote their own flux rates. Thus, Scala et al. (1968) illustrated nonlinear plots of permeability coefficient versus time for an anionic surfactant (sodium tetrapropylene benzene sulfonate), a cationic material (dodecyl trimethylammonium chloride), and soap.

Surfactants enhance the penetration of certain antimicrobial substances. The amounts of hexachlorophene and tetrachlorosalicylanilide that penetrate rat skin increase if the skin is washed with sodium lauryl sulfate (Sprott, 1965). Nickel salts compounded with anionic surfactants can cause eczema, but cationic or nonionic additives do not produce this dermatitis. This difference is probably due to the denaturing effect or acanthotic action of the anionic surfactant, which eases the passage of the metal sensitizer through the skin (Vinson and Choman, 1960).

Sprott (1965) correlates the effects which anionic surfactants have on the permeation of water-soluble substances with a protein-surfactant interaction. In this theory, the surfactant attaches to the protein and forces hydrophilic polar groups on the protein into the interior of the protein helices. In this configuration, there would be fewer charged groups on the surface of the helix available to interact with and to slow down the permeation of water, ions and hydrogen-bonding solutes.

Nonionic surfactants generally have little effect in promoting percutaneous absorption, although several reports discuss their influence (Stark et al., 1968; Stolar et al., 1960b; Mezei and Sager, 1967a; Stelzer et al., 1968; Aguiar and Weiner, 1969; Mezei and Ryan, 1972; Shen et al., 1976; Chowhan and Pritchard, 1978). For example, increasing concentrations of lauric diethanolamide up to 7% increase the permeation of hydrocortisone; above this figure, penetration reduces, probably because of micellar entrapment of the hydrocortisone (Shinkai and Tanaka, 1969). Polyoxyethylated materials may inhibit the penetration of sodium lauryl sulfate into isolated neonatal rat stratum corneum (Faucher et al., 1979).

Mezei and colleagues have used several methods to study the dermatitic effect of nonionic surfactants on rabbit skin (see Mezei et al., 1966; Mezei and Sager, 1967b; Mezei and White, 1969; Mezei and Lee, 1970). These studies suggest that in vivo nonionic surfactants change the biosynthetic rate, composition, and content of epidermal phospholipids. Such changes would presumably alter epidermal membrane structure since phospholipids form a major part of biological membranes. However, Dugard and Scheuplein (1973) concluded that such surfactants affect the protein rather than the lipid in the membrane.

The configuration of the nonionic surfactant, rather than its hydrophile-lipophile balance, appears to influence whether or not the surfactant promotes penetration. Drug absorption does not increase when the surfactant possesses several long hydrophilic chains (of more than five ethylene oxide units) rather than a single chain or several short chains. This suggests that the effectiveness of the surfactant depends on the facility with which its molecules penetrate lipid membranes (Gillian and Florence, 1973).

Long-chain derivatives of sulfoxides (such as decyl methyl sulfoxide) at low concentrations probably exert any penetration-enhancing effect they have via their surface active properties.

i. Miscellaneous materials From the viewpoint of safety and effectiveness, probably the best penetration enhancer of all is water. Nearly all substances penetrate better through hydrated stratum corneum than through the dry tissue. A corollary of this is that any chemical which is not pharmacologically active and which promotes stratum corneum hydration can be considered as a penetration enhancer. Examples include the natural moisturizing factor (NMF), its analogs, and urea (see Sec. III.B.1). Materials such as salicylic acid, which have a keratolytic action on the horny layer and which themselves are therapeutically active, are not conveniently considered as penetration under the definition used in this section.

Di-2-ethylhexylamine has also been shown to possess penetration-enhancing properties (Creasey et al., 1978).

D. Drug-Vehicle Interactions

In this section, we consider the situation in which the impermeability of the stratum corneum can be ignored in percutaneous absorption. Then the release rate of the drug from the topical vehicle provides the rate-limiting step in the overall diffusion process and the skin functions as a perfect sink. This could happen clinically if the horny layer severely disrupts or is absent because of disease or injury, or when diffusion of the drug in the vehicle is exceptionally slow. The vehicle also provides the rate-controlling mechanism in many of the in vitro release studies detailed in the literature, in which the investigators use an artificial permeable membrane or no membrane at all. Such experiments may correlate with the clinical usage of drugs only when the patient has severely damaged skin.

If we extend our definition of a topical vehicle to include a delivery device, we can consider in this section the Transdermal Therapeutic System (TTS; or Transiderm/Transderm) of the Alza Corporation. The device itself provides the rate-limiting step for percutaneous absorption leading to systemic therapy. The application site is the skin of the postauricular region as this area provides minimal resistance to the passage of drugs. The biopharmaceutical principles inherent in the design of the Transiderm will be discussed in Sec. III.D.4.

T. Higuchi (1960) formulated the mathematics which have proved to be of most practical use for describing conditions under which diffusion within the vehicle phase provides the rate-controlling step. The treatment assumes that the skin is a perfect sink which maintains essentially zero concentration of the penetrating material by rapidly dissipating it to the deeper tissues. Thus, the concentration gradient occurs solely in the applied material. Two general cases are absorption from a solution and absorption from a suspension.

1. Absorption from solution: skin a perfect sink

We can deduce an equation which applies to the release of a penetrant from one side of a layer of vehicle under the following conditions (T. Higuchi, 1960; W. I. Higuchi, 1961, 1962):

1. Only a single drug species is important in the vehicle; it is in true solution and the drug is initially uniformly distributed throughout the vehicle.
2. Only the drug diffuses out of the vehicle. Components other than the drug do not diffuse or evaporate, and skin secretions do not pass into the vehicle.
3. The diffusion coefficient of the drug in the vehicle is invariant with respect to time or position within the vehicle.
4. The penetrant, when it reaches the skin, absorbs instantaneously.

Under these limitations, we can apply Fickian diffusion theory to deduce (Crank, 1975)

$$M = hC_0 \left[1 - \frac{8}{\pi^2} \sum_{n=0}^{\infty} \frac{1}{(2n+1)^2} \exp\left(\frac{D_v t \pi^2}{4h^2} (2n+1)^2 \right) \right] \qquad (4.1)$$

where M is the quantity of drug released to the sink per unit area of application; h is the thickness of the vehicle layer; C_0 is the initial concentration of penetrating solute in the vehicle; D_v is the diffusion coefficient of the drug in the vehicle; t is the time after application; and n is an integer with values ranging from zero to infinity.

Various workers have used Eq. (4.1) in the simple form

$$M \simeq 2C_0 \left(\frac{D_v t}{\pi} \right)^{1/2} \qquad (4.2)$$

when the amount of drug released from the vehicle is not much greater than 30% (T. Higuchi, 1961), i.e., when t is short (Malone et al., 1974).

Figure 4.9 illustrates plots of a typical release experiment from homogeneous solution. The formulations consists of betamethasone-17-benzoate dissolved at various concentrations in a polar gel, diffusing into a chloroform sink (Barry and Woodford, 1978). Curves similar to those illustrated here been reported for many drugs and chemicals. For example, such curves have been obtained for the in vitro release of steroids from gels, creams,

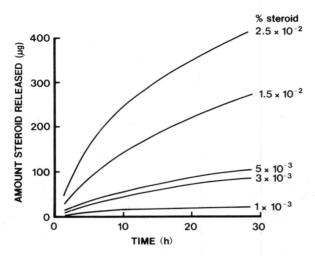

FIG. 4.9 In vitro release of betamethasone-17-benzoate from gel formulations as a function of time: steroid strength indicated on plots. (From Barry and Woodford, 1978.)

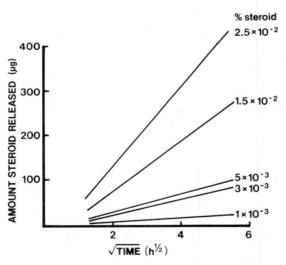

FIG. 4.10 In vitro release of betamethasone-17-benzoate from gel formulations as a function of the square root of time: steroid strength indicated on the plots. (From Barry and Woodford, 1978.)

and ointments (Poulsen et al., 1968; Ostrenga et al., 1971a,b; Malone et al., 1974; Horsch, 1975) and from silicone polymers (Roseman, 1972).

According to Eq. (4.2), a plot of the amount of drug released as a function of the square root of time should be a straight line. Figure 4.10 illustrates such a linear relationship for the betamethasone gels. Similar plots have been obtained for the release of steroids from semisolid formulations (Ayres and Laskar, 1974; Chowhan and Pritchard, 1975) and polymers (Roseman, 1972), as well as for the release of other substances from emulsions (Koizumi and Higuchi, 1968) and polymeric filsm (Borodkin and Tucker, 1974).

It appears that a relationship such as Eq. (4.2), or a modification of it in which the amount of drug released is still proportional to the square root of time, will often fit data outside the strict limits used originally to define Eqs. (4.1) and (4.2). For example, Barry and Woodford (1978) used a supporting membrane of cellulose acetate in the form of a bag which changed its mechanical properties with time. The bag became tough and rigid when immersed in chloroform and decreased in thickness. It is also probable that the nature of the polar gel altered when it was exposed to the chloroform. The amount of corticosteroid released after 28 hr of immersion in the chloro-

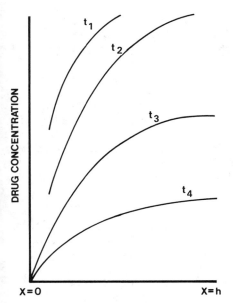

FIG. 4.11 Concentration profiles developed within an applied layer of vehicle for diffusion controlled release into skin acting as a perfect sink at x = 0: solution formulation. (From W. I. Higuchi, 1961, 1967.)

form was as much as 55% of the original amount in the gel. Similarly, calculating from the figures quoted by Poulsen et al. (1968), the quantity of
fluocinolone acetonide diffusing from a water-soluble gel into isopropyl
myristate is a linear function of $t^{1/2}$ up to about 65% release.

As a practical point, according to Eq. (4.2) under the conditions assumed, we may alter the release rate of a drug, and hence its bioavailability, by changing either the drug concentration or the diffusion coefficient
in the vehicle.

Figure 4.11 presents a diagrammatic representation of the concentration
profiles developed within an applied layer of vehicle for diffusion controlled
release into skin acting as a perfect sink (W. I. Higuchi, 1967). The diagram shows the variation of drug concentration across the vehicle layer at
four different time intervals, where $t_4 > t_3 > t_2 > t_1$.

2. Absorption from suspensions: skin a perfect sink

The amount released and the rate of release of materials suspended in
a topical vehicle such as an ointment or cream may be simply related to
time and to the variables of the system. The problem is one of the "moving
boundary" type, which was briefly considered in Chap. 2, Sec. II.D. We
derive our equations for a simple model system described as follows (T.
Higuchi, 1960, 1961):

1. The suspended drug is in a fine state of subdivision (micronized), so
   that the particle diameter is much smaller than the thickness of the
   applied layer of vehicle.
2. The particles are uniformly distributed throughout the vehicle and do
   not sediment.
3. The total amount of drug, soluble and suspended, per unit volume (A)
   is much greater than C_s, the saturation concentration (the solubility) of
   the drug in the matrix.
4. The surface to which the vehicle is applied is immiscible with the vehicle;
   i.e., skin secretions do not pass into the vehicle.
5. Only the drug diffuses out of the vehicle; vehicle components neither
   diffuse nor evaporate.
6. The receptor, i.e., the skin, functions as a perfect sink.

Just as we did for the solution case, we can draw concentration profiles
which exist within the vehicle after finite times of application to the skin
(see Fig. 4.12), where times after application, t, are in the order $t_4 > t_3 >
t_2 > t_1$. After any time, say t_1, the concentration plot shows a discontinuity,
as none of the suspended phase dissolves until the environmental concentration falls below C_s. The sharpness of the break depends largely on the
state of dispersion and the particle size of the solid phase. The concentration gradient immediately above the skin is essentially constant, provided
that A is very much greater than C_s. This follows from Fick's laws.

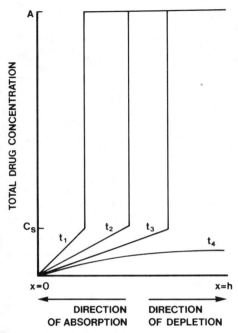

FIG. 4.12 Concentration profiles developed within an applied layer of vehicle for vehicle controlled release into skin acting as a perfect sink at x = 0: suspension formulation. (From W. I. Higuchi, 1961, 1967.)

Figure 4.13 illustrates the situation at a time t (full line) with h' representing the thickness of the zone of partial depletion. The amount of material absorbed by the skin (and depleted from the vehicle) corresponds to the shaded area of the diagram. After an increment of time, dt, the depletion zone increases by dh.

Based on this diagram for unit area in planar geometry the amount of drug, dM, additionally depleted by movement of the front by dh is

$$dM = A \, dh - \tfrac{1}{2} C_s \, dh \tag{4.3}$$

provided the concentration gradient is established and a quasi-steady state exists.

But according to Fick's law

$$\frac{dM}{dt} = \frac{D_v C_s}{h'} \tag{4.4}$$

or

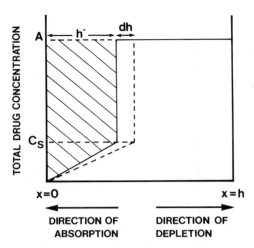

FIG. 4.13 Theoretical concentration profile existing in a vehicle containing suspended drug and in contact with a perfect sink at $x = 0$. (From T. Higuchi, 1961.)

$$A\frac{dh}{dt} - \frac{1}{2}C_s\frac{dh}{dt} = \frac{D_vC_s}{h'} \tag{4.5}$$

$$\frac{(2A - C_s)h'}{2D_vD_s}\,dh = dt \tag{4.6}$$

Integrating both sides

$$t = \frac{h'^2}{4D_vC_s}(2A - C_s) + K \tag{4.7}$$

where K is the integration constant. As $K = 0$ for t measured from zero

$$t = \frac{h'^2}{4D_vC_s}(2A - C_s) \tag{4.8}$$

and

$$h' = 2\left(\frac{D_vtC_s}{2A - C_s}\right)^{1/2} \tag{4.9}$$

From Fig. 4.13, the amount of drug depleted from vehicle, M, at time, t, is

$$M = h'A - \frac{h'C_s}{2} \tag{4.10}$$

Substituting for h' from Eq. (4.9)

$$M = \left(A - \frac{C_s}{2}\right) 2 \left(\frac{D_v t C_s}{2A - C_s}\right)^{1/2} = [D_v t (2A - C_s)C_s]^{1/2} \tag{4.11}$$

These equations hold essentially for all times less than that corresponding to complete depletion of the suspended phase.

The initial lag time, L, which is the time required to establish the quasi-steady state would in general be less than:

$$L = \frac{(n\alpha)^2}{6D_v} \tag{4.12}$$

where n is of the order of 2 or 3 and α is the mean distance between the suspended particles. Since α is assumed to be very small compared with the layer thickness in this model system, the lag time should be very short in comparison with the total depletion time.

If we differentiate Eq. (4.11) with respect to time, we obtain the instantaneous rate of absorption, or flux, at time t.

$$\frac{dM}{dt} = \frac{1}{2}\left(\frac{D_v(2A - C_s)C_s}{t}\right)^{1/2} \tag{4.13}$$

For the common condition in which the solubility of the drug in the vehicle is very small and A is appreciable (i.e., $A \gg C_s$), Eq. (4.11) simplifies to

$$M \simeq (2AD_v C_s t)^{1/2} \tag{4.14}$$

Equation (4.13) then becomes

$$\frac{dM}{dt} \simeq \left(\frac{AD_v C_s}{2t}\right)^{1/2} \tag{4.15}$$

In view of the physicochemical complexity of the dispersed systems considered here, Eqs. (4.14) and (4.15) are remarkably simple. The pharmaceutical formulator can manipulate the bioavailability of a drug from a topical semisolid suspension by altering the diffusion coefficent of the drug in the vehicle, the total drug concentration, or the drug solubility in the vehicle. However, Eq. (4.15) predicts that the release rate is proportional to the square root of the concentration. Thus, doubling the concentration of a drug in such a formulation only increases the release rate by about 40%. In vitro experiments with micronized dispersions of steroid at concentrations up to 0.1% show this to be true (Katz and Poulsen, 1971).

If the basic assumptions used to derive Eqs. (4.14) and (4.15) hold in
a particular experiment, good agreement between theory and practice
usually follows. However, as the relationships do not include a term for
particle size (only the requirement that particles should be "small" compared with the thickness of the applied vehicle layer), deviations do arise.
For example, Barrett et al. (1965) found that micronizing a fluocinolone
acetonide ointment improved its performance.

Chandrasekaran and Hillman (1980) have recently extended the Higuchi
treatment to develop a heterogeneous model of drug release from a polymer
matrix at high drug loading.

Katz and Poulsen (1971) have considered the question: Which of the
two systems discussed above (solution or suspension) provides the best
drug release? They conclude that, provided sink conditions prevail in the
skin, for identical initial concentrations and diffusion coefficients release
will ordinarily be faster from a formulation in which the drug is entirely
dissolved (Ostrenga et al., 1971a). This conclusion contrasts with the usual
situation in which the skin provides the rate-limiting step in percutaneous
absorption. Then only the thermodynamic activity of a drug in the base is
important. All saturated and suspension formulations of a drug in different
vehicles should provide the same flux rate, providing ideal conditions
exist.

3. Additional factors modifying release: skin a perfect sink

The previous two subsections have considered ideal, model systems.
Although these mathematical models have proved useful in formulation
studies, it will be appreciated that few practical topical semisolid vehicles
are simple, homogeneous phases. The closest approach to such a formulation is the polar gel. This usually consists of mixtures of polar liquids,
such as water, ethanol, propylene glycol, and polyethylene glycols, gelled
with a polymer such as Carbopol. For ointments, the most common base is
petrolatum (soft paraffin). This is a two-phase colloidal material which
contains liquid, microcrystalline, and crystalline paraffins. Batches of
petrolatum vary in their constituents and thus in their properties. These
variations arise from differences in the source of the crude material, different types and extents of refining, and differences in the blending processes which may be used after the petrolatum has been refined. Thus, the
release properties of petrolatum will not be simple and they may differ
from batch to batch. Barry and Grace (1971) have reviewed the structural
and rheological properties of petrolatum.

Topical vehicles may contain many ingredients. These include surfactants, solubilizers, buffers, chelating agents, preservatives, antioxidants,
humectants, emollients, thickeners, plasticizers, dyes, and perfumes.
Any one of these adjuvants may interact with the drug, the vehicle, or each
other, to modify the release characteristics of the preparation.

Many topical vehicles are multiphase systems, in which the drug
partitions between the phases. Wurster (1965) emphasized that the partition

coefficient of a drug between the phases in an emulsion vehicle, and not only the total concentration of drug in the vehicle, defines the actual diffusional concentration gradient. Of prime importance is the concentration of penetrant in the external phase of a cream, since this is the phase mainly in contact with the skin. This external phase concentration depends on the phase volumes and the solubilizing powers of the phases as they are affected by their chemical compositions and the presence of additives such as emulsifiers.

W. I. Higuchi and T. Higuchi (1960) provided a detailed analysis for drug diffusion through heterogeneous systems. They placed particular emphasis on the design of protective ointments and films, the release of drugs from such systems, and their passage through the skin. Section II. C of Chap. 2 considers the topic at greater length.

The drug may adsorb onto solid adjuvants in the dosage form, or it may complex with vehicle constituents. The drug solubility may be a function of vehicle pH, or it may depend on the presence of cosolvents or surfactants. The diffusion coefficient in the vehicle depends on the microviscosity. Such effects are discussed in Chap. 2, Sec. III.

Polymorphs are crystalline forms of a drug which differ in their physicochemical properties, including solubility. Thus, the particular polymorph used can affect drug availability from a suspension dosage form (Haleblian and McCrone, 1969).

Chapter 6 reviews in more detail the various types of vehicles which may be used to formulate dermatological preparations.

4. Transdermal therapeutic systems

A Transdermal Therapeutic System (TTS; also called Transiderm or Transderm) is a topical device designed to deliver drug to the surface of the skin at a controlled rate. This rate is well below the maximum that the skin can accept. In this sense, the device, not the stratum corneum, controls the rate at which the drug diffuses through the epidermis and passes into the general circulation via the capillaries.

The rationale for the use of such devices, and their design, have been discussed by Michaels (1975), Michaels et al. (1975), Shaw et al. (1975, 1977, 1980), Chandrasekaran et al. (1976, 1978a,b, 1979), Chandrasekaran and Shaw (1977), Shaw and Chandrasekaran (1978, 1981), and Heilmann (1978). However, much of the same basic information is repeated in these various publications.

A Transderm device aims to provide systemic therapy for acute or chronic conditions in a more convenient and effective way than methods currently available such as parenteral or oral therapy. In particular, at least in theory the percutaneous route could have the following advantages over the oral route [for general reviews which discuss the disadvantages of the traditional routes, see Wagner (1975), Gibaldi and Perrier (1975), and Gibaldi (1977)]:

1. The administration of a drug through the skin could eliminate the variables which influence gastrointestinal absorption. These variables include the drastic changes in environmental pH along the gastrointestinal tract (from stomach pH as low as 1 to intestinal pH of 8), food intake, stomach emptying time, and intestinal motility and transit time.

2. The drug diffuses into the systemic circulation without first entering the portal system and passing through the liver. This route eliminates the "first pass" effect by which the liver, the main metabolizing organ for most drugs, can drastically reduce the amount of drug which gets through intact to the systemic circulation.

3. Transdermal input of a drug may provide controlled, constant administration of a medicament by simple application to the skin surface. This controlled input may permit the display of only one pharmacological effect from a drug which, in a conventional dosage form, shows several effects. The continuity of input may allow drugs with short half-lives to be used; with other routes it may be difficult to ensure constant plasma concentrations. The prolonged, controlled delivery of a drug could improve patient compliance; the patient would not have the responsibility of frequent self-medication according to a prescribed regimen.

4. The percutaneous administration of drugs at a controlled rate could eliminate pulse entry into the systemic circulation. Peaks in plasma concentrations often cause undesirable side effects.

5. The transdermal route allows administration of drugs with a small therapeutic index, i.e., drugs for which the therapeutic concentration in the plasma lies close to the toxic level.

6. If we need to terminate therapy rapidly, simple removal of the device would interrupt absorption of the medicament.

In developing transdermal systems, we consider only drugs which are sufficiently potent that the dosage does not exceed about 2 mg per day. The compounds must not irritate or sensitize the skin. The medicament must have the correct physicochemical properties to partition into the stratum corneum and to permeate to the vascular region of the skin.

So far, the application of a TTS has been considered for ephedrine, chlorpheniramine, and scopolamine (hyoscine). As clinical trials have progressed with scopolamine, we will limit our consideration to this drug.

Chandrasekaran et al. (1976, 1980) and Chandrasekaran and Shaw (1978) demonstrated the validity of a dual-sorption model for the permeation of scopolamine through human skin in vitro. In this analysis, it is assumed that sorption occurs by two mechanisms. The first is simple dissolution to produce mobile, freely diffusible molecules. The second mechanism is an adsorption process which immobilizes molecules by binding them to the stratum corneum so that they do not diffuse. If we assume that the rate of exchange between mobile and immobile species is rapid compared with the diffusion process, then the two species are in local equilibrium. The drug concentration in the skin, with sink conditions on the dermal side, is then governed by

$$\left[1 + \frac{C_I^* b^*/K}{(1 + C_D b^*/K)^2}\right] \frac{\partial C_D}{\partial t} = D \frac{\partial^2 C_D}{\partial x^2} \tag{4.16}$$

where C_I^* is Langmuir's saturation constant; b^* is Langmuir's affinity constant; K is the partition coefficient; C_D is the mobile drug concentration; and x is the distance.

Equation (4.16) is a development of Fick's second law [see Chap. 2, Eq. (2.5)]. The second term within the brackets on the left-hand side of Eq. (4.16) arises as a consequence of drug immobilization. For mathematical simplicity so as to obtain an analytical solution it is assumed that, based on experimental data, this term is a constant.

To develop a suitable device, two main considerations have to be borne in mind. The device must rapidly provide scopolamine to saturate the binding sites in the skin so as to reduce the time lag required for steady state conditions to prevail. Then the rate-controlling element must dominate the drug input to the skin, so as to maintain the systemic concentration at the desired steady level.

Figure 4.14 is a schematic diagram of a TTS. The device is a multilayer laminate. It contains a drug reservoir holding scopolamine in a polymeric gel, sandwiched between an impermeable backing sheet and a rate-controlling, microporous membrane. A contact adhesive contains scopolamine; the adhesive secures the system to the skin behind the ear, and it also liberates a priming dose of drug to saturate the binding sites in the skin. The patient removes the protective strippable film before applying the device.

The contact adhesive comprises a polymeric gel saturated with scopolamine, with excess drug uniformly dispersed throughout the gel. Chandrasekaran and Shaw (1977) assume that the release kinetics for such a system

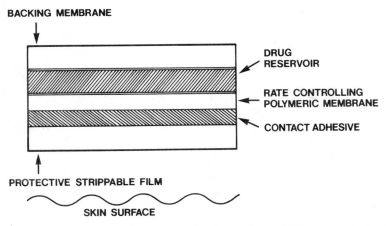

FIG. 4.14 Schematic diagram of a Transdermal Therapeutic System.

are those derived by T. Higuchi (1960, 1961), i.e., that the stratum corneum is here behaving as a perfect sink and the formulation is a simple suspension. These assumptions seem a little suspect, as the microporous membrane does not control the release of scopolamine from the contact adhesive. However, Candrasekaran and Shaw apply the conditions detailed in Sec. III.D.2 and use Eqs. (4.3) to (4.15). From Eq. (4.15), we see that the contribution of the drug in the contact adhesive to the overall scopolamine delivery kinetics varies as $t^{-1/2}$.

The polymeric drug reservoir provides scopolamine which is available for simple diffusion only through the pores of the microporous membrane. A suitable solvent, with the necessary solubility and diffusional characteristics for scopolamine, fills the pores. The fundamental equation is the simple flux expression with a modification for the porosity of the membrane (e) and a tortuosity factor τ (see Chap. 2, Sec. II.B):

$$\frac{dM}{dt} = \frac{eD \, \Delta C}{\tau h} \tag{4.17}$$

where dM/dt is the flux; ΔC is the concentration decrement across the microporous membrane; and h is the membrane thickness.

If the drug concentration in the contact adhesive is small compared with the saturated drug concentration in the drug reservoir (C_s), Eq. (4.17) becomes

$$\frac{dM}{dt} = \frac{eDC_s}{\tau h} \tag{4.18}$$

If we combine the effect of the priming dose from the contact adhesive (which dominates the temporal pattern of drug release) with the steady state delivery controlled by the microporous membrane, then we can approximate the scopolamine delivery rate from the TTS (R_s) by

$$R_s = G + H \exp(-at) \tag{4.19}$$

where G, H, and a are constants. The first term on the right-hand side of Eq. (4.19) represents the steady state delivery rate; the second term predicts the time dependent pattern of drug release during the priming dose period.

Figure 4.15 represents a typical in vitro release rate versus time profile for scopolamine liberated from a TTS into an infinite sink under isotonic and isothermal conditions (Chandrasekaran and Shaw, 1977). The line is the profile predicted by theory, using values for the constants in Eq. (4.19) of 3.8 and 150 $\mu g/cm^2$ hr for G and H, respectively, and 1.3 hr^{-1} for a. The data points are experimentally determined values. The agreement is good.

To measure the rate at which drug passes into the systemic circulation during the in vivo application of the device, we determine the urinary

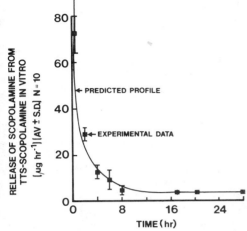

FIG. 4.15 In vitro release rate versus time profile for scopolamine released from a TTS; comparison of theory and experiment. (From Chandrasekaran and Shaw, 1977.)

excretion rate of scopolamine. From pharmacokinetic measurements, only about 10% of the scopolamine can be recovered in the urine in the free form after intramuscular or intravenous administration. Taking this into account and assuming that a similar recovery would be obtained during transdermal administration, we can compare in vitro experiments with in vivo results (Fig. 4.16). Although there are only two points on the in vivo graph, we see that after about 4 hr, the urinary excretion rate of scopolamine approaches 10% of the release rate of the drug from the TTS in vitro.

The user places the present TTS-scopolamine device behind the ear, a relatively permeable region of the skin. When the device is placed at other skin sites such as the back, which is less permeable than the postauricular area, the skin cannot accept the drug at the rate provided by the TTS. At such sites, the skin and not the system controls the input of scopolamine into the systemic circulation (Shaw et al., 1977).

One possible improvement to the device would be to include penetration enhancers (Sec. III.C.3) in the contact adhesive and the drug reservoir. These would increase the permeability of the skin and thereby possibly increase the number of drugs which could be administered this way. Skin sites other than behind the ear could also then be considered.

The scopolamine transdermal therapeutic system is 2.5 cm^2 in area; it provides a priming dose of 200 μg and a controlled release of 10 μg hr^{-1} for 72 hr. Clinical studies, trials at sea, and experiments in a vertical oscillator indicate that the device is a safe and effective dosage form for the systemic administration of scopolamine to prevent motion-induced

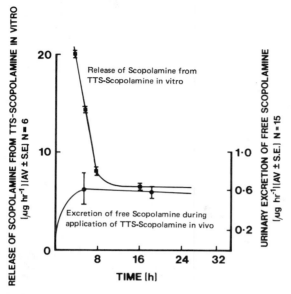

FIG. 4.16 Comparison of in vivo and in vitro data for the TTS-scopolamine device. Urinary excretion of free scopolamine = $9.5\% \pm 0.9\%$ (average $\pm$ SE) of total drug administered. (From Chandrasekaran and Shaw, 1977.)

nausea (Shaw et al., 1976; Shaw and Chandrasekaran, 1978). The controlled input to the systemic circulation allows the scopolamine to act as an anti-emetic without significant incidence of the parasympatholytic side effects of such drugs.

The TTS-scopolamine device presumably would also be useful to prevent the nausea and vomiting which are side effects of anticancer agents, and to treat vertigo. The basic technology of the appliance could be applied to a range of medicaments; for example, in cardiovascular therapy a suitable drug could be administered for the long-term treatment of hypertension. A device for delivering transdermal nitroglycerin is now ready for marketing.

E. Drug-Vehicle-Skin Interactions

In this section we consider the more usual situation in which we cannot ignore the impermeability of the stratum corneum; in fact, the horny layer provides the rate-limiting step in the overall percutaneous absorption process.

A valuable way to organize the discussion is to adopt the method pioneered by Poulsen (1972), who highlights the control which the vehicle may have over the diffusional flux of a drug through the skin. He considers several simple models which predict how the flux may change when the solubilizing power of the vehicle for the drug alters in specific ways. Although the models are simple compared with in vivo conditions, the predictions work well in clinical practice, particularly with topical steroids used as anti-inflammatory agents.

The models assume the following:

1. The horny layer of the skin provides the rate-limiting step in the absorption process.
2. The skin is a homogeneous, intact membrane; shunt routes, such as appendages, do not operate.
3. Unless otherwise specified, only a single drug species is important in the vehicle and it dissolves to form an ideal solution. (We can extend the treatment to mixtures of drugs, provided each behaves ideally and they do not interact). The penetrant is nonionic and it is unaffected by changes in pH of the vehicle.
4. Only the drug diffuses from the vehicle. Formulation components neither diffuse nor evaporate significantly and skin secretions do not dilute the vehicle.
5. The diffusion coefficient does not alter with time or position within the vehicle or in the stratum corneum.
6. Neither the vehicle nor the penetrant changes the diffusion coefficient within the horny layer during the absorption process.
7. Penetrant reaching the viable tissues immediately sweeps into the systemic circulation, so that sink conditions apply below the horny layer.
8. The drug concentration in the vehicle is constant during the diffusion process, i.e., the donor phase does not deplete significantly.
9. Unless specified, the vehicle does not damage the skin or otherwise alter its permeability during an experiment by, e.g., altering the hydration state of the stratum corneum or by functioning as a penetration enhancer
10. The drug remains unaltered and intact.
11. Flux estimates are steady state values.

Under these conditions, we use the diffusional model of simple zero-order flux (see Chap. 2, Sec. I.B).

$$\frac{dM}{dt} = \frac{KC_v D}{h} \tag{4.20}$$

where dM/dt is the steady state flux of penetrant per unit area of membrane; K is the partition coefficient of the drug between the stratum corneum and the vehicle (we also use the abbreviation PC in this section for direct comparison with published work); C_v is the concentration of drug dissolved in the vehicle; D is the diffusion coefficient of the drug in the horny layer; and h is the thickness of the stratum corneum.

For this analysis, we assume that h is constant and we estimate changes in the penetration rate from variations in the product KC_vD. The fundamental factors which control the magnitude of each of these parameters were discussed in Chap. 2, Sec. III.

The model consists of a vehicle which contains a specified total concentration of drug (dissolved and suspended) in contact with a skin surface of fixed thickness and area.

The vehicle is a primary solvent, such as water, to which we add a miscible cosolvent in amount ranging from 0 to 100%. This cosolvent may either solubilize or desolubilize the drug. Possible blends include water with propylene glycol, polyethylene glycols, hexylene glycol, propylene carbonate, methanol, or ethanol. Substances such as dimethyl sulfoxide, dimethyl formamide, dimethyl acetamide, longer-chain alkyl sulfoxides, and the pyrrolidones and their n-alkyl derivatives provide alternative solvents, but their penetration enhancing properties complicate the analysis of their effects. Blends of nonpolar solvents have seldom been rigorously investigated [an exception is the recent work of Turi et al. (1979) with polyoxypropylene 15 stearyl ether and mineral oil], even though clinicians often prefer to treat dermatoses with lipophilic vehicles such as petrolatum-based ointments. Mixtures of water and propylene glycol have proved to be the most useful blends, particularly when used to dissolve topical steroids. For example, fluocinonide is about 1,300 times more soluble in propylene glycol than in water (Poulsen, 1972).

A feature of the analysis is that we assume that the drug solubility in the vehicle varies in a first-order manner with the percentage, volume fraction, or weight fraction of cosolvent in the vehicle, as does the partition coefficient. Poulsen (1972) derived this concept intuitively, but the assumption is reasonable and it has been shown to apply for many semipolar nonelectrolytes in polar solvents (Flynn and Smith, 1972; Elworthy and Worthington, 1968; Peterson and Hopponen, 1953; Shihab et al., 1970; Poulsen et al., 1968; Yalkowsky et al., 1972; Yalkowsky and Flynn, 1974; Turi et al., 1979). Then

$$C_f = C_w \exp(\alpha f) \qquad (4.21)$$

or

$$\ln C_f = \ln C_w + \alpha f \qquad (4.22)$$

where C_f is the solute solubility in a mixed binary aqueous solvent with volume or weight fraction f of nonaqueous cosolvent, and C_w is the solubility in water. The constant α is characteristic of the system.

This relationship is sufficiently general to be useful in estimating or in predicting solubilities in binary systems, provided that the polarity of the drug is significantly lower than that of either solvent.

If we assume that the drug solubility in the membrane is independent of the composition of the binary solvent, the partition coefficient for a drug

K_f is equal to its constant solubility in the membrane C_m divided by its solubility in the binary solvent, as described by Eqs. (4.21) and (4.22). Then

$$K_f = \frac{C_m}{C_f} = \frac{C_m}{C_w \exp(\alpha f)} \tag{4.23}$$

$$K_f = K_w \exp(-\alpha f) \tag{4.24}$$

or

$$\ln K_f = \ln K_w - \alpha f \tag{4.25}$$

where K_w is the partition coefficient of drug relative to water. Substituting C_f from Eq. (4.21) and K_f from Eq. (4.24) into Eq. (4.20), we get

$$\frac{dM}{dt} = \frac{D}{h} C_w \exp(\alpha f) K_w \exp(-\alpha f) \tag{4.26}$$

and so

$$\frac{dM}{dt} = \frac{D}{h} C_w K_w \tag{4.27}$$

Thus, Eq. (4.27) states that the flux of a drug through the skin should be constant for saturated binary solvents which do not have a vehicle effect on the skin.

If the solvent blend does affect drug solubility in the skin (i.e., there is a vehicle effect), we express the partition coefficient as (Turi et al., 1979)

$$K_f = K_w \exp(-\beta f) \tag{4.28}$$

where β is another constant. In this situation

$$\frac{dM}{dt} = \frac{D}{h} C_w \exp(\alpha f) K_w \exp(-\beta f) \tag{4.29}$$

The flux rate of drug through the skin from saturated solution then depens on the particular values for the constants α and β.

In the different models, the total concentration of drug (dissolved and suspended) ranges from 0.05 to 10.00 mg g^{-1} of vehicle. The solubility of the drug in a specific vehicle determines the effective concentration for diffusional processes. Excess undissolved drug does not affect the penetration rate.

Hypothetical case 1: "ideal" behavior

In this model, we assume that the diffusion coefficient D is constant for all vehicle compositions and is therefore not a variable factor. Drug

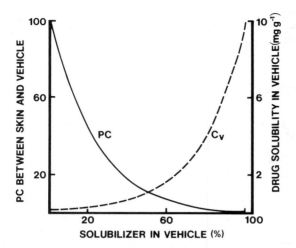

FIG. 4.17 Partition coefficient and solubility profiles for Case 1. (From Poulsen, 1972.)

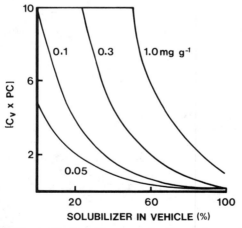

FIG. 4.18 Relative penetration rate profiles for Case 1. (From Poulsen, 1972.)

solubility in the vehicle relates to the concentration of solubilizer in a first-order manner. Changes in the vehicle composition do not affect the solubility of the drug in the stratum corneum. These conditions imply that changes in the drug solubility in the vehicle exactly oppose equal, opposite changes in the partition coefficient.

Figure 4.17 illustrates the relationship between the drug solubility in the vehicle (which ranges from 0.1 to 10.0 mg g^{-1}) and the partition coefficient (which changes from 100.0 to 1.0) as a function of the percentage of solubilizer in the vehicle (from 0 to 100%). We see that as we increase the solubility of the drug in the vehicle by adding more cosolvent, so the partition coefficient falls.

Figure 4.18 presents the data of Fig. 4.17 in the form of relative penetration rates, calculated from the product $C_V PC$. Note that C_V is the concentration of dissolved drug species. From these plots we see that if we formulate a series of gels of different solvent compositions but all of which contain 1 mg of drug per gram of vehicle then suspensions form in preparations containing up to 50% of solubilizer. For these gels, the product $C_V PC$ is constant and equals 10 units; thus the flux rate through the skin is constant.

Above 50% solubilizer, all the drug dissolves and C_V is constant at 1 mg g^{-1}. As the solubilizer concentration increases, the partition coefficient continues to fall and so does the flux rate. Thus, as far clinical activity is concerned, these gels should be less efficient, and considerably so at high solubilizer concentrations, even though the overall concentration of drug in the dosage form remains the same.

If we decrease the total amount of drug present in the gels, the penetration rate profile is similar but it shifts in the direction of lower percentage of solubilizer in the vehicle (see, for example, the graph for 0.3 mg/g in Fig. 4.18). At a concentration of 0.1 mg/g, the drug forms a saturated solution at zero percentage of solubilizer. There are no solid drug particles available to dissolve as the solubilizer concentration increases. Thus, C_V cannot increase to counterbalance the fall in the partition coefficient. The penetration rate profile shows a continuous decline with solubilizer concentration.

Systems containing 0.05 mg/g are always below saturation and the declining penetration profile begins at 5 units.

The most important feature of this model is that it predicts a decrease in penetration rate when the quantity of solubilizer in the vehicle exceeds the level required to just completely dissolve all the drug.

An alternative way to interpret the plots of Fig. 4.18 is in terms of thermodynamic activities. Equation (4.20) is equivalent to (T. Higuchi, 1960)

$$\frac{DM}{dt} = \frac{a}{\gamma} \frac{D}{h} \tag{4.30}$$

where a is the thermodynamic activity of the drug in its vehicle and γ is
the effective activity coefficient of the drug in the skin barrier phase. To
obtain the maximum rate of penetration, we must use the highest thermodynamic activity possible for the penetrating substance. The limiting value
for this activity is that of the pure form of the substance at the environmental temperature. Any higher activity represents supersaturation with
respect to the form. The conclusion, therefore, is that all vehicles which
contain the drug as a finely ground suspension (in which the activity is maximal and is equal to that of the solid drug) should produce the same rate of
penetration. Figure 4.18 indicates this penetration behavior, where the
plateau region represents suspensions with maximal thermodynamic
activities.

For materials which are not simple compounds, crystalline modifications (polymorphic forms) may exist at room temperature with different

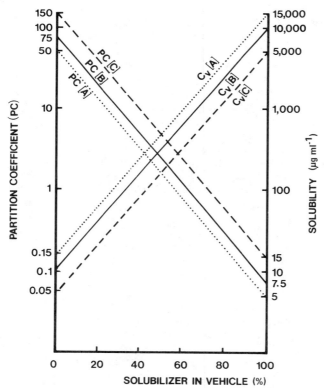

FIG. 4.19 Partition coefficient and solubility profiles for three hypothetical
compounds (A, B, C) for Case 1 behavior, log scales. (From Poulsen
et al., 1978.)

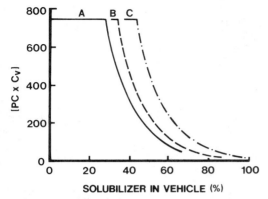

FIG. 4.20 Relative penetration rate profiles for compounds A, B, and C for Case 1 behavior. (From Poulsen et al., 1978.)

free energies and thermodynamic activities. In theory, by selecting the most energetic species to make the suspension, the formulator may increase the penetration rate. However, the more energetic the polymorph is, the lower is its stability. All higher energy states are metastable, and they change spontaneously to the stable form. Thus, when we try to formulate suspensions with high energy polymorphic forms, we meet problems with respect to the long-term stability of crystal habits.

The model also predicts the absorption control of solvents which contain mixtures of penetrating drugs (Poulsen et al., 1978). For three compounds (A, B, and C) which have solubilities in water of 15, 7.5, and 5 μg ml^{-1}, respectively, Fig. 4.19 illustrates the partition coefficient and solubility data (on logarithmic scales) as a function of the percentage of solubilizer in the vehicle. The same assumptions apply as before. In addition, we assume that the three drugs exhibit independent solubilities at low total (mixed) concentrations, they diffuse independently, and their diffusion coefficients in skin are identical.

Figure 4.20 illustrates relative steady state flux estimates calculated as before for three series of formulations (labeled—after the penetrant which each series contains—A, B, or C). The concentration of each drug in every preparation is 0.01% (100 μg ml^{-1}).

The thermodynamic activities of the diffusing species reach a limiting value at saturation, and each drug provides a plateau region. Suspended drug particles do not increase the penetration rate.

One can estimate steady state fluxes from any vehicle which contains from 0 to 100% solubilizer. For example, for a vehicle with 40% solubilizer, Fig. 4.21 illustrates relative penetration rates from formulations with the individual compounds and from preparations which contain a mixture of A, B, and C. These rates are plotted as functions of drug concentration in the vehicle. For the system labeled "Mixture," the optimum mixing ratio,

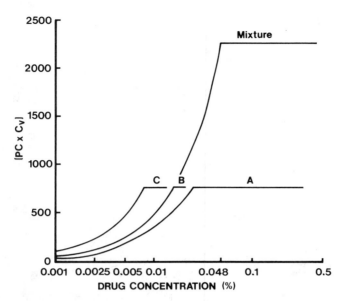

FIG. 4.21 Relative penetration rate profiles for compounds A, B, and C
and their mixture—for a vehicle with 40% solubilizer—for Case 1 behavior.
(From Poulsen et al., 1978.)

A:B:C of 3:2:1, comes from the individual solubilities illustrated in
Fig. 4.19.

The model predicts maximum fluxes for the series A, B, and C at
drug concentrations of 0.024, 0.016, and 0.008%, respectively. The maximum flux for the mixture which contains a total concentration of the three
drugs of 0.048% in the ratio of 3:2:1 is three times that which we can obtain
with a single drug at any concentration.

As before, this model predicts that we can achieve maximum penetration rates at any drug concentration (at or above the solubility in water) by
simply varying the cosolvent composition of the vehicle. Thus, if we reduce
the cosolvent concentration to 30% and the mixed drug concentration to
0.024%, we obtain the same flux rate as for the more concentrated mixture
discussed previously.

In practice, there are limitations to this approach. As the drug concentration in the vehicle falls, so the effect of depletion into the skin increases.
There are also practical problems with analysis and stability at low drug
concentrations.

Work with three of the esters of fluocinolone acetonide, in vivo and
in vitro, shows the value of this technique, as demonstrated by Poulsen
et al. (1978). These authors emphasize that the concept of using mixtures

of drugs in the way outlined above is useful only for compounds for which the skin is very impermeable and for which improved percutaneous absorption would be clinically beneficial. The medicaments should have similar and independent solubilities, comparable potencies and identical pharmacological properties. A further complication is that analytical techniques have to separate and quantitate low concentrations of drugs which were specifically chosen for their similar physicochemical properties, such as solubility.

Hypothetical case 2: "nonideal" behavior—drug solubility in skin increases with increase in solubilizer concentration in vehicle

In Case 2 behavior, we allow the solvent in the vehicle to influence the solubility of the drug in the skin, i.e., the vehicle affects the skin. This implies that the partition coefficient for the drug is not directly proportional to the reciprocal of the drug solubility in the vehicle but it depends on the vehicle composition. We assume that the solubility of the drug in the barrier phase increases with increase in the concentration of cosolvent in the vehicle. This means that, for finite concentrations of solubilizer, the partition coefficient profile as a function of percentage of solubilizer in the vehicle is higher than a Case 1 profile.

As before, we let increasing concentrations of solubilizer produce a first-order increase in vehicle solubility of a poorly water soluble drug. We specify that a 100-fold change in the solubility of the drug in the vehicle

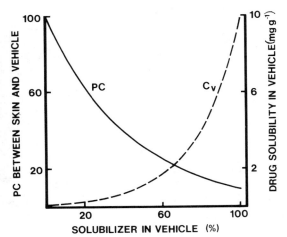

FIG. 4.22 Partition coefficient and solubility profiles for Case 2 behavior. (From Poulsen, 1972.)

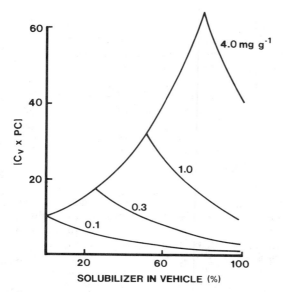

FIG. 4.23 Relative penetration rate profiles for Case 2. (From Poulsen, 1972.)

(from 0.1 to 10 mg g^{-1}) produces only a 10-fold change in the partition coefficient (from 100 to 10 units). The diffusion coefficient of the drug is constant for all conditions.

Figure 4.22 shows the relevant profiles: the partition coefficient and solubility plots are not mirror images.

We can construct theoretical penetration profiles as before, by plotting the product of the partition coefficient and the <u>dissolved</u> drug concentration in the vehicle as a function of the amount of solubilizer in the vehicle (Fig. 4.23).

We see that we now produce maxima in the penetration rates by increasing the amount of solubilizer. For example, for a sample of gels which each contain a total quantity of drug of 4 mg g^{-1}, the penetration rate increases to a maximum at 80% solubilizer. This is because, going from 0 to 80% solubilizer, the amount of dissolved drug increases but the partition coefficient does not fall as drastically as in Case 1. The product PCC$_V$ therefore increases. At saturation, with further increase in solubilizer concentration, the relative penetration rate falls: C$_V$ is constant, but PC continues to decline.

With less drug in the vehicle, the penetration profiles shift to lower maxima at lower concentrations of solubilizer. For a series of gels containing only 0.1 mg g^{-1} of drug, a saturated solution forms in pure water. Thus, only the declining phase of the penetration profile is apparent.

    Thus, in this model, drug penetrates the skin less effectively from
vehicles which contain either insufficient solubilizer to dissolve all the
drug, or solubilizer in excess of the amount required to produce a saturated
solution of drug.
    Workers at Syntex Research have shown practice that with a poorly
soluble corticosteroid such as fluocinonide the penetration rate from suspensions is much lower than the rate from vehicles which contain just sufficient solubilizer to completely dissolve the drug (Poulsen et al., 1968;
Katz and Poulsen, 1971; Ostrenga et al., 1971a; Katz and Poulsen, 1972).

    Hypothetical case 3: "nonideal" behavior—drug solubility
    in skin decreases with increase in cosolvent
    concentration in vehicle

    In this case, the added cosolvent is a desolubilizer and it produces a
first-order <u>decrease</u> in the vehicle solubility of a highly water soluble drug.
Also, the drug solubility in the skin reduces when we add cosolvent to the
vehicle; i.e., the vehicle affects the skin in a manner opposite to a Case 2
cosolvent. A 100-fold change in the solubility of the drug in the vehicle
(which decreases from 10.0 to 0.1 mg g^{-1}) produces a 10-fold increase in
the partition coefficient (from 0.1 to 1.0 unit). The diffusion coefficient is
again constant for all conditions.
    Figure 4.24 illustrates the solubility and partition coefficient plots.
In essence, after allowing for the different magnitudes of the partition coefficients, these plots are the reverse of the profiles in Case 2 (Fig. 4.22).
Thus, if in Fig. 4.24 we started the x axis at the left-hand side with pure
desolubilizer and we added water as a solubilizer, then, with a scaling

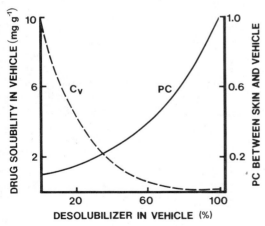

FIG. 4.24 Partition coefficient and solubility profiles for Case 3 behavior.
(From Poulsen, 1972.)

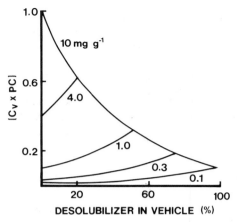

FIG. 4.25 Relative penetration rate profiles for Case 3. (From Poulsen, 1972.)

factor for the partition coefficient plot, we would obtain the same profiles as in Fig. 4.22.

Figure 4.25 illustrates the relative penetration rate profiles. For 10 mg g^{-1} formulations, as the percentage of desolubilizer increases, the solubility of the drug falls and C_V decreases. As the partition coefficient only increases at one-tenth the rate of the fall in C_V, then PCC$_V$ (the relative penetration rate) declines steadily.

Case 3 represents conditions where the drug is too soluble in a conventional aqueous vehicle for optimal penetration. For example, imagine that we wish to formulate a topical vehicle containing 4 mg g^{-1} of the drug. The relevant profile in Fig. 4.25 shows that we can increase the penetration rate by adding desolubilizer up to 20% (from 0 to 20% desolubilizer, C_V is constant but PC increases; see Fig. 4.24). Above 20% desolubilizer, C_V falls but at a rate faster than the increase in PC. The penetration rate profile therefore declines after the maximum for an optimum formulation for the vehicle of 20% desolubilizer and 80% water. Similar effects occur for 1.0 and for 0.3 mg g^{-1} of drug at higher concentrations of desolubilizer.

When the vehicle contains a concentration of drug equivalent to its solubility in pure desolubilizer (0.1 mg g^{-1}), then progressive additions of desolubilizer steadily increase the penetration rate as the partition coefficient increases, with no maximum in the plot.

Hypothetical case 4: "nonideal" behavior—diffusion coefficient in skin alters with cosolvent concentration in vehicle

So far, we have considered a variety of possible theoretical situations, in each of which we have assumed that the diffusion coefficient in the skin barrier does not alter when the vehicle composition changes. However, if we allow the vehicle to modify the properties of the stratum corneum in ways which change the solubility of the drug in the skin barrier (Cases 2 and 3), then we should also allow for consequent changes in the diffusion coefficient of the drug in the horny layer. We can readily appreciate situations in which we make D a specified function of vehicle composition by superimposing the effect of a varying D on the C_V and PC profiles previously considered.

As an example, we will consider the result of varying the diffusion coefficient in Case 2.

Case 4A We arbitrarily assume that the diffusion coefficient of the drug in the skin increases when we apply to the skin vehicles which contain more than a threshold concentration of solubilizer, e.g., 50%. Figure 4.26 shows the relative effective diffusion coefficient (D_1) as a function of solubilizer concentration, placed adjacent to the C_V and PC plots for Case 2.

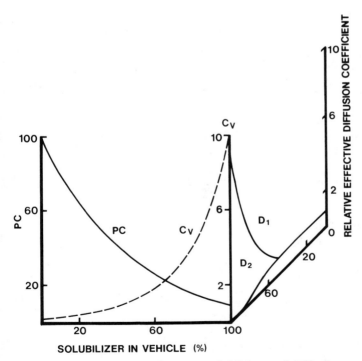

FIG. 4.26 Partition coefficient, solubility, and diffusion coefficient profiles for Case 4. (From Poulsen, 1972.)

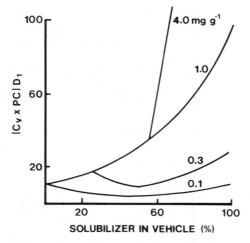

FIG. 4.27 Relative penetration rate profiles for Case 4A. (From Poulsen, 1972.)

Figure 4.27 illustrates the relative penetration rate ($C_V PCD_1$) as a function of solubilizer content in the vehicle.

The profiles are similar to those illustrated in Fig. 4.23, up to 50% solubilizer. Above this threshold, all penetration rates increase relatively as D_1 increases.

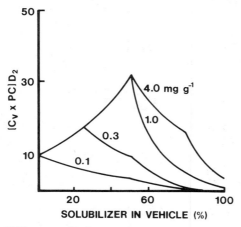

FIG. 4.28 Relative penetration rate profiles for Case 4B. (From Poulsen, 1972.)

Recently Turi et al. (1979) showed that propylene glycol decreases the resistance of the skin to the passage of diflurasone diacetate, i.e., D_1 increases. This decrease in skin resistance is proportional to the amount of propylene glycol in the vehicle.

Case 4B   Here we assume that the diffusion coefficient D_2 decreases steadily when the solubilizer concentration increases above 50% (see Fig. 4.26).

The resultant relative penetration rate profiles illustrated in Fig. 4.28 reveal the expected shape, identical to those in Fig. 4.23 up to 50% solubilizer content. For vehicles which contain more than 50% solubilizer, all penetration rates further decrease in proportion to the falling value of D_2.

Value, validity, and violations of the model approach
to skin permeation

In several parts of this book, and particularly in Secs. III.D and III.E of this chapter, we consider physicochemically ideal situations. Thus, mainly for the convenience of experimentation and for the analysis and interpretation of data, in the laboratory we often study only simple topical formulations of chemically ideal components applied to uniform, homogeneous membranes under closely controlled, invariable conditions. However, clinically orientated scientists are interested ultimately in what happens during topical therapy in patients with a diseased or damaged skin. In such therapeutic use, topical formulations are often multiphase, complex, and ill understood; the healthy skin is a diverse, laminated, specialized organ which becomes even more complex in disease; and the conditions under which drugs permeate the skin vary and are far from simple. The question therefore naturally arises: What is the value and relevance of a strict model approach to percutaneous absorption in the clinical treatment of a patient?

Model analysis has merit in the initial development and testing of topical delivery systems, provided that we appreciate its limitations. The discipline of thinking in strict physicochemical concepts also helps when we must analyze absorption phenomena in the richly varied diseased state. The alternative strategies, either of copycat formulations or of multiple, repetitive, empirical experiments, both in vitro and in vivo, followed by several clinical trials, do not advance fundamental scientific knowledge, waste time and money, and often lead to the marketing of suboptimal formulations. The crucial feature is that we should appreciate the rigorous assumptions employed in model analysis together with how clinical usage violates these suppositions. Then there is a reasonable probability that idealized in vitro experiments may lead to the formulation of bioavailable dermatologicals.

It is therefore useful, at the risk of some repetition, to summarize the main violations from the ideal conditions (see Sec. III.E, points 1 to 11) which can occur during skin permeation in vivo. Section III.D.3 of this chapter is also relevant to this discussion.

Previously, we assumed that, in general, the stratum corneum provides the rate-limiting step in the overall process of percutaneous absorption. However, the patient's skin may become permeable because of severe damage or disease. The vehicle used to apply the drug to the skin may occlude the tissue, raising its moisture content and temperature and thereby lessening both its resistance and its rate-determining role. As formulated in the laboratory, the vehicle may not retard significantly the release of a drug. In clinical use, following application to the skin, vehicle changes may reduce drug diffusion and release from the applied layer. In practice, such alterations may tend toward vehicle control of permeation.

The skin is not a simple, homogeneous, intact membrane but a laminated structure pieced by appendages. These appendages provide shunt routes for the permeation of electrolytes, large, polar molecules, and— of particular importance here—possibly many dermatological drugs (Scheuplein, 1978a,b).

Drugs are often nonideal, ionic, and affected by the initial pH of the vehicle and how the pH changes after application to the skin.

A single drug is seldom the only diffusing species—other drugs may diffuse and affect the permeation of the primary agent. Similarly, vehicle components, particularly low molecular weight solvents, may diffuse into the skin.

A significant source of confusion when interpreting percutaneous absorption processes arises from the assumption that the colloidal structure and composition of the vehicle remain constant after application to the skin. Violations to this stipulation include any phase changes and other alterations to the formulation which may occur as the patient rubs the base into the skin and any consequent changes during the time the vehicle remains on the surface. It is surprising how little we know about such changes as few investigations have been directed toward such crucial factors. Vehicle components must often evaporate or diffuse out of the vehicle, and skin secretions may penetrate the formulation. Both events may alter the physicochemical environment within the ointment or cream, compared to conditions within the container. For example, Coldman et al. (1969) used concentration changes arising from the loss of volatile components from a vehicle to promote steroid penetration through skin.

We have assumed that neither the penetrant nor the vehicle dynamically alters the diffusion coefficient of the drug in the barrier phase. However, during the permeation process, the pH of the stratum corneum and its hydration state may well change. The integrity of the barrier may decrease, even to the extent of frank, structural damage. The diffusivity of the drug may then not be independent of time or position within the barrier, or of drug concentration within the skin. These violations are both temporal and spatial, involving position within the skin and time of permeation.

The viable tissues may not function as a perfect sink, to sweep away diffusing molecules. Very nonpolar drugs may be so water insoluble that a negligible amount partitions from the stratum corneum into the epidermis and the flux across the horny layer becomes minimal. The stratum corneum may well absorb reasonable amounts of drug from the vehicle but not pass on the medicament to the site of action in, e.g., the dermis. This could happen with, say, some steroids, nicotinic acid esters, and the longer chain p-aminobenzoates, chemicals which are often used in laboratory investigations. The drug may also bind to components of the stratum corneum or induce vasoconstriction and thereby decrease the efficiency of the dermis as a sink.

A common postulate in skin permeation work, as it is one which is necessary for zero-order flux conditions to apply, is that the penetrant concentration or activity in the vehicle remains constant during the permeation process. However, in practice this assumption may often be infringed, and significant deviations probably occur in published work even when the authors assume compliance. Thus, finite amounts of drug may leave the vehicle to enter the skin, and the magnitude of this depletion effect will depend on the total amount of preparation applied. The skin may absorb vehicle components, or dilute the preparation with tissue fluids, with consequent effects on the drug's thermodynamic activity. Similarly, the drug may precipitate or supersaturate the vehicle as solvents leave, emulsions may invert, and pH changes may affect ionic drugs.

Unless the vehicle consists of an accepted penetration enhancer, or contains such an accelerant, it is tempting to assume that the vehicle is "inert" with respect to any effect it may have on the state of the skin. However, occlusive topicals such as ointments and pastes hydrate the skin, and high concentrations of, for example, glycols dehydrate the horny layer. A potentially more misleading concept is that most vehicle components do not affect the solubility of the drug in the skin barrier. In fact, many low molecular weight vehicle components such as propylene glycol (a good solvent for many drugs, e.g., steroids) probably pass rapidly into the stratum corneum. A "wick" effect may even operate. Once within the membrane, the solvent may increase the solubility of the drug in the layer of the stratum corneum in which the vehicle component concentrates. At the start of the diffusion process, this layer will be the topmost segment of the stratum corneum. The partition coefficient of the drug relative to this layer will increase, and this will lead to a raised concentration gradient for drugs across the stratum corneum. In vivo, it may well be that the solvent establishes steady state conditions both for its own diffusion and for the consequent increased flux of the drug. However, the vehicle may be depleted with respect to the solvent as time passes. The solvent concentration profile across the stratum corneum then alters and affects the flux of the drug. Thus, once again, temporal and spatial considerations further complicate any analysis of the permeation procedure. The effect of two or more mutually dependent diffusion processes occurring together in skin has seldom been thoroughly investigated. It is conceivable that the interpretation of some of the data in the

literature on drug permeation may be in error through neglecting the interaction of parallel permeation streams of vehicle components.

It is often assumed, without experimental verification, that the penetrant drug remains intact during permeation. However, the penetrant may
chemically degrade by, for example, hydrolysis or photolytic action, or
the skin may metabolize it. The vehicle or skin may sorb or complex with
the drug.

In a typical zero-order permeation experiment, flux estimates are
steady state values. In the clinic, steady state conditions may never be
achieved, as material is lost from the skin, dermatologicals are reapplied
several times daily, and the microenvironment of the skin changes dynamically.

From considerations such as those just detailed, we conclude that we
need an increased effort devoted to skin investigations under conditions
which more closely reflect clinical circumstances. Franz (1978) has recently moved towards this approach with his "finite dose" technique for
correlating in vitro skin diffusion with published in vivo work. A similar
technique has been used by Southwell and Barry (1981). During in vitro work
one could investigate systematically the effect of multiple application techniques with the skin at controlled hydration levels but not occluded. The
effect of vehicle changes after application to the skin and the role of vehicle
components in modifying skin could be studied. However, the design of the
experiment and the analysis of the results should still be as rigorous as
possible with respect to physicochemical theory. The requirement is therefore for a closer linking of the two main streams of investigation, which
we can designate as the biological and the physicochemical approach. A
synthesis of both outlooks is necessary for a successful attack on a dermatological problem which is to be approached via topical therapy.

F. Additional Comments on Diffusion Parameters
in Skin Permeation

In this section we briefly consider some additional influences on the diffusion coefficient and the partition coefficient with particular reference to
skin. Fundamental information on these parameters appears in Chaps. 2
and 3.

1. The diffusion coefficient

The diffusion coefficient was dealt with in some detail throughout
Chaps. 2 and 3, and specific factors which modify its value in homogeneous
liquids, aqueous and nonaqueous solutions, gels, and amorphous isotropic
polymers were considered in Chap. 2, Sec. III.D.

For typical small polar molecules such as water and the alcohols, the
reported diffusion coefficient in stratum corneum is of the order of 10^{-10} to

TABLE 4.4 Approximate Permeability Data for Various Homologous
Series Penetrating Through Skin

Penetrant	Diffusion coefficient (cm^2 sec^{-1})	Permeability coefficient (cm sec$^{-1} \times 10^7$)	Reference
C4 Series:			Blank and Scheuplein
Ethyl Ether	10^{-9}	42-48	(1969)
2-Butanone	10^{-9}	11-14	
1-Butanol	10^{-9}	5.6-11	
2-Ethoxyethanol	10^{-10}	0.56-0.84	
2-3-Butanediol	10^{-9}	0.14	
Alcohols—representative members:			Scheuplein and Blank (1973); Blank (1964); also see Table 3.3
Ethanol	10^{-9}	2.8	
Pentanol	10^{-9}	17	
Octanol	10^{-9}	146	
Steroids:			Scheuplein et al.
Progesterone	2×10^{-11}	4.2	(1969)
Cortexone	2×10^{-11}	1.3	
Cortexolone	4×10^{-12}	0.21	
Cortisone	1×10^{-12}	0.028	
Cortisol	3×10^{-13}	0.0084	

Source: Modified from Scheuplein (1978a).

10^{-9} cm^2 sec^{-1}, depending on the literature source (see Table 4.4; also
Table 3.3). At the other end of the spectrum, examples of values of diffusivities for steroids are aldosterone (4.9×10^{-13}), cortisone (1.3×10^{-12}),
testosterone (1.95×10^{-11}), and progesterone (1.6×10^{-11}) (Scheuplein
et al., 1969). Table 4.4 indicates that increased hydrogen bonding capacity
leads to decreased diffusivity through skin (Scheuplein, 1978a). Until now,
it has been generally assumed that the diffusivities of typical corticosteroids
which are used as topical anti-inflammatory agents are of the order of
10^{-13} cm^2 sec^{-1}. However, this value may be a significant underestimate,
and true estimates may be nearer 10^{-11} to 10^{-10} cm^2 sec^{-1} (Jones, 1979).
The evidence for this is twofold. Workers at Syntex Research, in California,
calculated D to be of the order of 10^{-11} cm^2 sec^{-1} from diffusive uptake
experiments with fluocinonide or fluocinolone acetonide penetrating human
skin in vitro. Jones (1979) also analyzed pharmacokinetically the vasoconstrictor data published by Barry and Woodford (1978) on betamethasone-
17-benzoate gels. He obtained an effective diffusivity of 1.1×10^{-11} cm^2 sec^{-1}

for this in vivo work. His analysis assumes that shunt diffusion is not important in triggering the vasoconstrictor response.

A possible explanation for the discrepancy between these results and those from older work depends on solvent effects which may not have been allowed for in the past. In some of the reported experiments with steroids in vitro, it is possible that the diffusivity slowly changed with time during the diffusion run as the solvent progressively conditioned the membrane. Thus, erroneously low values for D would be obtained from apparent lag times because no true steady state was established. If skin membranes are well conditioned with solvent before the flux experiment begins, then much shorter lag times, and hence higher diffusivities, are recorded. Additionally, the applicability of the lag-time method for determining diffusivities in heterogeneous membranes has been questioned (Flynn and Roseman, 1971).

In general, during any skin permeation process, the apparent diffusion coefficient determined may reflect influences other than the intrinsic mobility of the penetrant molecules. Such influences could include changes in drug mobility through the stratum corneum arising from plasticization by vehicle or penetrant, or deviations from ideal solution behavior. Internal chemical reactions within the tissue could immobilize a fraction of the penetrant molecules. All those factors may produce concentration dependent changes. However, regardless of the mechanisms which affect the magnitude of the diffusion coefficient, its value reflects the rate of penetration of a specific drug under specified conditions, and D is therefore a very useful parameter to know (Scheuplein, 1978a).

2. The partition coefficient

The basic physicochemical aspects of partition coefficient theory are dealt with in Chap. 2, Sec. III. B. Scheuplein (1978a) has considered the correlation between calculated and experimentally determined partition coefficients for stratum corneum.

At one time it was considered that an oil-water partition coefficient close to unity was required for good skin penetration (Cullumbine, 1948; Treherne, 1956). For example, Marzulli et al. (1965) found that, in the transport of phosphoric acid and various phosphates across isolated human stratum corneum, those compounds which were readily soluble in both benzene and water gave good steady state penetration rates. When the partition coefficient moved significantly from unity, the flux fell. Stoughton et al. (1960) recorded similar findings for nicotinic acid and its derivatives for the relationship between the "penetration index" (calculated from the minimum concentration required to produce erythema) and the partition coefficient between water and ether. Clendenning and Stoughton (1962) found an equivalent pattern of behavior between the water-benzene partition coefficients and the percentage absorption of various boronic acid derivatives.

However, the inference that a partition coefficient close to unity is necessary for good penetration for all homologous or congeneric series of compounds is incorrect, and the concept has led to erroneous conclusions (Katz and Poulsen, 1971). Many congeneric series display an optimal partition coefficient, well below the level of which the molecules are too water soluble to partition significantly into the stratum corneum. At higher values of the coefficient the compounds are so lipid soluble that they remain dissolved in the stratum corneum and will not readily pass into the water-rich viable tissues. This behavior leads to the well-known parabolic or bilinear relation between pharmacological activity and partition coefficient for a series of drugs. For many body tissues—for example, the gastrointestinal tract, the blood-aqueous barrier of the eye, and the skin—the optimal partition coefficient (n-octanol/water) at which maximum flux occurs is claimed to be 1,000 (Hansch and Dunn, 1972; Fujita et al., 1964).

The development of effective topic steroids to treat inflammatory diseases well exemplifies the importance of the partition coefficient. Thus, triamcinolone is five times more active systemically than hydrocortisone, yet it exhibits only one-tenth the topical activity. Conversion of the triamcinolone to its acetonide enhances its cutaneous activity 1,000-fold (McKenzie, 1962). Betamethasone possesses only 10 times the topical potency of hydrocortisone, although it is 30 times stronger systemically. Of 23 esters of betamethasone, the 17-valerate has the highest topical activity and this coincides with the most balanced lipid-water partition coefficient (McKenzie and Atkinson, 1964; Idson, 1975). The anti-inflammatory response to hydrocortisone and to its C-21 esters progressively develops as the ester side chain lengthens from zero to six carbon atoms and as the ether-water partition coefficient increases from 1.6 for hydrocortisone to 3,620 for hydrocortisone-21-caproate (Fig. 4.29). Thereafter the activity

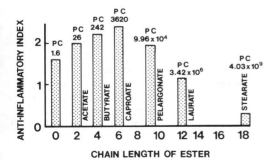

FIG. 4.29 Anti-inflammatory activity, ester chain length, and ether-water partition coefficients (P.C.) for hydrocortisone C-21 esters: P.C.'s above 3,620 were calculated. (From Schlagel and Northam, 1959; Schlagel, 1972.)

declines as the homologous series extends and the coefficient further
increases (Schlagel and Northam, 1959; Schlagel, 1972). Although molecular
modifications of the corticosteroids may change the anti-inflammatory
potency at least in part through alterations in the intrinsic activity at the
receptor site, the positive role of the partition coefficient in enhancing
transport through the skin to that site is undisputed.

All the foregoing examples use organic solvent/water distribution
measurements to correlate activity with partition coefficient. However,
realistically the only partition coefficient measurement for a drug that will
exactly relate to its permeation through the stratum corneum is the value
obtained for the equilibrium distribution of the penetrant between the topical
vehicle and the horny layer (Katz and Poulsen, 1971). But even when we
make equilibrium measurements for the drug between a solvent and isolated
stratum corneum, difficulties in interpretation still remain. In a typical
experiment, disks of stratum corneum may be immersed in a bathing solvent
containing the drug; the approach to equilibrium may take many days. If the
solvent is water, the tissue hydrates to a nonphysiological degree. Alternatively,
a glycol such as propylene glycol may dehydrate the membrane. Low molecular
weight solvents penetrate into the stratum corneum, possibly reaching high concentrations within the tissue. In extreme situations, e.g., for accelerants such
as DMSO, DMF, and DMAC, the stratum corneum may function almost like a
sponge. There may be so much solvent within the membrane that the drug does
not truly partition into the mosaic of the horny layer but dissolves in entrapped
solvent. Such conditions bear little resemblance to the usual in vivo use of topicals, where the vehicle is applied sparingly, penetrating molecules sweep into
the systemic circulation, and the stratum corneum is not saturated with solvent.

For convenience, even when workers determine partition coefficients
experimentally relative to stratum corneum, they often employ simple
solvents such as water or water/propylene glycol mixtures. Unless the
final marketed product is a simple gel, its components and structure may
bear little resemblance to the prototype test solvent. Thus, partition coefficients originally determined may not relate to the operative coefficient
when a patient applies an ointment or cream to a lesion. For severely
damaged skin, partitioning may not even be into the stratum corneum.

A final point is that experimentally determined partition coefficients
include any contributions that drug binding to stratum corneum components
makes. With extensive adsorption, it is possible to get high apparent partition coefficients yet have the penetration rate slower than for materials of
comparable molecular size and lipophilicity but which do not adsorb to
keratin.

3. Structure activity relationships

T. Higuchi (1977) recently discussed in a novel and interesting way the
relationship between the chemical structure of a drug and its optimal steady
state flux across the intact epidermal barrier. As he indicated, few funda-

mental experimental data exist on the effect of structural variation of chemical substances on their rates of percutaneous absorption. Scheuplein (1978a) and Scheuplein and Blank (1971) have summarized work on long-chain alcohols and steroids, and Feldman and Maibach (1970) considered some organic compounds. Scheuplein (1978a) speculated on how polar groups affect the route of penetration (see Chap. 3, Sec. II.D). However, such studies do not readily provide a systematic analysis of structure activity relationships.

In his discussion, T. Higuchi (1977) employs a model for the overall process of steady state percutaneous absorption that is a simplified version of Fig. 4.1. In his analysis, it is not necessary to consider specifically the follicular route, as it is often a minor pathway for percutaneous absorption and, anyway, the conclusions arrived at apply equally well to this route as to the bulk stratum corneum.

For the present discussion, we are particularly interested in the influence of drug structure on two steps in the overall process of absorption—the release of molecules from the solid state to the vehicle (e.g., for a suspension ointment) and the clearance of penetrant from the viable epidermis below the barrier layer of the stratum corneum.

a. Release of molecules to the vehicle If a drug substance has a finite solubility in its vehicle, the thermodynamic activity of the penetrant in the vehicle quickly reaches a common level following application to normal skin. Provided ideal conditions exist and the vehicle does not alter the skin barrier, the flux of drug through the stratum corneum relates directly to the thermodynamic activity of the drug immediately above the barrier; see Eq. (4.30). The pure drug substance, i.e., its crystals, usually provides the highest activity, which is maintained as long as any solid material remains in the applied layer.

Accepting that the maximum flux of drug through the skin will be closely controlled by the thermodynamic activity of the pure drug substance, we require a way of measuring or of predicting this maximal activity value for a wide variety of agents. If we could do this, we could in theory compare the relative maximal fluxes of a series of closely related or congeneric drugs. The problem is that classical thermodynamics does not apply to this situation. We cannot, for example, equate the activity of hydrocortisone with any concentration of betamethasone. There is no method in classical thermodynamics by which, for example, n molecules of hydrocortisone can equal m molecules of betamethasone.

We need to measure the relative ability of different drug molecules to escape from their neat states, which are usually crystalline. The usual convention is to choose, for organic materials, the pure solute at a given temperature and pressure as the standard state, with unit thermodynamic activity. For the present purposes, this approach has three basic weaknesses (Rytting et al., 1972; Davis et al., 1974; T. Higuchi, 1977):

1. The method confers the same numerical value for all pure substances. We require an approach which compares the escaping tendencies of a variety of substances in a quantitative fashion.
2. Most organic compounds exist in a number of crystalline forms (polymorphs) which may differ substantially in their energies.
3. Each drug in this reference state has a significantly different environment. The energetics of the escape depend not only on the kind of matrix which the molecules leave but also on the phase into which they pass. If we can select some common environment for the receptor phase, then we have selected a <u>reference state</u>, as it is known in chemical thermodynamics.

Following a detailed justification, Rytting et al. (1972) proposed that for the purpose of drug design it would be useful to designate an infinitely dilute solution of an alkane solvent as the reference state. Suitable aliphatic solvents would include hexane, cyclohexane, heptane, octane, and isooctane; all appear to yield approximately the same qualitative results. Among other advantages, the approach may be used to predict structure-activity relationships for systems essentially at equilibrium or quasi-equilibrium (T. Higuchi and Davis, 1970) such as steady state skin permeation. The thermodynamic activity of the drug, either in solution or in its pure state, is expressed in terms of the hypothetical concentration of the species in an infinitely dilute alkane solution such that

$$a_i = \gamma_i C_i \tag{4.31}$$

where a_i, γ_i, and C_i are the activity, activity coefficient, and concentration (moles/liter), respectively, of drug i; and γ approaches unity as C tends to zero. Thus, we accept as the standard reference state an infinitely dilute solution of the drug in an alkane solvent, and we set its hypothetical 1 M concentration to a thermodynamic activity of 1 (1 M or 1 mol fraction could also be used as the theoretical concentration).

This line of reasoning can lead to predictions with respect to the maximal rates of percutaneous absorption of different drugs. The basic concept or theorem can be expressed thus: "All other factors being equal, the maximal rate of transport of any chemical species is directly proportional to the thermodynamic activity of the pure form of the species defined in the terms given above" (T. Higuchi, 1977).

Table 4.5 lists a variety of substances, together with their approximate thermodynamic activities in the pure state, as defined above. Provided that all other factors are equal, the Higuchi theorem predicts that the maximal expected rate of percutaneous delivery should correlate with the values of the activities given. On this basis we would expect, for example, that chloroform and benzene would be delivered about a hundred times faster than the polar alcohols methanol and ethanol. Steroidal molecules (e.g., methyl testosterone or norethindrone and its acetate) should be delivered

TABLE 4.5 Approximate Thermodynamic Activities of Pure Compounds, for Correlation with Maximal Percutaneous Delivery

Compound	Activity of Pure State[a] (mol liter^{-1})	Compound	Activity of Pure State[a] (mol liter^{-1})
Methanol	0.1	Phenol	0.67
Ethanol	0.135	4-Iodophenol	1.56×10^{-2}
1-Butanol	0.20	4-Nitrophenol	3.6×10^{-4}
1-Hexanol	0.41	2,4,6-Triiodophenol	5×10^{-3}
Acetanilide	9×10^{-3}	Phthalic anhydride	5×10^{-4}
Benzene	11.2	Methyl testosterone	1.23×10^{-3}
Chloroform	12.4	Norethindrone	7.1×10^{-5}
Carbazole	1.5×10^{-3}	Norethindrone acetate	2.75×10^{-3}
Ethyl ether	9.55	Hydrocortisone	$< 2 \times 10^{-6}$
Picric acid	3×10^{-4}	Hydrocortisone acetate	$< 2 \times 10^{-6}$

[a]Estimated values at 25 °C with infinitely dilute solution in hexane, heptane, or octane having activity coefficient of unity (1 M concentration).
Source: T. Higuchi (1977).

much more slowly than such simple nonelectrolytes, and topical steroids such as hydrocortisone and hydrocortisone acetate should have low rates.

The basic theorem agrees with various empirical observations. These simple rules include such statements as:

1. Lipid molecules are more easily delivered to the skin than are hydrophilic molecules.
2. Polar substances are not as well absorbed as are nonpolar materials.
3. The lower the melting point of a solid, the more easily it is absorbed.
4. Organic liquids are better absorbed than solids.

The most important aspect of this approach is that it allows quantitative estimates as to the rate of percutaneous absorption of drugs in an area in which, because of experimental difficulties, including assay problems, experimental progress is usually slow and laborious.

b. Clearance of molecules from the stratum corneum barrier   After a molecule penetrates the stratum corneum, it suddenly meets the viable epidermis, which is an essentially aqueous phase. If the molecule is very

TABLE 4.6 Estimated Activity Coefficients of Organic Compounds in Water at 25 °C, for Correlation with Clearance from the Stratum Corneum Barrier

Compound	Activity coefficient[a]	Compound	Activity coefficient[a]
Alcohols		Phenol	0.70
Methanol	5.0×10^{-3}		
Ethanol	1.0×10^{-2}	Amines	
1-Propanol	4.3×10^{-2}	Butylamine	0.76
2-Propanol	2.7×10^{-2}	Pentylamine	3.1
1-Butanol	0.24	Hexylamine	13
2-Butanol	0.11	Octylamine	2.3×10^{2}
2-Methyl 1-Propanol	0.17	Decylamine	4.1×10^{3}
2-Methyl 2-Propanol	0.09	Alkanes	
1-Pentanol	0.98	Pentane	1.2×10^{4}
1-Hexanol	4.4	Hexane	6.2×10^{4}
1-Octanol	96	Heptane	2.5×10^{5}
1-Decanol	210	Octane	1.2×10^{6}

[a]Based on activity coefficients in infinitely dilute solution in isooctane to be unity with concentrations in mol liter^{-1}.
Source: T. Higuchi (1977).

lipophilic, with a low water solubility and a high affinity for the cornified tissue, its further transport toward the deeper tissues is adversely affected. For such molecules the thermodynamic activity of the diffusing species immediately below the horny layer barrier approaches that of the source and the rate-determining step is no longer the penetration of the barrier but rather clearance from the barrier.

We can arrive at some useful predictions with respect to those drugs for which barrier clearance may be important by considering the magnitudes of their activity coefficients in water (which are assumed to be similar to those in the water logged viable epidermis). If we use the same standard state for our drug substances as defined above, we can define the activity coefficient as

$$\gamma_{ik} = \frac{a_i}{C_{ik}} \tag{4.32}$$

where a_i is the activity of i in the system defined in terms of the unit molar hypothetically infinitely dilute reference system; γ_{ik} is the activity coefficient of i in a solvent, k, in equilibrium with the reference system; and C_{ik} is the concentration (moles per liter) of i in the solvent k.

For most lipophilic drugs in water, activity coefficients so defined are much greater than 1. Table 4.6 lists the estimated activity coefficients of some common substances in dilute aqueous solution. One way of appreciating the usefulness of these data is to realize that, for example, for a long-chain alcohol such as 1-octanol, a 0.01 M solution in water has the same thermodynamic driving tendency for octanol as its 1 M solution in an alkane solvent such as isooctant. Similarly, for methanol a theoretical 200 M solution in water would be needed to provide the same driving tendency as the unit molar solution in isooctane. This is a thermodynamic way for quantifying the concept that at the same concentration of drug polar materials are released to the skin better from nonpolar solvents than from polar solvents; for nonpolar materials the reverse is true. For the extreme case listed in the table (octane) a 8.3×10^{-7} M solution in water is equivalent to the 1 M isooctane solution.

T. Higuchi (1977) concludes that clearance from the barrier as the rate-determining process probably does not become significant for drugs until their activity coefficient in water becomes greater than about 10^3 to 10^5.

REFERENCES

Aguiar, A. J., and Weiner, M. A. (1969). J. Pharm. Sci. 58:210.

Allenby, A. C., Creasey, N. H., Edgington, J. A. G., Fletcher, J. A., and Schock, C. (1969a). Br. J. Dermatol. 81(Suppl. 4):47.

Allenby, A. C., Fletcher, J., Schock, C., and Tees, T. F. S. (1969b). Br. J. Dermatol. 81(Suppl. 4):31.

Almeyda, J., and Burt, B. W. (1974). Br. J. Dermatol. 91:579.

Almeyda, J., and Fry, L. (1973). Br. J. Dermatol. 88:493.

Amin, M. (1967). Ph.D. Thesis, University of Wisconsin, Madison.

Andersen, K. E., Maibach, H. I., and Anjo, M. D. (1980). Br. J. Dermatol. 102:447.

Anderson, R. L., Cassidy, J. M., Hansen, J. R., and Yellin, W. (1973). Biopolymers 12:2789.

Ando, H. Y., Ho, N. F. H., and Higuchi, W. I. (1977a). J. Pharm. Sci. 66:1977.

Ando, H. Y., Ho, N. F. H., and Higuchi, W. I. (1977b). J. Pharm. Sci. 66:1525.

Anonymous (1971). Drug. Ther. Bull. 9:29.

Anonymous (1973). Med. Lett. 15:104.

Arita, T., Hori, R., Anmo, T., Washitake, M., Akatsu, M., and Yajima, T. (1970). Chem. Pharm. Bull. 18:1045.

Armstrong, R. W., Eichner, E. R., Klein, D. E., Barthel, W. F., Bennett, J. V., Jonsson, V., Bruce, H., and Loveless, L. E. (1969). J. Pediat. 75:317.

Arno, I. C., Wapner, P. M., and Brownstein, I. E. (1967). Ann. N.Y. Acad. Sci. 141:403.

Ashton, H., Frenk, E., and Stevenson, C. J. (1970). Br. J. Dermatol. 84:194.

Association of the British Pharmaceutical Industry (1977). Guidelines for Preclinical and Clinical Testing of New Medicinal Products, Pt. 1: Laboratory Investigations, London, p. 1.

Astley, J. P., and Levine, M. (1975). J. Pharm. Sci. 65:210.

Ayres, P. J. W. (1977). In The Icthyoses, R. Marks and P. J. Dyke (Eds.). M.T.P. Press, Cardiff, Wales, p. 167.

Ayres, P. J. W., and Hooper, G. (1978). Br. J. Dermatol. 99:307.

Ayres, P. J. W., and Laskar, P. A. (1974). J. Pharm. Sci. 63:351.

Ayres, S. A., and Mihan, R. (1967). Cutis 3:139.

Baker, H. (1968). J. Invest. Dermatol. 50:283.

Barr, M. (1962). J. Pharm. Sci. 51:395.

Barrett, C. W., Hadgraft, J. W., Caron, G. A., and Sarkany, I. (1965). Br. J. Dermatol. 77:576.

Barry, B. W. (1976). Dermatologica 152(Suppl. 1):47.

Barry, B. W., and Grace, A. J. (1971). J. Texture Studies 2:259.

Barry, B. W., and Woodford, R. (1974). Br. J. Dermatol. 91:323.

Barry, B. W., and Woodford, R. (1975). Br. J. Dermatol. 93:563.

Barry, B. W., and Woodford, R. (1976). Br. J. Dermatol. 95:423.

Barry, B. W., and Woodford, R. (1977). Br. J. Dermatol. 97:555.

Barry, B. W., and Woodford, R. (1978). J. Clin. Pharm. 3:43.

Bartek, M. J., and La Budde, J. A. (1975). In Animal Models in Dermatology, H. Maibach (Ed.). Churchill Livingstone, Edinburgh and London, p. 103.

Bartek, M. J., La Budde, J. A., and Maibach, H. I. (1972). J. Invest. Dermatol. 58:114.

Beger, I., and Hauthal, H. G. (1976). In Dimethyl Sulfoxide, D. Martin and H. G. Hauthal (Eds.). Van Nostrand Reinhold, New York.

Behl, C. R., Flynn, G. L., Kurihara, T., Harper, N., Smith, W., Higuchi, W. I., Ho, N. F. H., and Pierson, C. L. (1980). J. Invest. Dermatol. 75:346.

Benson, P. F., and Pharoah, P. O. D. (1960). Guy Hosp. Rep. 109:212.

Berliner, D. L. (1972). Adv. Biol. Skin 12:357.

Bettley, F. R. (1961). Br. J. Dermatol. 73:448.

Bettley, F. R. (1963). Br. J. Dermatol. 75:113.

Bettley, F. R. (1965). Br. J. Dermatol. 77:98.

Bettley, F. R., and Donoghue, E. (1960). Nature 185:17.

Bickers, D. R. (1980). In Current Concepts in Cutaneous Toxicity, V. A. Drill and P. Lazar (Eds.). Academic Press, New York, p. 95.

Black, J. G., and Howes, D. (1979). J. Soc. Cosmetic Chemists 30:157.

Blank, I. H. (1952). J. Invest. Dermatol. 18:433.

Blank, I. H. (1953). J. Invest. Dermatol. 21:259.

Blank, I. H. (1964). J. Invest. Dermatol. 43:415.

Blank, I. H. (1965). J. Invest. Dermatol. 45:249.

Blank, I. H., and Gould, E. (1959). J. Invest. Dermatol. 33:327.

Blank, I. H., and Gould, E. (1961a). J. Invest. Dermatol. 37:311.

Blank, I. H., and Gould, E. (1961b). J. Invest. Dermatol. 37:485.

Blank, I. H., and Scheuplein, R. J. (1964). In Progress in the Biological Sciences in Relation to Dermatology. A. Rook and R. H. Champion (Eds.), Vol. 2. Cambridge Univ. Press, New York, p. 245.

Blank, I. H., and Scheuplein, R. J. (1969). Br. J. Dermatol. 81(Suppl. 4): 4.

Blank, I. H., and Shapiro, E. B. (1955). J. Invest. Dermatol. 25:391.

Blank, I. H., Gould, E., and Theobald, A. B. (1964). J. Invest. Dermatol. 42:363.

Blank, I. H., Scheuplein, R. J., and MacFarlane, D. J. (1967). J. Invest. Dermatol. 49:582.

Blois, M. S. (1972). Adv. Biol. Skin 12:153.

Blois, M. S., and Taskovitch, L. (1969). J. Invest. Dermatol. 53:344.

Borgstedt, H. H., and Di Stefano, V. (1967). Toxicol. Appl. Pharmacol. 10:523.

Borodkin, S., and Tucker, F. E. (1974). J. Pharm. Sci. 63:1359.

Bottari, F., Nannipieri, E., Saettone, M. F., Serafini, M. F., and Vitale, D. (1978). J. Soc. Cosmetic Chemists 29:353.

Braudé, M. C., and Monroe, R. R. (1965). Curr. Ther. Res. Clin. Exp. 7:502.

Brechner, V. L., Cohen, D. D., and Pretsky, I. (1967). Ann. N.Y. Acad. Sci. 141:524.

Breuer, M. M. (1979). J. Soc. Cosmetic Chemists 30:41.

Britz, M. B., Maibach, H. I., and Anjo, D. M. (1980). Arch. Dermatol. Res. 267:313.

Brobyn, R. D. (1975). In Biological Actions of Dimethyl Sulfoxide, S. W. Jacob and R. Herschler (Eds.). Ann. N.Y. Acad. Sci. 243:497.

Brode, E. (1968). Arzneim. Forsch. 18:580.

Brown, B. W. (1970). Am. J. Publ. Health 60:901.

Brown, J. H. (1967). Ann. N.Y. Acad. Sci. 141:496.

Brown, J., Winkelman, R. K., and Wolff, K. (1967). J. Invest. Dermatol. 49:386.

Burch, G. E., and Winsor, T. (1944). Arch. Intern. Med. 74:437.

Busse, M. J., Hunt, P., Lees, K. A., Maggs, P. N. D., and McCarthy, T. M. (1969). Br. J. Dermatol. 81(Suppl. 4):103.

Caccialanza, P., and Finzi, A. F. (1966). Farmaco [Prat.] 21:197.

Caldwell, I. W., Hall-Smith, S. P., Main, R. A., Ashurst, P. J., Kurton, V., Simpson, W. T., and Williams, G. W. (1968). Br. J. Dermatol. 80:11.

Campbell, P., Watanabe, T., and Chandrasekaran, S. K. (1976). Fed. Proc. 35:639.

Chandrasekaran, S. K., and Hillman, R. (1980). J. Pharm. Sci. 69:1311.
Chandrasekaran, S. K., and Shaw, J. E. (1977). Contemp. Topics Polymer
    Sci., 2:291.
Chandrasekaran, S. K., and Shaw, J. E. (1978). Curr. Probl. Dermatol.
    7:142.
Chandrasekaran, S. K., Michaels, A. S., Campbell, P., and Shaw, J. E.
    (1976). Am. Inst. Chem. Eng. 22:828.
Chandrasekaran, S. K., Campbell, P. S., and Michaels, A. S. (1977).
    Am. Inst. Chem. Eng. 23:810.
Chandrasekaran, S. K., Bayne, W., and Shaw, J. E. (1978a). J. Pharm.
    Sci. 67:1370.
Chandrasekaran, S. K., Benson, H., and Urquhart, J. (1978b). In Sustained
    and Controlled Release Drug Delivery Systems, J. R. Robinson (Ed.).
    Dekker, New York, p. 557.
Chandrasekaran, S. K., Theeuwes, F., and Yum, S. I. (1979). In Drug
    Design, E. J. Ariens (Ed.), Vol. 7. Academic Press, New York,
    p. 133.
Chandrasekaran, S. K., Campbell, P. S., and Watanabe, T. (1980).
    Polymer Eng. Sci. 20:36.
Chignell, C. F. (1971). In Handbook of Experimental Pharmacology, B. B.
    Brodie and J. Gillette (Eds.), Vol. 28, Pt. 1. Springer-Verlag, New
    York, p. 187.
Chowhan, Z. T., and Pritchard, R. (1975). J. Pharm. Sci. 64:754.
Chowhan, Z. T., and Pritchard, R. (1978). J. Pharm. Sci. 67:1272.
Chowhan, Z. T., Pritchard, R., Rooks, W. H., and Tomolonis, A. (1978).
    J. Pharm. Sci. 67:1645.
Christie, G. A., and Moore-Robinson, M. (1970). Br. J. Dermatol.
    Suppl. 6. 82:93.
Clendenning, W. E., and Stoughton, R. B. (1962). J. Invest. Dermatol.
    39:47.
Cohen, J. L., and Stoughton, R. B. (1974). J. Invest. Dermatol. 62:507.
Coldman, M. F., Poulsen, B. J., and Higuchi, T. (1969). J. Pharm. Sci.
    58:1098.
Coldman, M. F., Kalinovsky, T., and Poulsen, B. J. (1971). Br. J.
    Dermatol. 85:457.
Collom, W. D., and Winek, C. L. (1968). Clin. Tox. 1:309.
Conning, D. M., and Hayes, M. J. (1970). Br. J. Ind. Med. 27:155.
Cooperman, E. S. (1972). Cosmetics Perfumer 87:65.
Cortese, T. A. (1971). In Dimethyl Sulfoxide, Vol. 1: Basic Concepts of
    DMSO, S. W. Jacob, E. E. Rosenbaum, and D. C. Wood (Eds.). Dekker,
    New York, p. 337.
Craig, F. N., Cummings, E. G., and Sim, V. M. (1977). J. Invest.
    Dermatol. 68:357.
Cramer, M. B., and Cates, L. A. (1974). J. Pharm. Sci. 63:793.
Crank, J. (1975). In The Mathematics of Diffusion, 2nd ed. Oxford Univ.
    Press (Clarendon), New York.

Creasey, N. H., Battensby, J., and Fletcher, J. A. (1978). Curr. Probl. Dermatol. 7:95.
Cronin, E., and Stoughton, R. B. (1962). Br. J. Dermatol. 74:265.
Crown Zellerbach Corp. (S. W. Jacob and R. J. Herschler), Belgian Patent 644,613 (1964), U.S. Prior 1963; see Chem. Abstr. 63:9759b (1965).
Crown Zellerbach Corp., Dutch Claim 6,414,293 (1965), U.S. Prior 1963; see Chem. Abstr. 65:15167h (1966).
Csaky, T. Z., and Ho, P. M. (1966). Proc. Soc. Exp. Biol. Med. 122:860.
Cullumbine, H. (1948). Q. J. Exp. Physiol. 34:83.
Cumpelik, B. (1976). Cosmetics Toiletries 91:61.
Curri, S. B. (1967). Soap, Perfum. Cosmet. 40:109.
Davis, L. D. (1966). Clin. Med. 73:70.
Davis, S. S., Higuchi, T., and Rytting, J. H. (1974). Adv. Pharm. Sci. 4:73.
Dawber, R. P. R. (1972). Br. Med. J. iv:300.
Dawber, R. P. R. (1974). Br. Med. J. ii:526.
Dempski, R. E., Demarco, J. D., and Marcus, A. D. (1965). J. Invest. Dermatol. 44:361.
Desgroseilliers, J. P., Ling, G. M., Brisson, G., and Streter, J. (1969). J. Invest. Dermatol. 53:270.
Dienhuber, P., and Tregear, R. T. (1960). J. Physiol. 152:58.
Digiulio, D. N. (1977). U.S. Patent 4,017,641 (Apr. 12, 1977).
Dillaha, C. J., Jansen, G. T., and Honeycutt, M. W. (1966). Q. Bull. Dermatol. Found. (New York), p. 1.
Di Stefano, V., and Borgstedt, H. H. (1964). Science 144:1137.
Djan, T. I., and Grunberg, D. L. (1967). Ann. N.Y. Acad. Sci. 141:406.
Dobson, R. L., Jacob, S. W., and Herschler, R. J. (1970). U.S. Patent 3,499,961.
Dugard, P. H. (1977). Adv. Mod. Toxicol. 4:525.
Dugard, P. H., and Embery, G. (1969). Br. J. Dermatol. 81(Suppl. 4):69.
Dugard, P. H., and Scheuplein, R. J. (1973). J. Invest. Dermatol. 60:263.
Dugard, P. H., and Scott, R. C. (1978). I. C. I. Macclesfield, U.K. Personal Communication.
Durrheim, H., Flynn, G. L., Higuchi, W. I., and Behl, C. R. (1980). J. Pharm. Sci. 69:781.
Dutkiewicz, T., and Piotrowski, J. (1962). Prom. Toksikol. Klinika Prof. Zabolevanii Khim. Etiol. (Moscow: Gos. Izd. Med. Lit.) 5b 39:49.
Elfbaum, S. G., and Laden, K. (1968a). J. Soc. Cosmetic Chemists 19:119.
Elfbaum, S. G., and Laden, K. (1968b). J. Soc. Cosmetic Chemists 19:163.
Elfbaum, S. G., and Laden, K. (1968c). J. Soc. Cosmetic Chemists 19:841.
Elliott, J. A. Jr., and Odel, H. M. (1950). J. Invest. Dermatol. 15:389.

El-Shimi, A. F., Princen, H. M., and Risi, D. R. (1975). In Applied
Chemistry at Protein Interfaces (ACS Adv. Chem. No. 145), R. E.
Baier (Ed.). Washington, D.C., p. 125.
Elworthy, P. H., and Worthington, H. E. C. (1968). J. Pharm. Pharmacol.
20:830.
Embery, G., and Dugard, P. H. (1969). Br. J. Dermatol. 81(Suppl. 4):63.
Fabianek, J., and Herp, A. (1966). Proc. Soc. Exp. Biol. Med. 122:290.
Fanconi, V. G. (1962). Helv. Paediat. Acta 17:267.
Faucher, J. A., and Goddard, E. D. (1978a). J. Soc. Cosmetic Chemists
29:323.
Faucher, J. A., and Goddard, E. D. (1978b). J. Colloid Interface Sci.
65:444.
Faucher, J. A., and Goddard, E. D. (1978c). J. Soc. Cosmetic Chemists
29:339.
Faucher, J. A., Goddard, E. D., and Kulkarni, R. D. (1979). J. Am. Oil
Chem. Soc. 56:776.
Feiwel, M. (1969). Br. J. Dermatol. 81(Suppl. 4):113.
Feiwel, M., James, V. H. T., and Barnet, E. S. (1969). Lancet i:485.
Feldmann, R. J., and Maibach, H. I. (1966). Arch. Dermatol. 94:649.
Feldmann, R. J., and Maibach, H. I. (1967). J. Invest. Dermatol. 48:181.
Feldmann, R. J., and Maibach, H. I. (1969). J. Invest. Dermatol. 52:89.
Feldmann, R. J., and Maibach, H. I. (1970). J. Invest. Dermatol. 54:399.
Feldmann, R. J., and Maibach, H. I. (1974a). Toxicol. Appl. Pharmacol.
28:126.
Feldmann, R. J., and Maibach, H. I. (1974b). Arch. Dermatol. 109:58.
Felsher, Z., and Rothman, S. (1945). J. Invest. Dermatol. 6:271.
Fienblatt, B. I., Aceto, T., Beckhorn, G. (1966). Am. J. Dis. Child.
112:218.
Finkelstein, P., and Laden, K. (1971). Appl. Polymer Symp. No. 18:673.
Flesch, P., and Esoda, E. C. J. (1960). J. Invest. Dermatol. 35:43.
Flesch, P., and Esoda, E. C. J. (1963). Arch. Dermatol. 88:706.
Flesch, P., Esoda, E. C. J., and Roe, D. A. (1961). Arch. Dermatol.
84:213.
Flesch, P., Esoda, E. C. J., and Hodgson, C. (1962). Arch. Dermatol.
85:476.
Floden, C. H., Hagerman, G., Leczinsky, C. G., Skogh, M., and Swan-
beck, G. (1971). Läkartidningen 68:5160.
Flynn, G. L., and Roseman, T. J. (1971). J. Pharm. Sci. 60:1788.
Flynn, G. L., and Smith, R. G. (1972). J. Pharm. Sci. 61:61.
Forbes, P. D. (1969). Adv. Biol. Skin 9:419.
Foreman, M. I., Kelly, I., and Lukowiecki, G. A. (1977). J. Pharm.
Pharmacol. 29:108.
Foreman, M. I., Clanachan, I., and Kelly, I. P. (1978). J. Pharm.
Pharmacol. 30:152.
Fox, C., Tassof, J. A., Rieger, M. M., and Dean, J. E. (1962). J. Soc.
Cosmetic Chemists 13:263.

Fox, J. L., Yu, C.-D., Higuchi, W. I., and Ho, N. F. H. (1979). Int. J. Pharmaceutics 2:41.

Franz, T. J. (1978). Curr. Probl. Dermatol. 7:58.

Fredricksson, T. (1963). Acta Derm. Venereol. 43:91.

Fritsch, W. C., and Stoughton, R. B. (1963). J. Invest. Dermatol. 41:307.

Frosch, P. J., and Kligman, A. M. (1977). Br. J. Dermatol. 96:461.

Frosch, P. J., Duncan, S., and Kligman, A. M. (1980). Br. J. Dermatol. 102:263.

Fujita, T., Iwasa, J., and Hansch, C. (1964). J. Am. Chem. Soc. 86:5175.

Gabourel, J. (1972). Adv. Biol. Skin 12:51.

Garrett, H. E. (1965). Trans. St. John Hosp. Dermatol. Soc. 51:166.

General Practitioner Research Group (1973). Report No. 179. Practitioner 210:294.

Gibaldi, M. (1977). Biopharmaceutics and Clinical Pharmacokinetics, 2nd ed., Lea & Febiger, Philadelphia.

Gibaldi, M., and Perrier, D. (1975). Pharmacokinetics. Dekker, New York.

Gillian, J. M. N., and Florence, A. T. (1973). J. Pharm. Pharmacol. 25(Suppl.):137P.

Giorgi, G., and Segre, G. (1966). DMSO Symp. Vienna. G. Laudahn and K. Gertich (Eds.). (Publ. by Dolicur, Soladruck, Berlin.)

Goldman, L., Igelman, J. M., and Kitzmiller, K. (1967). Ann. N.Y. Acad. Sci. 141:428.

Goldstein, A. (1949). Pharmacol. Rev. 1:102.

Goldstein, A., Kalman, S. M., and Aronow, L. (1969). Principles of Drug Action. Harper & Row, New York, p. 106.

Gomez, E. C., and Prost, P. (1972). Adv. Biol. Skin 12:367.

Gomez, E. C., and Hsia, S. L. (1968). Biochemistry 7:24.

Greaves, M. S. (1971). J. Invest. Dermatol. 57:100.

Greeson, T. P., Levan, N. E., Freedman, R. I., and Wong, W. H. (1973). J. Invest. Dermatol. 61:242.

Grice, K., Sattar, H., and Baker, H. (1973). Acta Derm. Venereol. 53:114.

Groel, J. T. (1968). Arch. Dermatol. 97:110.

Gross, E., Kiese, M., and Resag, K. (1960). Arch. Toxikol. 18:331.

Hadgraft, J. (1980). Int. J. Pharmaceutics 4:229.

Haleblian, J., and McCrone, W. (1969). J. Pharm. Sci. 58:911.

Hall-Smith, S. P. (1962). Br. Med. J. 2:1233.

Hansch, C., and Dunn, W. J. (1972). J. Pharm. Sci. 61:1.

Hansen, M. S. (1978). Am. J. Cardiol. 42:1061.

Harrold, S. P., and Pethica, B. A. (1958). Trans. Faraday Soc. 54:1876.

Hausler, G., and Jahn, H. (1966). Arch. Int. Pharmacodyn. Ther. 159:386.

Heilmann, K. (1978). In Therapeutic Systems—Pattern-Specific Drug Delivery: Concept and Development. Thieme, Stuttgart, p. 52.

Henderson, T. R., Henderson, R. F., and York, J. L. (1975). In Biological Actions of Dimethyl Sulfoxide (Ann. N.Y. Acad. Sci. 243), S. W. Jacob and R. Herschler (Eds.), p. 38.

Hersle, K., and Gisslen, H. (1972). Z. Haut Geschlechtskr. 47:571.

Hey, M. J., Taylor, D. J., and Derbyshire, W. (1978). Biochem. Biophys. Acta 54:518.

Highman, B., and Altland, P. D. (1969). Life Sci. 8:673.

Higuchi, T. (1960). J. Soc. Cosmetic Chemists 11:85.

Higuchi, T. (1961). J. Pharm. Sci. 50:874.

Higuchi, T. (1977). In Design of Biopharmaceutical Properties through Prodrugs and Analogs, B. Roche (Ed.). American Pharmaceutical Association, Washington, D.C., p. 409.

Higuchi, T. (1979). Paper read at Postgraduate School on Optimisation of Drug Delivery, April. The School of Pharmacy, University of London. Publ. by the Pharmaceutical Society of Great Britain, p. 204.

Higuchi, T., and Davis, S. S. (1970). J. Pharm. Sci. 59:1376.

Higuchi, T., Richards, J. H., Davis, S. S., Kamada, A., Hou, J. P., Nakano, M., Nakamo, N. I., and Pitman, I. H. (1969). J. Pharm. Sci. 58:661.

Higuchi, W. I. (1961). Proc. Am. Soc. Coll. Pharm. Teachers Seminar 13:163.

Higuchi, W. I. (1962). J. Pharm. Sci. 51:802.

Higuchi, W. I. (1967). J. Pharm. Sci. 56:315.

Higuchi, W. I., and Higuchi, T. (1960). J. Am. Pharm. Assoc., Sci. Ed. 49:598.

Hindson, T. C. (1971). Arch. Dermatol. 104:284.

Holbrook, K. A., and Odland, G. F. (1974). J. Invest. Dermatol. 62:415.

Hooper, G. (1979). Pharm. J. p. 303.

Hooper, W. D., Bochner, F., Eadie, M. J., and Tyrer, J. H. (1974). Clin. Pharmacol. Ther. 15:276.

Hoppe, U. (1973). J. Soc. Cosmetic Chemists 24:317.

Horhota, S. T., and Fung, H.-L. (1978). J. Pharm. Sci. 67:1345.

Horita, A., and Weber, L. G. (1964). Life Sci. 3:1389.

Horsch, W. (1975). Pharm. Praxis Pharmazie 20:241.

Hsia, S. L. (1980). In Percutaneous Absorption of Steroids, P. Mauvais-Jarvis, C. F. H. Vickers, and J. Wepierre (Eds.). Academic Press, New York, p. 81.

Hsia, S. L., and Hao, Y. (1966). Biochemistry 5:1469.

Hsia, S. L., and Hao, Y. (1967). Steroids 10:489.

Hsia, S. L., Witten, V. H., and Hao, Y. L. (1964). J. Invest. Dermatol. 43:407.

Hsia, S. L., Mussallen, A. J., and Witten, V. H. (1965). J. Invest. Dermatol. 45:384.

Hucker, H. B., Miller, J. K., Hochberg, A., Brobyn, R. D., Riordan, F. H., and Calesnick, B. (1967). J. Pharmacol. Exp. Ther. 155:309.

Hunziker, N., Feldmann, R. J., and Maibach, H. I. (1978). Dermatologica 156:79.

Idson, B. (1967). J. Soc. Cosmetic Chemists 18:91.
Idson, B. (1969a). Drug Cosmet. Ind. 104(6):44.
Idson, B. (1969b). Drug Cosmet. Ind. 105(1):48.
Idson, B. (1971). In Absorption Phenomena (Topics in Medicinal Chemistry, Vol. 4), J. L. Rabinowitz and R. M. Myerson (Eds.). Wiley (Interscience), New York, p. 181.
Idson, B. (1975). J. Pharm. Sci. 64:901.
Idson, B. (1978a). J. Soc. Cosmetic Chemists 29:573.
Idson, B. (1978b). Curr. Probl. Dermatol. 7:132.
Imperial Chemical Industries Ltd. (J. S. D. Pearce and N. Senior), British Patent 1,040,635 (1964a); see Chem. Abstr. 65:18435c (1966).
Imperial Chemical Industries Ltd. (N. Senior), British Patent 1,043,012 (1964b); see Chem. Abstr. 66:14045t (1967).
Imperial Chemical Industries Ltd. (N. Senior and J. L. Madinaveitia), British Patent 1,043,104 (1964c); see Chem. Abstr. 66:5776h (1967).
Isherwood, P. A. (1963). J. Invest. Dermatol. 40:143.
Jacob, S. W. (1965). DMSO Symp., Berlin. G. Laudahn and H. J. Schlosshauer (Eds.). (Publ. by Dolicur, Soladruck, Berlin), p. 54.
Jacob, S. W., and Herschler, R. (1975). Editors for Biological Actions of Dimethyl Sulfoxide. Ann. N.Y. Acad. Sci. 243.
Jacob, S. W., and Rosenbaum, E. E. (1967). Ann. N.Y. Acad. Sci. 141:1.
Jacob, S. W., and Wood, D. C. (1967). Curr. Ther. Res. 9:299.
Jacob, S. W., Bischel, M., and Herschler, R. J. (1964). Curr. Ther. Res. 6:134.
Jacob, S. W., Rosenbaum, E. E., and Wood, D. C. (1971). Dimethyl Sulfoxide, Vol. 1: Basic Concepts. Dekker, New York, p. 479.
Jacobi, O. (1958). J. Appl. Physiol. 12:403.
Jacobi, O. (1959). Proc. Sci. Sect. Toilet Goods Assoc. 31:22.
Jacobi, O. (1972). Cosmetics Perfumer 87:35.
Jacoby, R. H., and Gilkes, J. J. H. (1974). Curr. Med. Res. Opinion 2:474.
Jolly, E. R., and Sloughfy, C. A. (1975). J. Soc. Cosmetic Chemists 26:227.
Jones, R. (1979). Syntex Research, Palo Alto, Calif., personal communication.
Juel-Jensen, B. E., and MacCallum, F. O. (1974). Br. Med. J. iii:41.
Kamiya, S., Wakao, T., and Nishioka, K. (1966). J. Clin. Ophthalmol. 20:143.
Kastin, A. J., Arimura, A., and Schally, A. V. (1966). Arch. Dermatol. 93:471.
Katz, M. (1973). In Drug Design (Medicinal Chemistry, Vol. 4), E. J. Ariens (Ed.). Academic Press, New York, p. 93.
Katz, M., and Poulsen, B. J. (1971). In Handbook of Experimental Pharmacology, B. B. Brodie and J. Gillette (Eds.), Vol. 28, Pt. 1. Springer-Verlag, New York, p. 103.

Katz, M., and Poulsen, B. J. (1972). J. Soc. Cosmetic Chemists 23:565.
Kedem, O., and Katchalska (1961). J. Gen. Physiol. 45:143.
Keen, C. L., and Eurley, L. S. (1977). Am. J. Clin. Nutr. 30:528.
Keen, P. (1971). In Handbook of Experimental Pharmacology, B. B. Brodie
    and J. Gillette (Eds.), Vol. 28, Pt. 1. Springer-Verlag, New York,
    p. 213.
Khan, S. A. (1978). The Practitioner 221:265.
Kinross-Wright, V. (1956). Psychiat. Res. Rep. 4:89.
Kitzmiller, K. W. (1967), cited in S. W. Jacob, Arzneim. Forsch. 17:
    1086.
Kjaersgaard, A. R. (1954). J. Invest. Dermatol. 22:135.
Kligman, A. M. (1964). In The Epidermis, W. Montagna and W. C. Lobitz
    (Eds.). Academic Press, New York, p. 387.
Kligman, A. M. (1965a). J. Am. Med. Assoc. 193:796, 923.
Kligman, A. M. (1965b). J. Am. Med. Assoc. 193:140, 151.
Kligman, A. M. (1978). Curr. Probl. Dermatol. 7:1.
Koizumi, T., and Higuchi, W. I. (1968). J. Pharm. Sci. 57:87.
Kolb, K. H., Jaenicke, G., Kramer, M., and Schulze, P. E. (1967).
    Ann. N.Y. Acad. Sci. 141:85.
Krasner, J., Giacoia, G. P., and Yaffe, S. J. (1973). Ann. N.Y. Acad.
    Sci. 226:101.
Kristensen, J. K., and Wadskov, S. (1977). J. Invest. Dermatol. 68:196.
Kristensen, J. K., Wadskov, S., and Henriksen, O. (1978). Acta Derm.
    Venereol. (Stockh.) 58:145.
Kuttenn, F., Mowszowicz, I., and Mauvais-Jarvis, P. (1979). In Percu-
    taneous Absorption of Steroids. P. Mauvais-Jarvis, C. F. H. Vickers,
    and J. Wepierre (Eds.). Academic Press, New York, p. 99.
Laboratoires Laroche Navarron, French Patent M4183 (1965a); see Chem.
    Abstr. 70:90758a (1969).
Laboratoires Laroche Navarron, French Patent M4253 (1965b); see Chem.
    Abstr. 68:6196u (1968).
Laden, K., and Spitzer, R. (1967). J. Soc. Cosmetic Chemists 18:351
    (British Patent 987,020).
Lansdown, A. B. G. (1978). Curr. Probl. Dermatol. 7:26.
Laudahn, G., and Gertich, K., Eds. (1966). DMSO Symp., Vienna. (Publ.
    by Dolicur, Soladruck, Berlin.)
Laudahn, G., and Schlosshauer, H. J. , Eds. (1965). DMSO Symp., Berlin.
    (Publ. by Dolicur, Soladruck, Berlin.)
Laurberg, G. (1975). Dermatologica 151:30.
Leake, C. D. (1966). Science 152:1646.
Leake, C. D. (1975). In Biological Actions of Dimethyl Sulfoxide (Ann.
    N.Y. Acad. Sci. 243), S. W. Jacob and R. Herschler (Eds.), p. 5.
Leung, L. C., and Ando, H. Y. (1979). J. Pharm. Sci. 68:571.
Levich, V. G. (1962). In Physicochemical Hydrodynamics. Prentice-Hall,
    Englewood Cliffs, N.J.

Liddle, G. W. (1956). J. Clin. Endocrinol. Metab. 16:557.

Loeffler, R. K., and Thomas, V. (1951). U.S. Atomic Energy Commission Rept. AD-225, B. Nucl. Sci. Abstr. 5, No. 323.

Longcope, C. (1980). In Percutaneous Absorption of Steroids, P. Mauvais-Jarvis, C. F. H. Vickers, and J. Wepierre (Eds.). Academic Press, New York, p. 89.

Loomis, T. A. (1980). In Current Concept in Cutaneous Toxicity, V. A. Drill and P. Lazar (Eds.). Academic Press, New York, p. 153.

Lorenzetti, O. J., Boltralik, J., Busby, E., and Fortenberry, B. (1975). J. Soc. Cosmetic Chemists 26:593.

Lunde, P. K. M., Rane, A., Yaffe, S. J., Lund, L., and Sjoqvest, F. (1970). Clin. Pharmacol. Ther. 11:846.

Lundell, E., and Nordman, R. (1973). Ann. Res. 5:404.

MacCallum, F. O., and Juel-Jensen, B. E. (1966). Br. Med. J. ii:805.

McClellan, W. S., and Comstock, C. (1949). Arch. Phys. Med. 30:29.

McCreesh, A. H. (1965). Toxicol. Appl. Pharmacol. 7(Suppl. 2):20.

McDermot, H. L., Murray, G. W., and Heggie, R. M. (1965). Can. J. Physiol. Pharmacol. 43:845.

MacKee, G. M., Sulzberger, M. B., Herrmann, F., and Baer, R. L. (1945). J. Invest. Dermatol. 6:43.

McKenzie, A. W. (1962). Arch. Dermatol. 86:611.

McKenzie, A. W., and Atkinson, R. M. (1964). Arch. Dermatol. 89:741.

McKenzie, A. W., and Stoughton, R. B. (1962). Arch. Dermatol. 86:608.

McKinivan, C. E. (1979). Abstr. Acad. Pharm. Sci., 26th National Meeting, Anaheim, Calif., Vol. 9, p. 22 (Apr.).

Magnusson, B. (1975). In Animal Models in Dermatology, H. I. Maibach (Ed.). Churchill Livingstone, Edinburgh and London, p. 76.

Magnusson, B., and Kligman, A. M. (1970). Allergic Contact Dermatitis in the Guinea Pig. Thomas, Springfield, Ill.

Maguire, H. C. (1973). J. Soc. Cosmetic Chemists 24:151.

Maibach, H. I., and Feldmann, R. J. (1967). Ann. N.Y. Acad. Sci. 141:423.

Maibach, H. I., Feldmann, R. J., Milby, T. H., and Serat, W. F. (1971). Arch. Environ. Health 23:208.

Mali, J. W. H. (1956). J. Invest. Dermatol. 27:451.

Malone, T., Haleblian, J. K., Poulsen, B. J., and Burdick, K. H. (1974). Br. J. Dermatol. 90:187.

Malkinson, F. D. (1958). J. Invest. Dermatol. 31:19.

Malkinson, F. D. (1964). In The Epidermis, W. Montagna and W. C. Lobitz, Jr. (Eds.). Academic Press, New York, Chap. 21.

Malkinson, F. D., and Ferguson, E. H. (1955). J. Invest. Dermatol. 25:281.

Malkinson, F. D., and Gehlmann, L. (1977). In Cutaneous Toxicity, V. A. Drill and P. Lazar (Eds.). Academic Press, New York, p. 63.

Malkinson, F. D., and Rothman, S. (1961). In Handbuch der Haut und
  Geschlechtskrankheiten, A. Marchionini and H. W. Spier (Eds.),
  Vol. 1, Pt. 3. Springer-Verlag, Berlin.
Malkinson, F. D., and Rothman, S. (1963). In Handbuch der Haut und
  Geschlectskrankheiten, J. Jadasohn (Ed.). Springer-Verlag, Berlin.
Malkinson, F. D., Lee, M. W., and Cutukovich, I. (1959). J. Invest.
  Dermatol. 32:101.
Malone, T., Haleblian, J. K. Poulsen, B. J., and Burdick, K. H. (1974).
  Br. J. Dermatol. 90:187.
Malten, K. E., Spruit, D., Balmaars, H. G. M., and De Keizer, M. J. M.
  (1968). Berufsdermatosen 16:11.
Marion-Landais, G., and Krum, R. J. (1979). Curr. Ther. Res. 25:56.
Markland, W. R. (1976). Cosmetics Toiletries 91:79.
Martin, D., and Hauthal, H. G. (1976). Dimethyl Sulfoxide. Van Nostrand
  Reinhold, New York.
Martindale: The Extra Pharmacopoeia, 27th ed. See Wade and Reynolds
  (1977).
Marzulli, F. N. (1962). J. Invest. Dermatol. 39:387.
Marzulli, F. N., and Maibach, H. I. (1975). In Animal Models in Derma-
  tology, H. Maibach (Ed.). Churchill Livingstone, Edinburgh and London,
  p. 156.
Marzulli, F. N., Callahan, J. F., and Brown, D. W. C. (1965). J. Invest.
  Dermatol. 44:339.
Marzulli, F. N., Brown, D. W. C., and Maibach, H. I. (1969). Toxicol.
  Appl. Pharmacol. Suppl. 3:76
Matheson, L. E., Wurster, D. E., and Ostrenga, J. A. (1979). J. Pharm.
  Sci. 68:1410.
Matheson, L. E., Wurster, D. E., and Ostrenga, J. A. (1980). Int. J.
  Pharmaceutics 4:309.
Matolsty, A. G., and Blank, I. H. (1955). J. Invest. Dermatol. 25:2.
Matoltsy, A. G., Matoltsy, M., and Schrogger, A. (1962). J. Invest.
  Dermatol. 38:251.
Matolsty, A. G., Downes, A. M., and Sweeney, T. M. (1968). J. Invest.
  Dermatol. 50:19.
May, R. H., Selymes, P., Weekley, R. D., and Potts, A. M. (1960).
  J. Nerv. Mental Dis. 130:331.
Memschel, H. (1925). Arch. Exp. Pathol. Pharmakol. 110:1.
Meyer, W., and Neurand, K. (1976). Lab. Animals 10:237.
Meyer, W., Schwarz, R., and Neurand, K. (1978). Curr. Probl. Dermatol.
  7:39.
Mezei, M., and Lee, A. K. Y. (1970). J. Pharm. Sci. 59:858.
Mezei, M., and Ryan, K. (1972). J. Pharm. Sci. 61:1329.
Mezei, M., and Sager, R. W. (1967a). J. Pharm. Sci. 56:12.
Mezei, M., and Sager, R. W. (1967b). J. Pharm. Sci. 56:1604.
Mezei, M., and White, C. N. (1969). J. Pharm. Sci. 58:1209.

Mezei, M., Sagar, R. W., Stewart, W. D., and Deruyter, A. I. (1966). J. Pharm. Sci. 55:584.

Michaels, A. (1975). In Permeability of Plastic Films and Coatings (Polymer Sci. Technol., 6), H. Hopfenburg (Ed.). Plenum, New York, p. 409.

Michaels, A. S., Chandrasekaran, S. K., and Shaw, J. E. (1975). Am. Inst. Chem. Eng. 21:985.

Michelfelder, T. T., and Peck, S. M. (1952). J. Invest. Dermatol. 19: 237.

Middleton, J. D. (1968). Br. J. Dermatol. 80:437.

Middleton, J. D., and Roberts, M. E. (1978). J. Soc. Cosmetic Chemists 29:201.

Minato, A., Fukuzawa, H., Seiiju, H., and Yasuko, K. (1967). Chem. Pharm. Bull. 15:470.

Monash, S. (1957). J. Invest. Dermatol. 29:367.

Monash, S., and Blank, H. (1958). Arch. Dermatol. 78:710.

Montagna, W. (1963). Arch. Dermatol. 88:53.

Montagna, W. (1967). Arch. Dermatol. 96:357.

Montagna, W., and Ellis, R. A. (1961). Adv. Biol. Skin 2:2, 117.

Montagna, W., and Yun, J. S. (1961). J. Invest. Dermatol. 43:11.

Montes, L. F., Day, J. L., Wand, C. J., and Kennedy, L. (1967). J. Invest. Dermatol. 48:184.

Moore, D. H., Chasseaud, L. F., Bucke, D., and Risdall, P. C. E. (1976). Food Drug Cosmet. Toxicol. 14:189.

Morain, W. D., Replogle, C. A., and Curran, P. F. (1966). J. Pharmacol. Exp. Ther. 154:298.

Munro, D. D. (1969). Br. J. Dermatol. 81(Suppl. 4):92.

Munro, D. D. (1976). Br. J. Dermatol. 94:67.

Munro, D. D., and Stoughton, R. B. (1965). Arch. Dermatol. 92:585.

Mustakallio, K. K., Kiistala, U., Piha, H. J., and Nieminen, E. (1967). Scand. J. Clin. Lab. Invest. 19(Suppl. 95):50.

Nachman, R. L., and Esterly, N. B. (1971). J. Pediat. 79:628.

National Academy of Sciences Report (1973). Dimethyl Sulfoxide as a Therapeutic Agent. NAS, Washington, D.C.

Nelson, M. F., Jr., and Stewart, D., Jr. (1956). J. Soc. Cosmetic Chemists 7:122.

Nelson Research and Development Co. (1976). Belgian Patent 843,140. See also U.S. Patents 588,248, 588,234, 3,989,815, 3,989,816, 3,991,203, 3,937,823.

Newhouse, M. L. (1964). Br. J. Ind. Med. 21:287.

Noonan, P. K., and Wester, R. C. (1980). J. Pharm. Sci. 69:365.

Olin Mathieson Chemical Corp., Belgian Patent 670,560 (1965a); see Chem. Abstr. 65:8684b (1966).

Olin Mathieson Chemical Corp. (1965b). Belgian Patent 668075; see Chem. Abstr. 65:10436g (1966).

Olin Mathieson Chemical Corp. (1966). Dutch Claim 6,512,940; U.S. Prior 1964; see Chem. Abstr. 65:688b (1966).

O'Neill, R. C., and Carless, J. C. (1980a). J. Pharm. Pharmacol. 32 (Suppl.):10P.

O'Neill, R. C., and Carless, J. C. (1980b). J. Pharm. Pharmacol. 32 (Suppl.):11P.

Onken, H. D., and Moyer, C. A. (1963). Arch. Dermatol. 87:584.

Orr, N. A., Smith, J. F., and Hill, E. A. (1979). Br. J. Dermatol. 100: 736.

Ostrenga, J. A. (1967). Ph.D. Thesis, University of Wisconsin, Madison, p. 77.

Ostrenga, J., Haleblian, J., Poulsen, B., Ferrell, B., Mueller, N., and Shastri, S. (1971a). J. Invest. Dermatol. 56:392.

Ostrenga, J., Steinmetz, C., and Poulsen, B. (1971b). J. Pharm. Sci. 60:1175.

Padberg, G. (1967). Arch. Klin. Exper. Dermatol. 229:33.

Padberg, G. (1969). J. Soc. Cosmetic Chemists 20:719.

Padberg, G. (1972). J. Soc. Cosmetic Chemists 23:271.

Perlman, F., and Wolfe, H. F. (1966). J. Allergy 38:299.

Peterson, C. F., and Hopponen, R. E. (1953). J. Am. Pharm. Ass., Sci. Ed. 42:540.

Pfizer, Inc. (1976). U.S. Patent 4,018,889; see also U.S. Patent 646,295.

Pictrowski, J. (1957). J. Hyg. Epidemiol. Microbiol. Immunol. (Praha) 1:23.

Pontio, M., and Karki, N. T. (1965). Arch. Interam. Rheumatol. 8:133.

Pope, F. M., Rees, J. K., Wells, R. S., and Lewis, K. G. S. (1972). Br. J. Dermatol. 86:291.

Portnoy, B. (1965). Br. J. Dermatol. 77:579.

Poulsen, B. J. (1972). Adv. Biol. Skin 12:495.

Poulsen, B. J. (1973). In Drug Design (Medicinal Chemistry, Vol. 4), E. J. Ariens (Ed.). Academic Press, New York, p. 93.

Poulsen, B. J., Young, E., Coquilla, V., and Katz, M. (1968). J. Pharm. Sci. 57:928.

Poulsen, B. J., Chowhan, Z. T., Pritchard, R., and Katz, M. (1978). Curr. Prob. Dermatol. 7:107.

Powers, D. H., and Fox, C. (1959). J. Soc. Cosmetic Chemists 10:109.

Prakongpan, S., Higuchi, W. I., Kwan, K. H., and Malokhia, A. M. (1976). J. Pharm. Sci. 65:685.

Proctor & Gamble Co. (1976). U.S. Patent 3,952,099; see also U.S. Patents 3,527,864, 3,839,566, 3,903,256, 3,678,156, 3,896,238, 3,953,599; and Dutch Patent 7,304,699.

Prottey, C. (1976). Br. J. Dermatol. 94:579.

Pugh, C. (1976). Cosmetics Toiletries 91:57.

Putterman, G. J., Wolejska, N. F., Wolfram, M. A., and Laden, K. (1977). J. Soc. Cosmetic Chemists 28:521.

Rammler, D. H., and Zaffaroni, A. (1967). Ann. N.Y. Acad. Sci. 141:13.
Rasmussen, J. E. (1978). Arch. Dermatol. 114:1165.
Rasmussen, J. E. (1979). In The Year Book of Dermatology 1979, R. L.
    Dobson (Ed.). Year Book Med. Publ., Chicago, p. 15.
Reid, J., and Brookes, D. B. (1968). Br. J. Dermatol. 80:328.
Resh, W., and Stoughton, R. B. (1976). Arch. Dermatol. 112:182.
Rieger, M., and Deem, D. E. (1974). J. Soc. Cosmetic Chemists 25:253.
Ritschel, W. A. (1969). Angew. Chem., Int. Ed. 8:699; Angew. Chem.
    81:757.
Roseman, T. J. (1972). J. Pharm. Sci. 61:46.
Rosen, H., Blumenthal, A., Panasvich, R., and McCallum, J. (1965).
    Proc. Soc. Exp. Biol. Med. 120:511.
Rosten, M. (1970). Aust. J. Dermatol. 11:142.
Roth, H. L., and Gellin, G. A. (1973). Cutis 11:237.
Rushmer, R. F., Buettner, K. J. K., Short, J. M., and Odland, G. F.
    (1966). Science 154:343.
Rytting, H., Davis, S. S., and Higuchi, T. (1972). J. Pharm. Sci. 61:817.
Sams, W. M., Carroll, N. V., and Crantz, K. (1966). Proc. Soc. Exp.
    Biol. Med. 122:103.
Sansone, G., and Reisner, R. M. (1971). J. Invest. Dermatol. 56:166.
Sansone-Bazzano, G., Reisner, R. M., and Bazzano, G. (1972). J. Clin.
    Endocrinol. Metab. 34:512.
Sansone-Bazzano, G., Seeler, A. K., Cummings, B., and Reisner, R. M.
    (1979). J. Invest. Dermatol. 73:118.
Sarkany, I., Hadgraft, J. W., Caron, G. A., and Barrett, C. W. (1965).
    Br. J. Dermatol. 77:569.
Scala, J., McOsker, D. E., and Reller, H. H. (1968). J. Invest. Dermatol.
    50:371.
Schaefer, H. (1979). Percutaneous Absorption of Steroids. International
    Symp., Paris, Apr. 1979.
Scherbel, A. L., McCormack, L. J., and Layle, J. K. (1967). Ann. N.Y.
    Acad. Sci. 141:613.
Schering, A. G., French Patent M4,190 (1965); see Chem. Abstr. 67:
    94001j (1967).
Scheuplein, R. J. (1965). J. Invest. Dermatol. 45:334.
Scheuplein, R. J. (1966). Final Comprehensive Report, Contract No.
    AD822655. Clearing House for Federal Scientific and Technical Infor-
    mation, National Bureau of Standards, Washington, D.C.
Scheuplein, R. J. (1978a). In The Physiology and Pathophysiology of the
    Skin, A. Jarrett (Ed.), Vol. 5. Academic Press, New York, pp. 1669,
    1692, 1730.
Scheuplein, R. J. (1978b). Curr. Probl. Dermatol. 7:172.
Scheuplein, R. J., and Blank, I. H. (1971). Physiol. Reviews 51:702.
Scheuplein, R. J., and Blank, I. H. (1973). J. Invest. Dermatol. 60:286.
Scheuplein, R. J., and Ross, L. (1970). J. Soc. Cosmetic Chemists 21:853.

Scheuplein, R. J., Blank, I. H., Brauner, G. J., and MacFarlane, D. J.
(1969). J. Invest. Dermatol. 52:63.

Schlagel, C. A. (1972). Adv. Biol. Skin 12:339.

Schlagel, C. A., and Northam, J. I. (1959). Proc. Soc. Exp. Biol. Med.
101:629.

Schneider, W., and Schuleit, H. (1951). Arch. Dermatol. Syphilol. 193:
434.

Scholtz, J. R. (1961). Arch. Dermatol. 84:91.

Schroer, R. A. (1976). U.S. Patent 3,957,994.

Schumacher, G. E. (1967). Drug Intelligence 1:188.

Scott, A. (1959). Br. J. Dermatol. 71:181.

Scott, G. V., Robbins, C. R., and Barnhurst, J. D. (1969). J. Soc.
Cosmetic Chemists 20:135.

Sears, P. G., Lester, G. R., and Dawson, L. R. (1956). J. Phys. Chem.
60:1433.

Sejrsen, P. (1966). Scand. J. Clin. Lab. Invest. Suppl. 99:52.

Sejrsen, P. (1969). Circ. Res. 25:215.

Sejrsen, P. (1971). Measurement of cutaneous blood flow by freely diffusible radioactive isotopes. Thesis, Copenhagen. Dan. Med. Bull. Suppl.
18.

Sekura, D. L., and Scala, J. (1972). Adv. Biol. Skin 12:257.

Sellers, E. M., and Koch-Weser, J. (1974). Biochem. Pharmacol. 25:553.

Settle, W. Hegeman, S., and Featherston, R. M. (1971). In Handbook of
Experimental Pharmacology, B. B. Brodie and J. Gillette (Eds.),
Vol. 28, Pt. 1. Springer-Verlag, New York, p. 175.

Shaw, J. E., and Chandrasekaran, S. K. (1978). Drug Metab. Rev. 8(2):
223.

Shaw, J. E., and Chandrasekaran, S. K. (1981). In Drug Absorption:
Proceedings of the International Conference on Drug Absorption, Edin-
burgh, 1979, L. F. Prescott and W. S. Nimmo (Eds.). Adis Press,
New York, p. 186.

Shaw, J. E., Chandrasekaran, S. K., Michaels, A. S., and Taskovitch,
L. (1975). In Animal Models in Human Dermatology, H. Maibach (Ed.).
Churchill Livingstone, Edinburgh and London, p. 138.

Shaw, J. E., Bayne, W., and Schmitt, L. (1976). Clin. Pharmacol. Ther.
19:115.

Shaw, J. E., Chandrasekaran, S. K., Campbell, P. S., and Schmitt, L. G.
(1977). In Cutaneous Toxicity, V. A. Drill and P. Lazer (Eds.). Academic Press, New York, p. 83.

Shaw, J. E., Taskovich, L., and Chandrasekaran, S. K. (1980). In Current Concept in Cutaneous Toxicity, V. A. Drill and P. Lazar (Eds.).
Academic Press, New York, London, p. 127.

Shelley, W. B., and Melton, F. M. (1949). J. Invest. Dermatol. 13:61.

Shen, W., Danti, A. G., and Bruscato, F. N. (1976). J. Pharm. Sci. 65:
1780.

Shihab, F., Sheffield, W., Sprowls, J., and Nematollahi, J. (1970). J. Pharm. Sci. 59:1574.
Shinkai, H., and Tanaka, I. (1969). J. Pharm. Soc. Jap. 89:1283.
Siddiq, E. A., and Majid, R. (1969). Current Sci. (Bangalore). 38:215.
Simpson, J. R. (1975). Practitioner 215:226.
Singer, E. J., and Vinson, L. J. (1966). Proc. Sci. Sect. Toilet Goods Assoc. 46:29.
Skog, E., and Wahlberg, J. F. (1967). Acta Derm. Venereol. (Stockh.) 47:426.
Smith Kline & French Laboratories Ltd., British Patent 1,072,014 (1965); see Chem. Abstr. 67:76313h (1967); Dutch Claim 6,602,139 (1966); see Chem. Abstr. 66:57779f (1967).
Smith, Q. T., and Allison, D. J. (1967). Acta Derm. Venereol. (Stockh.) 47:435.
Smith, H. W., Clawes, H. A., and Marshall, E. K. (1919). J. Pharmacol. 13:1.
Smith, J. G., Fischer, R. W., and Blank, H. (1961). J. Invest. Dermatol. 36:337.
Société Pluripharm (1964). French Patent 1,447,946; see Chem. Abstr. 66:58838h (1967).
Solomon, A. E., and Lowe, N. J. (1978). Arch. Dermatol. 114:1029.
Solomon, A. E., and Lowe, N. J. (1979). Br. J. Dermatol. 100:717.
Solomon, H. M. (1971). In Handbook of Experimental Pharmacology, B. B. Brodie and J. Gillette (Eds.), Vol. 28, Pt. 1. Springer-Verlag, New York, p. 234.
Southwell, D., and Barry, B. W. (1981). Proc. 1st Int. Symp. on Dermal and Transdermal Absorption, Munich.
Southwell, D., Barry, B. W., Evans, R., and Fildes, F. J. T. (1980). Br. Pharm. Conf. Commun. No. 9P.
Spencer, T. S., Linamen, C. E., Akers, W. A., and Jones, H. E. (1975). Br. J. Dermatol. 93:159.
Spiegel, A. J., and Noseworthy, M. M. (1963). J. Pharm. Sci. 52:17.
Spiegel, A. J., and Noseworthy, M. M. (1966). J. Am. Med. Ass. 197: A36.
Spier, H. W., and Pascher, G. (1955a). Arch. Klin. Exp. Dermatol. 199: 411.
Spier, H. W., and Pascher, G. (1955b). Arch. Klin. Exp. Dermatol. 201: 181.
Spier, H. W., and Pascher, G. (1956). Arch. Klin. Exp. Dermatol. 203: 234.
Spier, H. W., and Pascher, G. (1957). Arch. Klin. Exp. Dermatol. 204: 140.
Sprott, W. E. (1965). Trans. St. John's Hosp. Dermatol. Soc. 51:186.
Spruitt, D. (1961). Am. Perfumer Cosmet. 37:69.
Spruitt, D., and Malten, K. E. (1965). J. Invest. Dermatol. 45:6.

Stankoff, E. (1962). Soap Perfumery Cosmetics 35:341.
Stark, J. F., Christian, J. E., and Dekay, H. G. (1968). J. Am. Pharm. Ass. Sci. Ed. 47:223.
Steigleder, G. K. (1962). Klin. Wochenschr. 40:1154.
Steinberg, A. (1967). Ann. N.Y. Acad. Sci. 141:532.
Stelzer, J. M., Colaizzi, J. L., and Wurdack, P. J. (1968). J. Pharm. Sci. 57:1732.
Sternberg, T. H., Levan, P., and Wright, E. T. (1961). Curr. Ther. Res. 3:349.
Steward, W. D., Danto, J. L., and Maddin, W. S. (1969). Cutis 5:1241.
Stjernvall, L. (1969). Naturwissenschaften 56:465.
Stolar, M. E., Rossi, G. V., and Barr, M. (1960a). J. Am. Pharm. Assoc., Sci. Ed. 49:144.
Stolar, M. E., Rossi, G. V., and Barr, M. (1960b). J. Am. Pharm. Assoc., Sci. Ed. 49:148.
Stoughton, R. B. (1964). In Progress in Biological Sciences in Relation to Dermatology, Vol. 2. A. Rook and R. H. Champion (Eds.). Cambridge University Press, New York, p. 263.
Stoughton, R. B. (1965a). Toxicol. Appl. Pharmacol. 7:1.
Stoughton, R. B. (1965b). Arch. Dermatol. 91:657.
Stoughton, R. B. (1966). Arch. Dermatol. 94:646.
Stoughton, R. B. (1969). U.S. Patent 3,472,931.
Stoughton, R. B. (1972). Adv. Biol. Skin 12:535.
Stoughton, R. B. (1975). In Animal Models in Dermatology, H. Maibach (Ed.). Churchill Livingstone, Edinburgh and London, p. 121.
Stoughton, R. B. (1976a). U.S. Patent 3,932,653.
Stoughton, R. B. (1976b). U.S. Patent 3,969,516.
Stoughton, R. B. (1977). U.S. Patent 4,039,664.
Stoughton, R. B., and Fritsch, W. (1964). Arch. Dermatol. 90:512.
Stoughton, R. B., Clendenning, W. E., and Kruse, D. (1960). J. Invest. Dermatol. 35:337.
Stringer, H., and Engel, G. B. (1966). Lancet 1:825.
Sulzberger, M. B., and Witten, V. H. (1961). Arch. Dermatol. 84:1027.
Sulzberger, M. B., Cortese, T. A., Fishman, L., Wiley, H. S., and Peyakovich, P. (1967). Ann. N.Y. Acad. Sci. 141:437.
Swanbeck, G. (1968). Acta Derm. Venereol. (Stockh.) 48:123.
Sweeney, T. M., and Downing, D. T. (1970). J. Invest. Dermatol. 55:135.
Sweeney, T. M., Downer, A. M., and Matolsty, A. G. (1966). J. Invest. Dermatol. 46:300.
Szakall, A. (1955). Arch. Klin. Dermatol. 201:331.
Szakall, A. (1957). Arzneim. Forsch. 7:408.
Szmant, H. H. (1975). In Biological Actions of Dimethyl Sulfoxide (Ann. N.Y. Acad. Sci. 243), S. W. Jacob and R. Herschley (Eds.), p. 20.
Tartarini, S., Morganti, P., and Muscardin, L. (1976). Dragoco Rept. 26:1493.

Taskovitch, L., and Shaw, J. E. (1978). J. Invest. Dermatol. 70:217.

Tauber, U. (1976). Arzneim. Forsch. 26:1484.

Thorne, N. (1979). Pharm. J., p. 395.

Tissot, J., and Osmundsen, P. E. (1966). Acta Derm. Venereol. (Stockh.) 46:447.

Tregear, R. T. (1964). In Progress in the Biological Sciences in Relation to Dermatology, A. Rook and R. H. Champion (Eds.), Vol. 2. Cambridge Univ. Press, New York, p. 275.

Tregear, R. T. (1966). Physical Functions of Skin. Academic Press, New York.

Treherne, J. E. (1956). J. Physiol. 133:171.

Turi, J. S., Danielson, D., and Woltersom, J. W. (1979). J. Pharm. Sci. 68:275.

Tyrala, E. T., Hillman, L. S., Hillman, R. E., and Dodson, W. E. (1977). J. Pediat. 91:481.

Vickers, C. F. H. (1963). Arch. Dermatol. 88:20.

Vickers, C. F. H. (1966). In Modern Trends in Dermatology, R. B. McKenna (Ed.), Vol. 3. Butterworths, London, Chap. 4.

Vickers, C. F. H. (1969). Br. J. Dermatol. 81:902.

Vinson, L. J., and Choman, B. R. (1960). J. Soc. Cosmetic Chemists 11:127.

Vinson, L. J., Singer, E. W., Koehler, W. R.,Lehman, M. D., and Masurat, T. (1965). Toxicol. Appl. Pharmacol. 7:7.

Vogel, J., Ache, M., and Seyferth, E. (1967). Arzneim. Forsch. 17:640.

Wade, A., and Reynolds, J. E. F., Eds. (1977). Martindale: The Extra Pharmacopoeia, 27th ed. Pharmaceutical Press, London, p. 912.

Wagner, J. G. (1975). Fundamentals of Clinical Pharmacokinetics. Drug Intelligence Publns., Hamilton, Illinois.

Wahlberg, J. E. (1968). Acta Derm. Venereol. (Stockh.) 48:549.

Watson, P. G. (1973). The Practitioner 211:829.

Weber, W. W. (1972). Adv. Biol. Skin 12:153.

Wechsler, H. L., Kirk, J., and Slowe, J. (1978). Int. J. Dermatol. 17:237.

Weekley, R. D., Potts, A. M., Reboton, J., and May, R. H. (1960). A.M.A. Arch. Ophthalmol. 64:65.

Weigand, D. A., Haywood, C., and Gaylor, J. R. (1974). J. Invest. Dermatol. 62:563.

Weigand, D. A., Haywood, C., Gaylor, J. R., and Anglin, J. H. (1980). In Current Concepts in Cutaneous Toxicity. V. A. Drill and P. Lazar (Eds.). Academic Press, New York, p. 221.

Wepierre, J., Nouvel, G., Cabanne, F., and James, M. (1966). Thérapie 21:1531.

Wester, R. C., and Maibach, H. I. (1975a). Toxicol. Appl. Pharmacol. 32:394.

Wester, R. C., and Maibach, H. I. (1975b). In Animal Models in Dermatology, H. Maibach (Ed.). Churchill Livingstone, Edinburgh and London, p. 133.

Wester, R. C., and Maibach, H. I. (1976). J. Invest. Dermatol. 67:518.

Wester, R. C., and Maibach, H. I. (1977). In Cutaneous Toxicity, V. A. Drill and P. Lazer (Eds.). Academic Press, New York, p. 111.

Wester, R. C., and Noonan, P. K. (1980). Int. J. Pharmaceutics 7:99.

Wester, R. C., Noonan, P. K., Cole, M. P., and Maibach, H. I. (1977). Pediat. Res. 11:737.

Wester, R. C., Noonan, P. K., and Maibach, H. I. (1979). J. Soc. Cosmetic Chemists 30:297.

Wester, R. C., Noonan, P. K., and Maibach, H. I. (1980). Arch. Dermatol. Res. 267:229.

Whitefield, M. (1979). Br. J. Dermatol. 100:736.

Wickrema Sinha, A., Shaw, S. R., and Weber, D. J. (1978). J. Invest. Dermatol. 71:372.

Wilkinson, J. B. (1973). Harry's Cosmeticology, Vol. 1. Leonard Hill Books, Aylesbury, England, p. 64.

Willis, I., and Kligman, A. M. (1970). Arch. Dermatol. 102:405.

Wilson, J. D., and Walker, J. D. (1969). J. Clin. Invest. 48:371.

Winkelmann, R. K. (1969). Br. J. Dermatol. 81(Suppl. 4):11.

Winter, G. D., and Wilson, L. (1976). In Mechanisms of Topical Corticosteroid Activity. L. C. Wilson and R. Marks (Eds.). Churchill Livingstone, Edinburgh and London, p. 77.

Witten, V. H., Brauer, E. W., Loeninger, R., and Holmstrom, V. (1956). J. Invest. Dermatol. 26:437.

Witten, V. H., Stein, S. J., and Michaelides, P. (1963). Arch. Dermatol. 87:458.

Wolff, K., and Winkelmann, R. K. (1967). Adv. Biol. Skin 8:135.

Woodford, R., and Barry, B. W. (1974). Curr. Ther. Res. 16:338.

Woodford, R., and Barry, B. W. (1977a). J. Pharm. Sci. 66:99.

Woodford, R., and Barry, B. W. (1977b). Curr. Ther. Res. 21:877.

Wotiz, H. H., Mescon, H., Doppel, H., and Lemon, H. M. (1956). J. Invest. Dermatol. 26:113.

Wurster, D. E. (1965). Am. Perfumer Cosmet. 80:21.

Wurster, D. E. (1972). Adv. Biol. Skin 12:153.

Wurster, D. E. (1978). Curr. Probl. Dermatol. 7:156.

Wurster, D. E., and Dempski, R. E. (1960). J. Am. Pharm. Assoc., Sci. Ed. 49:305.

Wurster, D. E., and Dempski, R. E. (1961). J. Pharm. Sci. 50:588.

Wurster, D. E., and Kramer, S. F. (1961). J. Pharm. Sci. 50:288.

Wurster, D. E., and Munies, R. (1965). J. Pharm. Sci. 54:554.

Wurster, D. E., Ostrenga, J. A., and Matheson, L. E. (1979). J. Pharm. Sci. 68:1406.

Yalkowsky, S. H., and Flynn, G. L. (1974). J. Pharm. Sci. 63:1276.

Yalkowsky, S. H., Flynn, G. L., and Amidon, G. L. (1972). J. Pharm. Sci. 61:983.

Yarrow, H. (1979). Pharm. J.:413.

Yu, C.-D. (1978). Prodrug-based topical delivery: Simultaneous skin transport and bioconversion. Ph.D. thesis, University of Michigan, Ann Arbor.

Yu, C. D., Fox, J. L., Ho, N. F. H., and Higuchi, W. I. (1979a). J. Pharm. Sci. 68:1341.

Yu, C. D., Fox, J. L., Ho, N. F. H., and Higuchi, W. I. (1979b). J. Pharm. Sci. 68:1347.

Yu, C. D., Fox, J. L., Higuchi, W. I., and Ho, N. F. H. (1980a). J. Pharm. Sci. 69:772.

Yu, C. D., Gordon, N. A., Fox, J. L., Higuchi, W. I., and Ho, N. F. H. (1980b). J. Pharm. Sci. 69:775.

Yu, C. D., Higuchi, W. I., Ho, N. F. H., Fox, J. L., and Flynn, G. L. (1980c). J. Pharm. Sci. 69:770.

Zuckner, J., Uddin, J., and Gantner, G. E. (1967). Ann. N.Y. Acad. Sci. 141:555.

— 5 —

METHODS FOR STUDYING
PERCUTANEOUS ABSORPTION

I. INTRODUCTION

An experiment which monitors the percutaneous absorption of a drug from a topical formulation may be designed to provide answers to one or more questions from an extensive list of problems. Some of the puzzles which a bioavailability study may seek to resolve include:

1. What is the flux of the drug through the skin and how is this governed by the partition coefficient, the apparent diffusion coefficient, and structure-activity relationships?
2. What is the dominant route of penetration through the skin—the stratum corneum or the appendages (pilosebaceous unit or eccrine sweat gland)?
3. Which is more important in clinical use or as a toxic hazard—transient diffusion (possibly down the shunt route) or steady state permeation (usually across the intact stratum corneum)?
4. Does the drug bind to components within the stratum corneum, the viable epidermis or the dermis; or does it form a depot in the subcutaneous fat?
5. What is the rate-limiting step in the percutaneous absorption of the penetrant—drug dissolution or diffusion within the vehicle, partitioning into the various skin layers, diffusion through these strata, or removal by the blood, lymph, or tissue fluids?
6. How do skin age, condition, site, blood flow, and metabolism affect topical bioavailability? Do differences between species need to be considered?
7. How do various vehicles modify the release and absorption of the medicament? Specifically, is an aerosol spray, solution, suspension, gel, powder, ointment, cream, paste, tape, or possibly a delivery device the optimum formulation for a specific drug?

8. Are the vehicle components truly inert or do they affect the permeability of the stratum corneum, if only by hydrating it?
9. If we need to increase the flux of the drug, should we include penetration enhancers within the formulation; on the other hand, does a too potent drug need retarding?
10. Is the formulation correctly designed for treating intact stratum corneum, thickened epidermis, or damaged skin?
11. Should the experimental design provide a full pharmacokinetic profile for the drug and so measure absorption, distribution, metabolism, and excretion?

To answer such questions many different techniques have been developed, but no single method can yield a full picture of the complex process of percutaneous absorption; the myriad procedures reported in the literature may obscure rather than clarify our understanding (Katz and Poulsen, 1971; Idson, 1971, 1975; Nugent and Wood, 1980). Therefore, this chapter deals only with some of the more important methods of general applicability [and so excludes, for example, the measurement of nail plate permeability (see Walters et al., 1981)]. The primary division is into in vivo (Sec. II) and in vitro (Sec. III) procedures: the former class uses the skins of living humans or experimental animals in situ, whereas the latter employs isolated membranes (biological or artificial) and includes simple release studies. Finally, Sec. IV deals with the specialized topic of steroid bioassays. Katz and Poulsen (1971) have tabulated a selection of the many studies in percutaneous absorption undertaken up until 1970, classified according to the compounds used.

II. IN VITRO METHODS

The general advantage of using, for example, an excised skin technique is that the investigator may control the laboratory environment and so elucidate individual factors which modify drug penetration. Thus, in vitro methods are valuable for screening procedures and for deducing physicochemical parameters such as fluxes, partition coefficients, and diffusion coefficients. A theoretical disadvantage of such a technique is that the method does not exactly duplicate the behavior of living tissue in situ, particularly with respect to a capricious blood supply and metabolism. A minor problem with topical steroids is that they constrict the capillaries in vivo and may decrease their own clearances; in vitro this would not happen. However, provided it can be established that the rate-limiting step in the percutaneous absorption of a compound in vivo is diffusion through the dead horny layer, then a well-designed in vitro methodology should produce results which correlate reasonably well with in vivo studies (Marzulli et al., 1969; Franz, 1975, 1978). The inherent assumption that the stratum corneum functions as a permeability barrier in the same way in vivo and in vitro has been tested mainly for

transepidermal water loss because of its relative ease of measurement
(Blank, 1952; Baker and Kligman, 1967a; Bettley and Grice, 1965; Mailli,
1956; Onken and Moyer, 1963; Rosenberg et al., 1962; Rutter and Hull,
1979; Örsmark et al., 1980; Oishi et al., 1976; Nilsson, 1977; Lamke
et al., 1977; Elias et al., 1980).

When human skin is available, the biological diversity in its permeability between specimens and within samples from one specimen or individual
poses a problem. Even with close control of laboratory conditions and experimental technique, the variability for replicate experiments may exceed
that for a well-designed in vivo procedure. If possible, the experimental
design should make each skin sample function as its own control. Section II
of Chap. 4 details the factors implicated in regional and individual variations, such as age, sex, race, anatomic site, condition, and circulatory
effects. Southwell and Barry (1982) quantified the biological and experimental variability within and between specimens of human skin in terms of
solute penetrability in vivo and in vitro, from their own data and from published results. In vivo, the intraspecimen variation calculated as percent
standard deviation (coefficient of variation) was about 30% and the inter-
specimen variation was 45%; the in vitro parameters were 45 and 65%,
respectively.

Any suitable assay technique may be used to measure the penetrant
concentration, but scintillation counting, gas chromatography (GC), or high-
performance liquid chromatography (HPLC) methods predominate because
of their ease of use and sensitivity. They usually monitor the delivery rate
of the chemical into the receptor solution or its rate of loss from the donor
phase. A few workers determine the radioactive drug concentrations within
discrete skin layers by serial removal of the stratum corneum with adhesive
tape and by sectioning the remaining epidermis and dermis with a micro-
tome. The tapes with adherent horny layers and the sections are analyzed by
scintillation counting (Kammerau et al., 1976; Schalla et al., 1976; Schaeffer
et al., 1978; Gazith et al., 1978; Von Kotwas et al., 1979). However, the
technique provides only a "snapshot in time" of the tissue distribution of the
drug, with the danger also that material may dislodge during manipulation.

When chemical analytical techniques are not feasible, punch biopsies of
tissue may be mounted on a medium inoculated with bacteria or fungi and
the segments assayed for antimicrobial activity (Stoughton, 1975).

Many methods are common to in vitro and in vivo procedures (Sec. III.B
provides further information).

A. Release Methods Without a Rate-Limiting Membrane

These procedures record the kinetics of drug release from a formulation to
a simple immiscible phase which is supposed to correspond in properties
with human skin. The limitations of this assumption are evident in light of

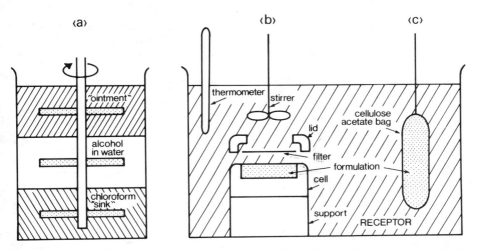

FIG. 5.1 Release methods without a rate-limiting membrane (not to scale).
(a) Stirrer agitates three phases which represent the formulation, the skin
and the blood supply. (From Busse et al., 1969.) (b) Release from an open
container to a stirred immiscible receptor phase. (c) Release through a
simple dialysis membrane.

the biological and physicochemical complexity of mammalian skin. Such
techniques measure drug-vehicle interactions and the release characteristics
of the formulation, and as such they are valuable but have little direct relevance to the process of percutaneous absorption. Solvents which have been
used include simple aqueous media such as water, agar, and gelatin (Gemmell
and Morrison, 1957) and isopropyl myristate, an organic solvent with a blend
of polar and nonpolar characteristics which make it more like skin (Schutz,
1957; Poulsen et al., 1968; Coldman et al., 1969; Poulsen, 1970).

One arrangement used to study the release of a corticosteroid from
model ointment systems had a liquid oily composition (the "ointment"),
containing betamethason 17-valerate, floating on aqueous alcohol (representing skin) on top of a chloroform sink which simulated the blood supply
(Busse et al., 1969). A stirrer with three vanes agitated the layers, and
the amount of steroid delivered to the chloroform was measured as a function of time (Fig. 5.1).

A simpler arrangement exposes the open neck of a glass vessel filled
with a formulation to a stirred immiscible receptor phase; the orientation
of the container depends on the relative densities of its contents and the
receptor fluid. Filter paper or a similar material may hold the product in
place and prevent bulk transfer of the vehicle to the solvent (see, e.g.,
Malone et al., 1974; Takehara and Koike, 1977a,b, 1979a; Shima et al.,
1981). Sometimes a simple dialysis membrane such as cellulose acetate

may close the receptacle (Howze and Billups, 1960; Billups and Patel, 1970; Nambu et al., 1971; Nambu et al., 1975; Ayers and Laskar, 1974; Mériaux-Brochu and Paiement, 1975), or a simple bag of the membrane may be used (Barry and Woodford, 1978).

The most useful practical equations for such experimental results are the "square root of time" relationships.

For solutions

$$M \simeq 2C_0 \left(\frac{D_v t}{\pi}\right)^{\frac{1}{2}} \tag{5.1}$$

where M is the quantity of drug released to the sink per unit area of application; C_0 is the initial concentration of penetrating solute in the vehicle; D_v is the diffusion coefficient of drug in the vehicle; and t is the time elapsed since the start of the solute release.

For suspensions

$$M \simeq (2AD_v C_s t)^{\frac{1}{2}} \tag{5.2}$$

where A is the total concentration of drug in the vehicle and C_s is its solubility in the formulation.

Section III. D of Chap. 4 provides a fuller account of the relevant physicochemical theory together with some plots as examples.

B. Diffusion Methods with a Rate-Controlling Membrane

1. Simulated skin membrane

Because human skin may be difficult to obtain and varies in its permeability, many workers use other materials to simulate it. Thus, a cellulose acetate membrane can be sandwiched in a diffusion cell (Gary-Bobo et al., 1969; Dipolo et al., 1970). However, in most circumstances the membrane simply hinders the penetrant as it diffuses through its channels and the transport process correlates at best with molecular permeation across porous capillary endothelium; the transfer mechanism is dialysis or passage through macroscopic ducts filled with solvent. For example, permeation parameters for hydrocortisone, dexamethasone, testosterone, progesterone, estrone, estradiol, and estriol have been deduced for cellulose acetate transport (Barry and El Eini, 1976; Barry and Brace, 1977). Evidence that diffusion may occur mainly through hydrated regions of co(polyether)polyurethane membranes has been presented (Hunke and Matheson, 1982).

Polydimethylsiloxane membranes [silicone rubber, Silastic (Dow Corning Corporation)] have been much used for drug transport studies because they are hydrophobic, relatively highly permeable, and are easy to prepare (Most, 1970; Garrett and Chemburkar, 1968a,b; Roseman and Higuchi, 1970; Haleblian et al., 1971; Flynn and Smith, 1972; Lovering et al., 1974;

Bottari et al., 1977; Di Colo et al., 1980; Flynn et al., 1981). The permeant dissolves in the barrier matrix and diffuses across it; silicone rubber is highly permeable to many drugs compared with a thermoplastic resin like polyethylene because the high segmental chain mobility readily forms passages for diffusion. Thus, the diffusion coefficients of many steroids are about 10^{-6} cm^2 sec^{-1}, and the flux through an 0.1 mm thick membrane ranges from 6 μg cm^{-2} day^{-1} for cortisol to 1,350 μg cm^{-2} day^{-1} for 19-norprogesterone (Kincl et al., 1968). The commercial product may contain some 20 to 30% of a dispersed phase of fumed silica filler (Flynn and Roseman, 1971), which provides an obstructive effect to diffusion; thus, membranes from a single batch should be used throughout an experiment. Takehara and Koike (1979b) included glass beads in their membranes to assess this obstructive influence. Lovering and Black (1974) investigated the diffusion layer effect which operated during the passage of phenylbutazone through polydimethylsiloxane and showed non-Fickian behavior. Nakano and Patel (1970) used silicone rubber and reported that their results agreed with the in vivo data of Stolar et al. (1960). Recent work which employs these membranes to correlate in vitro data with in vivo skin permeation experiments includes that of Davis and Khanderia (1977) and of Al-Khamis (1981).

Diffusion coefficients of materials in organic phases, such as isopropyl myristate, can be estimated in a special cell. This produces the hydrodynamic pattern of a rotating disk so as to impose a set convective diffusion pattern in an aqueous phase on both sides of a Millipore filter soaked in oil (Riddiford, 1966). Good correlation was claimed with in vivo percutaneous absorption data (Albery et al., 1974, 1976; Albery and Hadgraft, 1979; Guy and Fleming, 1979). Tanaka et al. (1978) also used a Millipore filter saturated with oil in their studies.

The Transderm Therapeutic System (TTS) employs a microporous membrane (exact composition undisclosed) to control the permeation rate of scopolamine into human skin in vivo; the device has also been tested in vitro on cadaver skin (see Chap. 4, Sec. III.D.4).

An interesting concept is to use, as a model membrane, synthetic zeolites (aluminosilicates with a rigid three-dimensional structure) incorporated into a polystyrene matrix. The composite is claimed to be useful for examining effects such as the dependence of permeation on pH and the action of penetration enhancers (Dyer et al., 1979).

Membranes may also be obtained from biological materials, such as collagen (Nakano et al., 1976). A promising approach uses egg shell membranes, since like the stratum corneum they consist mainly of keratin. For salicylic acid permeation at various pH values, this membrane behaves as a dialysis medium similar to cellulose acetate; treated with isopropyl myristate to simulate the lipid phase of the horny layer, the system acts like a polyamide lipoid membrane (Washitake et al., 1980).

O'Neill (1980) has written a comprehensive review of 213 references concerned with membrane systems, with the emphasis on the controlled release of pharmacological agents. He deals with the principles of barrier permeation and the physicochemistry and applications of silicone rubber, ethylene-vinyl acetate copolymers, polyurethanes and other dense polymers, hydrogels, and microporous membranes. Used together with Chap. 2 of the present volume and the references cited therein, his paper provides an introduction to the basic principles of diffusion through membranes.

2. Natural skin membranes

Excised skin from a variety of animals, including rats, mice (normal and hairless), rabbits, guinea pigs, hamsters, pigs, hairless dogs, and monkeys, has been used in diffusion cells. However, as explained in Chap. 4, Sec. II.F, mammalian skin varies widely in characteristics such as stratum corneum thickness and the number density of sweat glands and hair follicles. Cattle and sheep develop skin which is even more dissimilar to that of man. Thus, Pitman and Rostas (1981, 1982) speculate that in these animals the bulk transport of neutral molecules of small to medium size is via skin appendages and that the composition and properties of the sebum-sweat emulsion associated with the skin is important. If at all possible, investigative problems should not be made more complex by selection of an animal tissue to represent human skin.

If human skin specimens from surgical procedures or from cadavers are unavailable, a pressure-sensitive tape can be applied to remove sheets of stratum corneum of about 15 μm thick (Marzulli, 1962). Cantharidin- or suction-blistered skin may be used provided that it is examined with a dissecting microscope to ensure the absence of holes (Idson, 1975).

Undoubtedly, however, the most satisfactory procedure is to obtain human skin from autopsies or amputations. This skin may be used immediately or stored at -24 °C for a long time, and it may be subjected to greater extremes of heat, humidity, pH, and various fluids than other biological tissues without irreversibly changing its barrier properties. Dead skin retains its impermeability remarkably well (Stoughton, 1964; Tregear, 1966). Thus, stratum corneum clearly resists cold damage better than most other tissues since cryobiologists assume that the critical temperature for cellular destruction is -18° to -20 °C (Zaccarian and Adham, 1967). Water flux does not alter significantly for several days after death or if the tissue is frozen and thawed (Berenson and Burch, 1951). Freezing rat skin does not affect phenol penetration (Roberts et al., 1974); storage for up to 6 months at -20 °C leaves human skin permeability unaffected (Astley and Levine, 1976); and Elias (1981) claims that a temperature as low as -70 °C does not affect barrier properties. However, Swarbrick et al. (1982) advise that, for chromone acids used as penetrants, frozen samples of excised skin should be avoided since the extent of permeation exceeds that obtained with fresh skin.

With reference to the preparation of stratum corneum membranes, Rietschel and Akers (1978) showed that there were no significant differences

between specimens attributable to the harvest method in terms of hygro-
scopicity from cantharidin blisters, heat, trypsin, heat plus trypsin, or
ammonia fume separation. A typical procedure which we use is to store
autopsy strips of abdominal skin at -24 °C in heat-sealed, evacuated plastic
bags. When required for an experiment we trim off excess fat and remove
the stratum corneum by the heat treatment method of Kligman and Christophers (1963). The skin is clamped between metal plates previously warmed
to 58-60 °C and kept at this temperature for 2 min in a water bath; then, the
skin is removed and dried. The end of the stratum corneum is cut across,
the membrane is lifted and rolled onto a glass rod, and then onto tin foil for
wrapping and storing flat at -24 °C. It is preferable to reject specimens with
long hairs as these may tear the membrane during preparation or interfere
with the smooth action of a dermatome (see below). (We avoid trypsinization
so as not to damage the membrane, except when preparing stratum corneum
disks for partition studies.) Then we lay the separated tissue epidermal side
down on filter paper soaked in 0.0001% trypsin in 0.5% sodium bicarbonate
solution, incubate overnight at 37 °C, press onto tin foil, rub with a cotton
wool applicator to remove mushy epidermis, rinse with distilled water, and
air-dry on a Teflon surface.

Epidermal sheets may also be obtained from 1- to 2-day-old mice by
subcutaneous injection of exfoliative fractions derived from culture super-
natants of certain phage group 2 staphylococci. Two hours later, the animals
are killed and upper epidermal sheets may be rubbed off (Elias et al.,
1974a, 1977). In an analogous technique, human skin freed from fat may be
floated dermis side down for 4 hr at 37 °C on an antibiotic solution containing
a partially purified fraction of staphylococcal exfoliatin, when sheets composed of stratum corneum and stratum granulosum may be peeled away
(Elias et al., 1974b, 1981).

To prepare full-thickness human skin membranes (composed of stratum
corneum, epidermis, and some dermis) a suitable procedure is to trim away
excess fat to provide strips of uniform thickness. These are clamped between metal plates at -24 °C for an hour, and then the upper plate is warmed
to ease its removal from the horny layer; the still frozen subcutaneous fat
adheres firmly to the lower plate. When the free surface becomes warm
enough to be just movable when subjected to light finger pressure, a Davies
Dermatome 7 (Duplex Electro Dermatome) slices a strip of desired thickness
(we use 430 μm).

Nearly all investigators clamp such membranes in a diffusion cell and
measure the passage of a compound from the stratum corneum side through
to a fluid bath. However, it is important that the tissue be equilibrated with
receptor solution before it is fastened in the cell. If it is mounted dry and
then donor and receptor solutions are applied, the stratum corneum hydrates
and swells and the shunt route may constrict. This closure would lead to
erroneous results for experiments which measure the permeation of drugs
entering via this pathway.

Many types of diffusion cells have been described, often differing in nonessential details; relevant reviews are those of Flynn and Smith (1971) and Nugent and Wood (1980). This chapter surveys only representative examples divided into two main groups—those methods designed to satisfy physical criteria for steady state diffusion or zero-order flux, and those which simulate more closely the in vivo condition.

3. Diffusion cells: zero-order or steady state flux

A well-stirred donor solution at constant concentration delivers penetrant across a membrane to be received by an agitated "sink" receptor liquid which may simulate the blood supply in skin. The receptor fluid can be water, saline, buffer (all with or without preservatives), or, for poorly water-soluble compounds, 50% ethanol in water. In light of the biological variability of skin, it is permissible to have up to 10% depletion of the donor phase and a similar level of buildup in the receptor phase (provided that saturation is not approached). Zero-order flux conditions are not significantly violated.

Perspex diffusion cells (Fig. 5.2a) similar to those of Patel and Foss (1964), when used with a readily available synthetic membrane such as cellulose acetate, can have large compartment and membrane areas (Barry and El Eini, 1976; Barry and Brace, 1977). Brass bolts with winged nuts clamp the membrane between the two halves of the cell, and stoppers close the sampling channels. Teflon-coated bar magnets, controlled by immersible stirring units, agitate the donor and receptor solutions and so minimize stagnant layers. Samples for analysis may be withdrawn by pipette at suitable time intervals, their volumes being replaced with the appropriate solvent.

Garrett and Chemburkar (1968a) modified a design of Lyman et al. (1964) so that membranes closed both ends of a T-joint cell. The cell was filled with penetrant solution recycled from a reservoir and was inverted in a beaker containing the receptor medium.

Figure 5.2b illustrates a smaller glass apparatus of the type we use with human skin membranes that are limited in area. A disk cut from a stainless steel Millipore filter supports delicate stratum corneum sheets without, for most substances, significantly adding to the diffusional resistance; Parafilm or a glass tube may seal the sampling port.

Bettley (1961) built an immersible cell which rotated about a central axis like a wheel. As it revolved, an air bubble rushed through each chamber producing turbulence and so mixed the fluids without imposing a mechanical strain on the epidermis.

A cell with continuously circulating donor and receptor solutions, and therefore efficient mixing, is illustrated in Fig. 5.2c. If required, the liquids can pass through a flow cell located in a spectrophotometer.

Such vertical membrane designs have the following advantages: the receptor and donor compartments may be immersed in a constant temperature water bath; air bubbles do not readily lodge under the membrane and

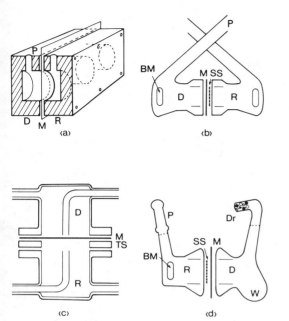

FIG. 5.2 Diffusion cells for zero-order or steady state flux experiments (not to scale). (a) Bank of three cells drilled from a Perspex block. (b) Simple glass diffusion cell suitable for human skin. (c) Glass cell with continuously circulating donor and receptor solutions. (d) Glass cell used for determining vapor diffusion through skin. Key: D, donor compartment; R, receptor compartment; M, membrane; P, sampling port; BM, bar magnet; SS, stainless steel support; TS, Teflon support; W, well; Dr, drierite.

thus decrease the diffusional flux; and no hydrostatic head distorts and possibly ruptures the flexible membrane. A more complex cell with these advantages is that of Flynn and Smith (1971), which can also pump the solution to a spectrophotometer.

As a final example for this section, Fig. 5.2d illustrates another vertical membrane arrangement which we use to examine the diffusion of vapors through the skin. The "well" in the donor section holds the volatile penetrant, either neat or dissolved in a vehicle; the tube sealing this part can hold a desiccant such as drierite to minimize hydration of the stratum corneum.

When using simple zero order flux conditions, as discussed in Chapter 2, investigators are interested in how three amounts vary with time (Scheuplein, 1978):

1. The quantity which enters the membrane up to any time t, $Q^i(t)$
2. The quantity which passes through the membrane and reaches the sink, $Q^o(t)$
3. The quantity which remains in the membrane, $Q^m(t)$

Only two of these amounts are independent because mass balance requires that $Q^i(t) = Q^o(t) + Q^m(t)$. These portions are given by

$$\frac{Q^i(t)}{KhC'_0} = \frac{Dt}{h^2} + \frac{1}{3} - \frac{2}{\pi^2} \sum_{n=1}^{\infty} \frac{1}{n^2} \exp\left(-\frac{Dn^2 \pi^2 t}{h^2}\right) \tag{5.3}$$

$$\frac{Q^o(t)}{KhC'_0} = \frac{Dt}{h^2} - \frac{1}{6} - \frac{2}{\pi^2} \sum_{n=1}^{\infty} \frac{(-1)^n}{n^2} \exp\left(-\frac{Dn^2 \pi^2 t}{h^2}\right) \tag{5.4}$$

$$\frac{2Q^m(t)}{KhC_0} = 1 - \frac{8}{\pi^2} \sum_{n=0}^{\infty} \frac{1}{(2n+1)^2} \exp\left[-\frac{(2n+1)^2 D^2 \pi^2}{h^2}\right] \tag{5.5}$$

where K is the partition coefficient; h is the membrane thickness; C'_0 is the donor concentration; and D is the diffusion coefficient.

As t approaches infinity the exponential terms become negligible, and therefore at long times the linear steady state expressions are

$$Q^i(t) = \frac{KDC'_0}{h}\left(t + \frac{h^2}{3D}\right) \tag{5.6}$$

$$Q^o(t) = \frac{KDC'_0}{h}\left(t - \frac{h^2}{6D}\right) \tag{5.7}$$

$$Q^m = \frac{KhC'_0}{2}$$

Figure 5.3 shows all three quantities plotted as functions of time in a dimensionless form (compare Chap. 2, Sec. I.B.6). The hyperbolic graph of Q^m represents the sorption of the penetrant by the membrane; the graph of Q^o shows the delay period (responsible for the lag time) until steady state develops; and the Q^i graph depicts the quantity measured indirectly when the disappearance is monitored of a substance from a bathing solution. The slopes of Q^i and Q^o become linear and equal in steady state.

With reference to such treatments, Lee (1980) has published a refined integral method for approximate analytical solutions for sorption from a constant, finite volume. These solutions provide simple accurate ways for determining diffusion coefficients from sorption experiments.

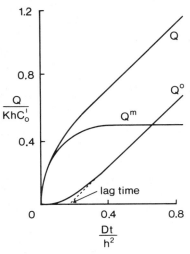

FIG. 5.3 Amount of penetrant entering the membrane (Q^i), diffusing through (Q^o), and being sorbed (Q^m) under zero order flux conditions. The curves are based on Eqs. (5.3) to (5.5). (From Scheuplein, 1978.)

4. Diffusion cells: simulation of in vivo conditions

In general, diffusion cells designed to mimic topical therapy use a stirred or flow-through receptor solution to correspond to the blood supply and an unmixed donor phase to represent a formulation applied to the skin. The material may be a solid deposited from a volatile solvent, a liquid, a semisolid (ointment, cream, paste, or gel), a film, or even a drug device such as the TTS. The donor compartment may be closed or open to ambient conditions or to a controlled humidity, and additional materials may be added or the skin washed during a permeation experiment. Results may still be analyzed using Eqs. (5.3) to (5.8), insofar as these apply to skin, provided the donor concentration does not deplete significantly and stationary layers are not rate limiting with respect to skin diffusion. However, the use of such an "infinite source" and steady state conditions does not parallel normal therapy in man. Section III.E.5 of Chap. 4 discusses this dilemma in more detail, and Franz (1978) has summarized some important objections to the infinite dose technique when used as a predictive model for living man. Of major significance is the presence of a fully hydrated membrane because under normal in vivo conditions the stratum corneum is not macerated and therefore is not as permeable to many penetrants (see Chap. 4, Secs. III.B.1 and III.C.1). Also, in man, a dermatological product may not be a steady source of penetrant, as the drug concentration may increase as solvents evaporate, decrease as the chemical diffuses, or material may be rubbed

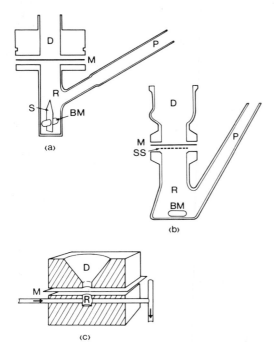

FIG. 5.4 Diffusion cells for simulation of in vivo conditions (not to scale).
(a) Teflon and glass cell similar to the design of Coldman et al. (1969).
(b) Glass cell with stainless steel support for the membrane. (c) Stainless
steel cell with flow through receptor solution. (Based on a design of Cooper,
1982.) Key: D, donor compartment; R, receptor compartment; M, membrane; P, sampling port; BM, bar magnet; S, polyethylene sail; SS, stainless
steel support.

off, washed off, or shed with desquamating scales. Alternatively, a patient
may apply replicate doses to the same area of skin.

        Figure 5.4 illustrates typical cell designs. The first example is an
improved version of the simple cell of Samitz et al. (1967) as used by workers at Syntex Research. It has a lower glass chamber, with a side arm for
sampling, which holds receptor fluid (heated and cooled to expel dissolved
gases). The height of the liquid is adjusted to match the position of the horizontal membrane (Coldman et al., 1969). A polyethylene sail attached to a
Teflon-coated bar magnet stirs the solution. A Teflon upper chamber, open
or closed with a cover slip, clamps the skin onto the ground glass surface
at the top of the receptor chamber, and two metal rings with screws and a
rubber washer hold the parts together. The side port may be sealed with
Parafilm, and any air bubbles which collect under the skin may be dislodged

by tipping. Eight cells can be mounted radially around a Plexiglas holder which fits over a magnetic stirrer, in a room where constant temperature and humidity are maintained. One minor problem with this design is the relative fragility, i.e., uneven pressure through the screws readily shatters the glass.

ᚴ A similar design used in our laboratories has glass chambers with ground faces enclosing the skin membrane which, for fragile stratum corneum, may be supported with a stainless steel mesh disk cut from a Millipore support screen (Fig. 5.4b). A clamp holds the chambers together, and a small well in the side of the donor compartment catches the contents and prevents spillage during air bubble displacement. We routinely immerse the lower half (containing physiological buffer at pH 7.4) in water at 37°C, stir the receptor solution with a bar magnet, and expose the upper chamber to 22°C and 60% relative humidity. Thus, water and temperature gradients develop across the skin similar to those in vivo. The donor section may also be covered to simulate steady state conditions. A comparable design has recently been used by Bronaugh et al. (1981).

One experimental difficulty encountered with such cells is the repetitive nature of multiple sampling and receptor replacement, which we have done, on occasion, every few hours for up to two weeks; a continuous flow-through cell with automatic fraction collection avoids this tedium. Figure 5.4c illustrates one of our answers, a stainless steel cell in which flat surfaces provide a pressure seal for the skin after the two compartments are bolted together (Cooper, 1982). The design is economical in the use of skin, with a donor chamber volume of only about 0.1 cm^3 and membrane area of 0.1 cm^2 A multichannel peristaltic pump drives solution through the lower section (volume 35 μl) at about 3.5 ml hr^{-1}, thus replacing the receptor about 100 times per hour, maintaining sink conditions. Bubble traps prevent air from collecting under the skin. The apparatus automatically collects radioactive samples in scintillation vials from 24 such cells arranged in four lines of six spaced at right angles above a specially constructed large fraction collector table. Alternatively, when appropriate, the cells could be linked to a spectrophotometer.

Many other designs exist, including U-shaped glass vessels with skin draped over one arm (Stoughton and Fritsch, 1964; Stoughton, 1970, 1975) and modifications in which glass rods recessed in a Teflon washer support the delicate membrane (Foreman et al., 1977).

One particular use for the "in vivo mimic" approach is to examine drug diffusion from dry films deposited on the skin. Variations in dose size, hydration, or the addition of other materials to the film may also be investigated. It is useful to identify two modes of application—the "finite dose" and the "infinite dose." In considering these, we will assume that the dissolution rate of the precipitated drug is not the rate-limiting step for the permeation process.

a. Finite dose technique: depleting donor concentration A small volume of drug dissolved in a volatile solvent and applied to the skin readily evaporates to leave a thin solid film of penetrant. The profile of flux versus time from such a thin layer of finite thickness, δ, passes through a maximum of a size and a position defined by equations derived from the general solution for the simple membrane problem (Scheuplein and Ross, 1974; Crank, 1975). Thus, the position of maximum flux is

$$T_{max} = \frac{h^2 - \delta^2}{6D} \simeq \frac{h^2}{6D} \tag{5.9}$$

and the size of maximum flux is

$$J_{max} = \frac{1.85 D C_0 \delta}{h^2} \tag{5.10}$$

where C_0 is the concentration of the penetrant within the first layer of the stratum corneum; ideally, this should be a maximum at equilibrium when solid drug contacts the surface. Provided the solid film is very thin compared with the stratum corneum, its thickness may be neglected. Thus, for example, Eq. (5.9) provides an estimate of the diffusion coefficient, D, for a solid drug delivered to the skin from an aerosol under ambient conditions. Since C_0 is in general unknown, only a qualitative verification has been made of the D-dependence of the size of the maximum flux; see Eq. (5.10).

It would be convenient if we could use Eq. (5.9) to examine the effect on the diffusion coefficient of applying treatments to the solid film, such as adding penetration enhancers (discussed later). However, the determination of D under such conditions would be invalid on at least three counts:

1. Typical accelerants are good solvents and would usually dissolve the film, thereby reducing the thermodynamic activity of the drug in the skin surface, at least until the solvent penetrates the skin and redeposits the film.
2. The enhancer dynamically alters the permeability as it penetrates so that the membrane changes its properties during the experiment.
3. The accelerant may change the membrane thickness as it passes through.

b. Infinite dose technique: constant donor concentration With a suitably thick dry film, the drug depletes negligibly and the physical and mathematical description changes from that of a thin finite layer to an essentially infinite source which maintains a constant donor concentration of dissolved drug on the stratum corneum surface. With sink conditions in the receptor, after the initial transient period the concentration gradient across the skin, and hence the flux through the skin, should remain constant.

Franz (1978) used an open cell and a washing technique to compare the penetration characteristics, in vitro with those in vivo, of hippuric, nicotinic, acetylsalicylic, salicylic, and benzoic acids and also thiourea, chloramphenicol, phenol, urea, nicotinamide, caffeine, and dinitrochlorobenzene.

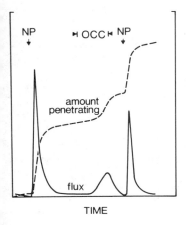

TIME

FIG. 5.5 Diagrammatic representation of the amount penetrating and the flux through human skin of Flurbiprofen deposited from acetone and treated sequentially with N-methylpyrrolidone (NP), occlusion (occ), and NP. Cells used were of the design illustrated in Figure 5.4b.

He found good agreement between the two sets of data in respect of the kinetics and the total amount absorbed.

We have also used the in vivo mimic approach with aspirin, caffeine, mannitol, Flurbiprofen, and Ibuprofen to examine the effects of hydration, solvents and penetration enhancers. For example, Figure 5.5 shows some results obtained when 5 mg of radioactive Flurbiprofen (a nonsteroidal anti-inflammatory drug) was deposited from acetone onto full-thickness cadaver skin. The plot of cumulative amount penetrated against time indicates low permeation until N-methylpyrrolidone (NP), a penetration enhancer, was added to the film. The graph suddenly increases, only returning to its original slope some hours later when most of the NP has passed through the skin. The peak in the flux plot (obtained from gradients to the line) emphasizes the accelerant activity. For Flurbiprofen, hydration of the stratum corneum caused by occluding the donor chamber had little effect on the amount penetrating and the flux. A second application of NP produced another dramatic effect. The experiment was run for 10 days, after which the stratum corneum still maintained its integrity, illustrating how degradation resistant this biological tissue is.

The technique has the advantage that sequential treatments may readily be applied to the same sample of skin, which therefore acts as its own control. This feature is particularly useful because of the great variability of human skin.

C. Partition Coefficient Determinations

The dominant role which the partition coefficient may play in controlling the flux of a penetrant through the skin has been emphasized in this book, particularly in Chap. 2, Sec. III.B and Chap. 4, Sec. III.F.2. However, the ideal thermodynamic treatment of partitioning considers the activity of one molecular species distributing between immiscible phases at equilibrium with no significant chemical interactions. Real situations, of course, deviate from this ideal, and the partitioning process of a drug from a complex vehicle to stratum corneum diverges more than most. The horny layer absorbs greater than its own weight of many liquids and interacts extensively with most materials of medicinal interest. However, many workers, including Scheuplein and Blank (1971), Scheuplein (1978), and Dürrheim et al. (1980), have amply demonstrated the value of partition measurements for predicting the permeability characteristics of solutes in skin and for deducing thermodynamic parameters to probe the physicochemical nature of the stratum corneum.

A general method which we use to derive partition coefficients is to weigh small disks of dry stratum corneum (approximately 3.5 mg) and to equilibrate them with radioactive drug solution (1 ml) in sealed glass vials in a shaking water bath. The disks are removed, quickly rinsed, blotted with tissue paper, and weighed wet. They are dissolved in 1 ml Soluene 350; then 1 ml water and 10 ml of a scintillation fluid (such as FisoFluor-1) are added, and the vials are stored overnight to allow chemiluminescence to subside. Radioactivity may then be measured using [^{14}C]toluene as an internal standard for quench correction. Volumes (0.1 to 0.2 ml) of the vehicle at equilibrium are made up to 1 ml with water, 10 ml FisoFluor-1 is added, and the radioactivity is counted. The ratio of penetrant amount per wet weight or per dry weight of stratum corneum to drug concentration in the bathing vehicle provides the wet or dry partition coefficient, respectively.

III. IN VIVO METHODS

In the final analysis, to gain a full insight into the percutaneous absorption process of a drug in a living animal we must determine the permeation in that species. However, particularly in man, this approach is often fraught with experimental and ethical difficulties. Many in vitro procedures monitor steady state fluxes across the intact stratum corneum, whereas in vivo methods often employ physiological end points. These may be sensitive to minute amounts of the penetrant entering the skin during the transient phase of diffusion and particularly down the shunt routes. A further complication is that many drug molecules probably penetrate the living skin mainly through the shunt routes, and an in vitro procedure which neglects this aspect is potentially misleading (see Chap. 3, Sec. II.D). Another severe difficulty with human subjects or living experimental animals is that the techniques determine the extent of absorption indirectly. In a typical experiment, the investigator applies a radioactive drug in an ointment to the animal's skin and assesses the kinetics of skin permeation from the rate of excretion in the urine. However, the drug may be partially metabolized while crossing the viable tissues of the skin (see Chap. 4, Sec. II.D). Body organs may take up a fraction of the penetrant, and a correction for this has sometimes been made by the worker injecting intravenously a single dose and determining urinary excretion (Feldmann and Maibach, 1970). However, sufficient time must be allowed for collection of all the excreted drug; otherwise the organ storage value may include a sizeable error (Franz, 1978). For some compounds, binding, slow metabolism and distribution of the medicament to a "deep compartment" may rate limit the excretion (Garrett, 1973).

When experimental animals are used as models for man, in addition to species differences we must allow for increased permeation because of shaving and we must prevent the animal from ingesting or inhaling part of the dose.

This section will deal only with techniques of general applicability. More specialized methods such as the human skin window and dermal perfusion have been dealt with briefly by Katz and Poulsen (1971).

A. Animal Models

A persistent theme in work on percutaneous absorption is the development of suitable animal models which correlate adequately with man. However, most experimental animals differ significantly from man in the features which affect percutaneous absorption: the thickness and nature of the stratum corneum, the density of hair follicles and sweat glands, the nature of the pelt, the papillary blood supply, and subtle biochemical aspects. Section II.F of Chap. 4 discussed such differences between species as they affect percutaneous absorption.

An additional limitation arises when the investigation aims primarily to assess the therapeutic activity of a drug as well as its bioavailability from a formulation; few techniques produce disease states in animals which are similar to human afflictions (Newcomer and Landau, 1964; Chase, 1969; Van Scott, 1972; Jones, 1975). However, several diseases are common to dog and man (Muller and Kirk, 1969). Manna et al. (1982) developed an animal model for chronic ulceration, and various workers have produced several types of "clean" wounds using, e.g., cantharidin or suction blisters, adhesive tape stripping, scalpel blade abrasion and sand papering (Krawczyk and Wilgram, 1975; Devitt et al., 1978; Pang et al., 1978; Eaglstein and Mertz, 1978; Scott and Dugard, 1981; for a review, see Scott, 1982). A new model for a scaling dermatosis induces hyperproliferation in hairless mice (Nguyen et al., 1981). Even when simulated disease states can be developed, their response to drugs may mislead in an extrapolation to man (Scott, 1965).

Prediction methods for possible toxic hazards use animals routinely.
The subject has been reviewed by Draize (1959) and Idson (1968), and a
report on a symposium on animal models in dermatology includes several
contributions to this subject (Maibach, 1975).

The situation as summarized by Katz and Poulsen (1971) still holds today: animal models are invaluable for the more detailed study of the anatomy,
physiology, and biochemistry of the skin, for screening topical agents, and
for detecting possible toxic hazards. We can add that they are also useful
in biopharmaceutical studies. However, experience gained with experimental animals is not a substitute for detailed, careful studies in man.

B. Techniques

1. Observation of a physiological or pharmacological response

If the penetrant stimulates a biological reaction when it reaches the
viable tissues, then this response may provide the basis for determining
the penetration kinetics. At least in theory, local allergic, toxic, or physiological reactions may be used and various topical agents affect such skin
functions as sweat gland secretion, pigmentation, sebaceous gland activity,
vasodilatation, vasoconstriction, vascular permeability, epidermal proliferation, and keratinization. The most productive technique in terms of biopharmaceutical application is the vasoconstrictor or blanching response to
topical steroids, which Sec. IV.C discusses in more detail. Other methods
include determination of changes in blood pressure to monitor, for example,
topical application of nitroglycerin (Francis and Hagan, 1977), reduction in
pain threshold, production of convulsions, and the red tear response (Katz
and Poulsen, 1971). Frewin (1969) studied microscopically the influences of
physical, cosmetic, and medicinal therapy on human cutaneous circulation.

2. Physical properties of the skin

A wealth of information is available on methods for measuring diverse
physical properties of skin, in vivo and in vitro, much of it presented in the
bioengineering literature. A list of just some of the methods includes the
measurement of transepidermal water loss, thermal determinations (conductivity, differential scanning calorimetry, surface sorption), mechanical
analysis (linear and nonlinear viscoelastic techniques), use of ultrasound,
classification of function and dimension, spectral analysis (visible, UV, IR—
including attenuated total reflectance IR, UV fluorescence, and multiple
internal reflection spectroscopy), and use of photoacoustic and electrical
properties. Quatrone and Laden (1976) have reviewed in vitro methods for
the evaluation of emollients, and Wueper et al. (1981) have edited a symposium on photobiology and photomedicine. Tregear (1966) wrote a classic
review text, and Wilkes et al. (1973) summarize additional information. A

recent symposium on bioengineering and the skin provided a modern introduction and a useful summary of many of these practices (Marks and Payne,
1981). Many of these procedures reveal information which may be relevant
to a specific aspect of percutaneous absorption, but an exhaustive treatment
is out of place here.

3. Analysis of body tissues or fluids

Urinary analysis is often used to study percutaneous absorption, and
the work of Wurster and Kramer (1961), Butler (1966), and particularly
Feldmann and Maibach (1965, 1966, 1967, 1968, 1969, 1970) illustrates its
value. However, as emphasized earlier, all the drug which penetrates the
skin should be accounted for by a "calibration" of the subject with a slow
intravenous injection and a simultaneous determination of blood levels. The
aim is to allow for all the pharmacokinetic factors inherent in drug absorption, distribution, storage, metabolism, and excretion. This combined procedure is a good method for in vivo assessment of topical bioavailability
(Blank, 1960a; Griesemer et al., 1958).

Analysis of the penetrant in the circulating blood can present difficulties
with dilution, extraction, and detection, although modern analytical techniques are developing so rapidly that, for example, nanogram quantities of
the psoralens (Neild and Scott, 1982) and nitroglycerin (Sved et al., 1982)
may be detected. Some of the relevant earlier attempts at plasma analysis
include those of Gemmell and Morrison (1958a,b), Stolar et al. (1960), and
Stelzer et al. (1968). More modern work has established the pharmacokinetics of topically applied lindane (Hosler et al., 1979), and Horhota and
Fung (1978) measured nitroglycerin absorbed in the shaved rat.

Feces analysis alone has limited use (Inman et al., 1956; Malkinson
and Kirschenbaum, 1963).

A combination of blood, urine, and feces analysis was used with rats,
monkeys, and human volunteers to examine the percutaneous absorption and
excretion of tritium-labeled diflorasone diacetate, a novel topical steroid
(Wickrema Sinha et al., 1978). For a topical antiacne agent, the cumulative
excretion in urine and feces, together with determinations of the areas under
the plasma concentration-time curves, showed that in the monkey the free
base was twice as bioavailable as the salt form (Webster and Noonan, 1978).

Sometimes the drug has a particular affinity for a specific animal organ,
which can be removed and the drug content analyzed. Iodine, iodides, and
mercury have been investigated in this manner (Miller and Selle, 1949; Tas
and Feige, 1958; Cyr et al., 1959; Laug et al., 1947a,b). Biopsies of
organs and skin tissue may be analyzed and even individual sections measured
(see Sec. II).

Section II of Chap. 4 provides references which give further details of
the methods used for drug analysis during in vivo work.

4. Surface loss

Equation (5.3) and Fig. 5.3 suggest that measurements of the rate of loss of a penetrant from an applied vehicle should lead to a determination of the flux of the material into the skin. Thus, chambers could be filled with the formulation, attached to the skin, and the absorption rate calculated from loss measurements. However, because of the general impermeability of the skin, the concentration decrease would generally be small and analytical techniques would have to be very accurate to measure tiny differences. Such concentration differences as could be detected would most likely arise from the vehicle composition changing by evaporation or by dilution with sweat or transepidermal water. Alternatively, any drug decrease may only reflect deposition on the skin surface or combination with the stratum corneum, rather than penetration to the systemic circulation (Blank, 1960b).

The main use of a loss technique has been to monitor the decrease in radioactivity at the skin surface (Malkinson, 1956, 1958, 1964; Ainsworth, 1960; Wahlberg, 1965). As Katz and Poulsen (1971) indicate, for use with a Geiger counter the isotope should emit medium- or high-energy beta particles; if they have too low an energy, the particles absorb within the epidermis. Highly penetrating gamma particles may yield false positive results after the penetrant has passed the skin.

5. Histology

It is tempting for an experimenter to try to locate the routes through which materials penetrate the skin by examining microscopic sections. However, such an approach can mislead because the drastic treatment applied in preparing the skin sections encourages leaching and translocation of diffusible materials away from their original sites.

Histochemical techniques have elucidated absorption profiles and penetration routes for those few compounds which produce colored end products after chemical reaction. For example, certain drugs change epidermal sulfhydryl groups in an easily detectable way (Duemling, 1941; Strakosch, 1944; MacKee et al., 1945; J. W. Goldzieher et al., 1952; Sobel et al., 1958; Bradshaw, 1961; Calman, 1970; Chayen et al., 1970). In earlier days workers colored a penetrant with a dye and then examined skin sections to locate the penetrant. However, physicochemical theory emphasizes that membrane transport occurs at the molecular level with each species partitioning and diffusing separately. Thus the dyed complex dissociates and results are valid only for the dye itself (Malkinson, 1964). The use of an added dye, or any other different tracer molecule, should be avoided.

A few compounds fluoresce, and their behavior in skin may be revealed by microscopy [for vitamin A, see Montagna (1954); for tetracycline and benzpyrene, see Meyer (1966)]. Baker and Kligman (1967b) used tetrachlorosalicylanilide to determine the permeability of the stratum corneum. An examination of UV fluorescence photomicrographs of hairless hamster skin treated with crude coal tar suggests that the hair follicles in this species provide an important route for the penetration of tar components. In unfixed sections, the follicle, sebaceous gland, and fat cells underlying the dermis contained high concentrations of material (Foreman et al., 1979).

A crude measurement of skin penetration examines tissue sections for physiological changes such as those caused by keratolytics and emollients (Strakosch, 1943; Marks, 1978) and sex hormones (M. A. Goldzieher, 1946; J. W. Goldzieher, 1949; Homburger et al., 1961).

Microscopic autoradiography, another useful procedure, cannot be applied to diffusible substances without modification. To do so can lead to a self-deception which almost guarantees that the recorded anatomic site of the penetrant is artificial because of translocation (Roth, 1971). The substance emits alpha and beta rays (Choman, 1960), and there may be considerable scattering on the autoradiogram; reducing substances reacting with the photographic emulsion—or an incorrect technique—can produce shadowing (Blank, 1960b; Rogers, 1967). Tritium-labeled isotopes are useful because of their weak emissions; strong beta emitters can darken areas as much as 2 or 3 mm away from the particle location, a great distance on the cellular scale. As for other histological techniques, the cutting, handling, and development of the tissue may displace or remove the penetrant and produce false results (Stoughton, 1964).

IV. BIOASSAYS FOR TOPICAL STEROIDS

Topical corticosteroid bioassays are the most sophisticated and refined of all bioassays which we use to develop and to assess dermatological formulations (Haleblian, 1976). In particular, we may not only employ the vasoconstrictor assay to evaluate the intrinsic activity of a topical steroid for correlation with possible clinical anti-inflammatory action, but we may use it also as a test in fundamental biopharmaceutical studies. Thus, the blanching test occupies a unique position among topical bioassays, and in this chapter we will consider its use in some detail. For completeness, we will also briefly deal with other bioassays for topical glucocorticoids. There are, of course, many other types of bioassay used to screen various topical formulations prior to clinical trial. Because of their specialized nature we will not consider them here. The interested reader may consult Haleblian (1976), who has reviewed bioassays for topical corticosteroids, antibacterials, antifungals, antiyeast preparations, antimitotics, antiperspirants, sunscreen agents, antidandruff, anesthetic-analgesic formulations, antipruritics, antiwart, poison oak/ivy dermatitis, and psoriasis. Mills and Kligman (1975) discuss comedolytic agents; Kligman and Wong (1979) present an improved bioassay for assessing comedogenic substances; Pochi (1975) considers the assessment of sebaceous gland activity as a useful model for developing antiacne formulations; and Gomez and Frost (1975) deal with the relevance of the hamster flank organ as a model of the human sebaceous gland and its response to antiandrogens. Gellin (1975) reviews chemically induced depigmentation in animal models. Leyden et al. (1979) present updated and expanded in vivo methods for determining the efficacy of topical antimicrobial agents.

A. Antigranuloma

The effect of systemic corticosteroids on the generation of granulation tissue was evaluated by Ragan et al. (1949) and Selye (1953). Hershberger and Calhoun (1957) developed the standard antigranuloma bioassay, and several variants have been used to evaluate the relative potencies of topical gluco-corticoids (Ringler, 1964; Lerner et al., 1964a,b; Dipasquale et al., 1970; Dorfman, 1970). The standard procedure implants subcutaneous control cotton pellets and pellets impregnated with steroid into adrenalectomized rats the day after their operations. The implants are removed after 6 days and dried to constant weight. From log dose-log response curves, the relative inhibition of granuloma formation assesses the relative potencies of the test compounds. This bioassay measures local activity rather than topical action, although a simultaneous assessment of thymus involution determines systemic activity (see the next subsection).

B. Thymus Involution

Some investigators have employed the thymolytic anti-inflammatory activity of corticosteroids to predict their possible value as topical steroids. One standard thymolytic test uses bilaterally adrenalectomized rats with cotton pellets inserted subcutaneously. The test steroid is injected subcutaneously daily for 6 days. After a further day, the thymus is removed and weighed; log dose-response curves allow the inhibition of the thymus to indicate the relative potencies of the experimental steroids (Lerner et al., 1964a; Ringler, 1964; Dorfman, 1970).

C. Inflammation

Since the clinical value of topical corticosteroids lies in their anti-inflammatory properties, several important bioassays develop and then treat inflammatory responses in experimental animals and in man. We can discuss these assays in categories of the type of agent or process used to induce the inflammation.

1. Croton oil

Although early workers concluded that the application of croton oil as an irritant gave unpredictable results (Sidi and Bourgeois-Gavardin, 1953), more careful attention to test design has yielded some useful information. The topical rat ear assay, designed by Tonelli et al. (1965) and used by Witkowski and Kligman (1956, 1959) and Banfi et al. (1976), has been modified by Dorfman (1970) and Fregnan and Torsello (1975) to study the relative potencies of anti-inflammatory compounds. A blend of 20% pyridine, 5% water, 74% ether, and 1% croton oil is applied to one ear, and a solution of the test steroid in this irritant-solvent vehicle is applied to the other. After 6 hr, the ears are removed and weighed or small biopsies are weighed. The anti-inflammatory effect of the test compounds may be determined from the relative suppression of the croton-oil-induced inflammation.

This bioassay has several advantages as a preliminary screening process. It is simple, nonocclusive, and it provides dose-response data; the test is highly sensitive and reasonably specific for anti-inflammatory activity; the procedure yields clues regarding the potential dissociation of topical and systemic drug action, and it is one of the few topical animal screening models (Schlagel, 1975).

Because the results which the bioassay produces may vary with the animal species (Harman et al., 1971), and since croton oil irritation in human skin mimics clinical inflammatory conditions (Witkowski and Kligman, 1959), the technique was adapted to human skin. In studies which used croton oil applied to the forearm, followed by steroid application, readings were taken on a 0 to 5 scale based on the degree of erythema, induration, and vesiculation. The scores were subtracted from those of untreated croton oil sites so as to obtain the relative potencies of commercially available corticosteroid preparations (Burdick, 1972a,b; Ortega et al., 1972).

A rank order of corticosteroids evaluated by the suppression of croton-oil-induced pustules or kerosene-provoked blisters correlated reasonably well with clinical judgements of comparative efficacy, although the grading was not always the same in both inflammatory tests (Kaidbey and Kligman, 1974).

Recently, Lorenzetti (1975, 1979) presented data derived from his own experiments or abstracted from the literature on the relative potencies of topically applied steroids in the rat croton oil-erythema assay as well as in the human vasoconstrictor assay. A total of 34 steroids were considered, including hydrocortisone, dexamethasone, prednisolone, betamethasone, fluorometholone, fluprednisolone, and their esters; flurandrenolone, triamcinolone, fluocinolone, and their derivatives; also beclomethosone propionate, fluprednylidene 21-acetate, flumethasone pivalate, halcinonide, and desonide. The author concluded that for these assays there is an excellent animal-to-human clinical correlation in anti-inflammatory potency.

Japanese workers have compared the croton oil assay with a new technique (homologous passive cutaneous anaphylaxis) for evaluating steroidal ointments (Iizuka et al., 1981).

2. Mustard oil and nitric acid

Various concentrations of mustard oil in liquid petrolatum (mainly 80%) and nitric acid in water (usually 15%) were kept in contact with the normal skin of volunteers. Corticosteroid ointments were rubbed into the insulted sites at time intervals ranging from 24 hr before to 24 hr after the application of the two primary irritants. The time of appearance of the inflammatory reaction, its rate of progress, and the final degree of response were noted. The inflammatory reaction was graded as erythema, erythema plus obvious edema, additional formation of papules or vesicles, or necrosis (Scott and Kalz, 1956b). The major factors which influenced the results were the relationship between the time of steroid application and the induction of inflammation, the duration of steroid contact with the skin site, the concentration of the corticosteroid, the intensity of the inflammatory stimulus, and the thickness of the epidermis.

3. Tetrahydrofurfuryl alcohol

Tetrahydrofurfuryl alcohol moderately irritates human skin. It also has the practical advantage that it is an excellent solvent for a wide range of compounds, including steroids. Solutions of the test compounds are applied to the skin under occlusion, and the erythema produced is scored on a 0 to 6 scale. When the erythema reduces in the presence of a steroid, the compound is rated as an anti-inflammatory agent. The investigators who used this bioassay concluded that fluorometholone was 40 times more active topically than hydrocortisone, even though the systemic activities were equal; flurandrenolide was more effective than hydrocortisone acetate (see Schlagel and Northam, 1959; Schlagel, 1965; also Brunner and Finkelstein, 1960; Gray et al., 1961).

4. Kerosene

As previously mentioned in the croton oil section, kerosene-induced inflammation in human skin has been used to evaluate commercial steroid preparations (Kaidbey and Kligman, 1974). Steroid preparations were applied under occlusion for 6 hr, and the resulting blanching was scored 1 hr later. The sites were then challenged with irritant patches of kerosene applied for 20 hr, and the responses were graded on a 5-point scale which ranged from 0 for complete absence of pustules or vesicles to 4 for bullae. The rank order of steroid anti-inflammatory efficacy correlated reasonably well with clinicians' judgements of comparative effectiveness. Zaynoun and Kurban (1974) used the same technique to evaluate steroid creams and to correlate the results with double-blind clinical studies.

5. Lipopolysaccharide

Heite et al. (1964) evaluated five steroid ointments and two controls for their abilities to suppress the erythema produced by a subcutaneous injection

of bacterial lipopolysaccharide into human skin. Hydrocortisone was ineffec-
tive in this bioassay.

6. Histamine

Reddy and Singh (1976) assessed the abilities of previously applied
alcoholic solutions of steroids to reduce the size of histamine wheals induced
in human skin by the pinprick method. The authors claimed that the method
was simple, easy, and reliable and that the test could be used with white-
or dark-skinned subjects.

7. Experimentally produced eczematous reactions: allergens

Several early attempts to produce useful models of allergic contact
eczema so as to simulate clinical syndromes were only partially successful;
induction of the lesions and their control by steroids were inconsistent and
unreliable (Schlagel, 1975). Modern work has been more successful, both
in the way in which the techniques produced standard lesions and their subsequent treatment. Bielicky and Döring (1974) extended the electrophoretic
studies of Haxthausen (1955, 1956) and Novak and Bartak (1971; see also
Novak, 1972) and used a variety of steroids in neomycin-sensitized persons.
Go (1969) investigated the performance of fluocinolone acetonide cream in
alleviating the eczema produced by a variety of substances.

Scott (1965) induced eczematous lesions in guinea pigs by sensitizing
them with dinitrochlorobenzene and then evaluated the efficacy of six commercial steroid ointments. Burrows and Stoughton (1976) found that the prior
application of potent steroids inhibited the development of sensitization to
this allergen.

Evans et al. (1971) sensitized mice by painting the abdomen with oxazolone in olive oil (Asherson and Ptak, 1968; Dietrich and Hess, 1970). Seven
days later the animals were challenged on one ear with oxazolone in acetone.
Graded doses of steroids (hydrocortisone, betamethasone 17-valerate, triamcinolone acetonide, and fluocinolone acetonide) dissolved in the oxazolone
solution were applied to the opposite ear. Activity of the corticosteroids was
expressed as percentage of inhibition of ear weight gain in treated versus
control ears, or as relative ear weight among the ears treated with various
steroids. The data revealed a disproportionately low activity for betamethasone 17-valerate relative to the acetonide compounds. Young et al. (1978a)
concluded that betamethasone valerate acted as an anticorticosteroid in this
assay in the rat, as well as in the antilymphocyte bioassay (see also Sec.
IV.D.3). They concluded that this steroid behaves uniquely in the rat; in
mouse and in man the compound behaves as a normal corticosteroid.

Rhus (poison oak/ivy) dermatitis is common in the United States. In a
human bioassay, the oleoresin was applied to the forearms of human volunteers and when lesions formed the sites were treated (Frank et al., 1955);
interpretation of the results is difficult. As an alternative method we can

establish lesions in guinea pigs by sensitizing them with multiple injections
of a poison ivy/oak extract in complete Freund's adjuvant (Bowser and Baer,
1963; Kepel et al., 1974). The sensitized animals are challenged at the ear
by rubbing in undiluted antigen. After 24 hr the developed lesion is treated
with a steroid gel. The end point is the reduction in weight of a biopsy from
the treated ear with reference to the contralateral control ear. The model
may be useful in screening agents and formulations for treating human Rhus
dermatitis and related lesions of delayed hypersensitivity.

8. Tape stripping

After Wolf (1939) observed that stripping the epidermis with adhesive
tape damaged local tissue, Wells (1957) suggested that this technique could
be used to study the anti-inflammatory activity of topical steroids. He found
that hydrocortisone inhibited the vasodilatation normally produced by 30
strippings of the stratum corneum. The Wells technique was further investigated as a bioassay by Shelmire (1958), Möller and Rorsman (1960), and
Heseltine et al. (1962) for hydrocortisone and triamcinolone acetonide. Although tape stripping essentially removes the barrier to steroid penetration
through the skin, with all that this implies with respect to biopharmaceutical
studies, the method has been employed more recently during the development of corticosteroid formulations (Bagatell and Augustine, 1974; Liebsohn
and Bagatell, 1974; Maibach, 1976; Goldlust et al., 1976; Täuber, 1976;
Täuber et al., 1976; Wendt and Reckers, 1976).

9. UV erythema

Ultraviolet (UV) light injures the skin in a complex fashion which involves
epidermal cell death, increased mitotic index, hyperplasia, cellular exuda-
tion, and vasodilatation (Snyder, 1975). Since most steroid responsive diseases are inflammatory, a UV erythema suppression bioassay is at least
potentially useful for evaluating the relative activities of corticosteroids and
their formulations.

Erythema produced in dog skin (Chimoskey et al., 1975) and in rat skin
(Lewis, 1976) was inhibited by topical steroids; experiments with guinea
pigs yielded contradictory results (Winder et al., 1958; Gupta and Levy,
1973; Chimoskey et al., 1975). Jarvinen (1951) discovered that massive
oral doses of cortisone reduced somewhat the intensity of erythema produced
in human skin by UV, and this work led to investigations which employed
topical steroids in human volunteers. Everall and Fisher (1952) were the
first to evaluate a topical corticosteroid (cortisone acetate) in preventing
the effects of UV rays on human skin.

Among the variables in human volunteer studies have been the UV dose
used and whether the steroid was applied before or after irradiation.

When corticosteroids were applied before exposure to UV (Kanof, 1955;
Scott and Kalz, 1956a,b; Ljunggren and Möller, 1973) or grenz rays (Kalz

and Scott, 1956), the erythema decreased. When investigators claimed prevention of erythema with steroid applied after UV irradiation, usually the effect was not shown with light levels greater than three minimum erythema doses, i.e., 3 MED (Burdick et al., 1973). However, Stoughton (1971) suppressed 5 MED by using occluded steroid preparations. Other investigations have used 1 MED (Burdick et al., 1973; Lewis and Fox, 1976) and 2 MED (Kaidbey and Kurban, 1976). Burdick (1972a,b), Burdick et al. (1973), and Haleblian et al. (1977) used a combination of the vasoconstrictor test and UV erythema suppression as human bioassays for corticosteroids.

Woodford (1977) found that the MED varied with the volunteer, the day of testing, and the site of application. Because of these factors, together with the lack of precision of the test, reluctance of volunteers to participate in repeated UV trials, and possible adverse effects of such repeated skin exposure to UV irradiation (Snyder and May, 1975; Urbach et al., 1976; Magnus, 1976; Warin, 1978; Kaidbey and Kligman, 1978, 1981; Parrish et al., 1978, 1981), the test should be abandoned for assessing topical steroid activity and bioavailability in humans in favor of the vasoconstrictor assay.

D. Cytological Techniques

The activity of corticosteroids may be assessed by their effects on the growth of skin, its components, or its appendages.

1. Fibroblast inhibition

Corticosteroids act on many different types of cell. In particular, the fibroblasts of connective tissue respond to an inflammatory stimulus via a series of reactions which glucocorticoids inhibit (Dougherty and Schneebeli, 1955; Ruhmann and Berliner, 1965). Within the inflammatory process fibroblasts manufacture connective tissue components, and they are the cells of origin or transformation for many other cell types. On exposure to steroids, fibroblasts react morphologically, e.g., the cytoplasm and nucleus disintegrate and cell replication is inhibited. We can directly correlate both these reactions with the anti-inflammatory activity of corticosteroids (Berliner and Ruhmann, 1967). Thus, the potencies of topical steroids have been measured using a sensitive assay based on the in vitro inhibition of fibroblast growth when incubated with propylene glycol solutions of the steroids. A plot of fibroblast growth (logarithm of the number of cells) versus log dose of steroid provides a measure of the relative potencies of steroids such as hydrocortisone and fluocinolone acetonide (Berliner, 1964; Berliner and Ruhmann, 1966; Berliner et al., 1966, 1967, 1970; Ruhmann and Berliner, 1967; Berliner and Nabors, 1967). The effects of glucocorticosteroids on primary human skin fibroblasts have been studied by Ponec et al. (1977a,b, 1980).

We can reasonably expect that those steroids which exhibit the greatest
lytic action against fibroblasts in culture would also do the same in vivo and
thus increase the danger of skin atrophy (Harman et al., 1971).

Haleblian (1976) tabulated the relative potencies of steroids such as
corticosterone, hydrocortisone, prednisolone, dexamethasone, parametha-
sone, triamincinolone acetonide, and fluocinolone acetonide as determined
by the antigranuloma bioassay, thymus involution, and fibroblast inhibition.

Further information concerning the effects of glucocorticoids on the
growth of fibroblasts has been given by Priestley (1978), Priestley and
Brown (1980), Platt (1978), Runikis et al. (1978), and Saarni et al. (1980).

2. Reduction of mitotic rate

Corticosteroids reduce the mitotic rate in normal human skin (Reaven
and Cox, 1968; Marks et al., 1971; Stoughton, 1972a) and in psoriatic skin
(Kalkoff et al., 1966; Fry and McMinn, 1968; Baxter and Stoughton, 1970).
Therefore, Fisher and Maibach (1971) suggested that this reduction in the
mitotic rate might be employed as a bioassay for topical steroids. Chaudhury
et al. (1956) and Hennings and Elgjo (1971) demonstrated a similar effect on
the normal and stripped skin of the mouse. Marks et al. (1973) developed
this tape-stripping technique to stimulate mitosis in the dorsal skin of the
hairless mouse. Topical steroid creams were applied under occlusion for
5 to 196 hr; the mice were injected intraperitoneally with Colcemid (deme-
colcine) to block cell division during metaphase; and 4 hr later they were
sacrificed. The dorsal skin was removed, fixed, and the mitotic index was
established. It was found that hydrocortisone had a significant antimitotic
effect at a concentration of $10^{-2}\%$; betamethasone 17-valerate was much
more active (detectable effect at $10^{-4}\%$). It is noteworthy that even bland
topical applications, with no added pharmacological agents, can have an
antimitotic effect on the epidermis of the stripped dorsal skin of hairless
mice (Tree and Marks, 1975).

3. Skin thinning

Spearman and Jarrett (1975) considered that, because thinning of the
epidermis follows an inhibition of epidermal mitosis, measurement of the
epidermal thickness of the mouse tail in the presence and absence of steroids
should prove to be a useful bioassay. These investigators applied various
steroid preparations to the tail skin of mice, sacrificed them, fixed and
stained the skin, and measured the epidermal thickness; the mouse tail is
particularly suitable for this purpose because the dermoepidermal junction
is virtually flat and lies parallel to the surface. The results obtained with
five marketed preparations closely corresponded to their clinical activities
in proliferating skin diseases. Winter and Wilson (1976a) considered that
the back skin of the domestic pig was more like human skin than was mouse

skin, and they used the epidermal thinning technique in both pig and man
(Winter and Wilson, 1976a,b; Winter and Burton, 1976).

Certain ointment bases, when applied to guinea pig skin, produce measurable and reproducible epidermal thickening (Schaaf and Gross, 1953;
Sarkany and Gaylarde, 1973), which may be suppressed by topical steroids.
A bioassay was developed on the reduction of the epidermal thickening
caused by the ointment base alone. The effect was related to the molecular
structure of the corticosteroid, its concentration, and the base used (Barnes
et al., 1975).

Delforno et al. (1978) showed that corticosteroids reduced viable epidermal cell size, not the number of cell layers.

In addition to epidermal measurements, investigators have experimented
with atrophy of the dermis or of the entire skin. Weirich and Longauer (1974)
monitored steroid effects on guinea pig dermis, and Wilson Jones (1976) extended that work to include whole skin thickness in man. Marks (1976), Dykes
and Marks (1979), and Brogden et al. (1976) discussed methods for the measurement of skin atrophogenicity of topical steroids. Kirby and Munro (1976)
used a micrometer to measure the total skin thickness in the mouse ear and
the human forearm and found that the magnitude of steroid-induced thinning
depended on the formulation applied. Stevanovic (1976) has attempted to
elucidate the mechanism of skin atrophy. Jablonska et al. (1979), using a
histological technique, evaluated skin atrophy in man induced by topical
corticosteroids; other workers have employed xeroradiographic, ultrasonic,
and stereomicroscopic methods (Marks et al., 1975; Alexander and Miller,
1979; Tan et al., 1981a,b; Frosch et al., 1981).

It is interesting that betamethasone 17-valerate acts as an anticorticosteroid in the rat as judged in dermal atrophy, anti-inflammatory, and antilymphocyte bioassays (Young et al., 1978a,b).

4. Inhibition of hair growth

Corticosteroids inhibit hair growth in the rat when they are applied
directly to the skin. The bioassay of Whitaker and Baker (1951) uses this
phenomenon by recording the extent and the pattern of regrowth of hair in
the clipped, dorsal region of the neck after treatment with steroids (Whitaker
and Baker, 1948; Baker, 1951; Fukuyama and Baker, 1958). This bioassay
was used to study the effect of molecular changes in a series of seven hydrocortisone analogs.

5. Leukocyte challenge

Corticosteroids inhibit the release of lysosomal enzymes from human
and rodent neutrophils. Watson et al. (1979) therefore tested seven corticosteroids for their effect on the release of β-glucuronidase when human white
cells were challenged with zymosan. The resultant ranking of the steroids
correlated quite well with published vasoconstrictor assays.

E. Psoriasis Bioassay

Most bioassays fail to deal with spontaneously occurring skin diseases
(Haleblian, 1976). The psoriasis bioassay was developed for treatment of
the disease lesion, and as such it is the nearest approximation to a clinical
trial. Chronic stabilized psoriatic patients are selected as test subjects,
and steroid preparations are applied under occlusion to the psoriasis plaque.
The area is read as either unchanged or converted to normal skin, and the
results may be presented as log dose versus percent cleared (probit) graphs.
A ranking was obtained of the relative potencies of fluocinonide, fluocinolone
acetonide, betamethasone valerate, and fluandrenolide (Scholtz and Dumas,
1968; Dumas and Scholtz, 1972; Burdick, 1972a).

F. The Vasoconstrictor Test

It has been known for more than 30 years that certain steroids make human
tissues pale. For example, Hollander et al. (1950) discovered that intra-
arterial steroids blanched engorged synovial membranes in rheumatoid
arthritis; Ashton and Cook (1952) reported vasoconstriction in superficial
corneal vascularization treated with subconjunctival steroids. For the skin,
Stüttgen (1961) showed that intracutaneous injection of hydrocortisone derivatives induced pallor. The blanching produced by topical application of anti-
inflammatory steroids has been used as a valuable bioassay since the early
1960s. McKenzie and Stoughton (1962), observing that treating psoriasis with
steroids under plastic wrap blanched the lesion and also normal skin, considered that this effect might be used to assess the percutaneous penetration
of corticosteroids. Their assay technique was to apply corticosteroid solutions or suspensions in 95% ethanol to healthy, unbroken forearm skin of
volunteers. One arm was protected with a perforated metal guard and left
unoccluded, while the other arm was wrapped with an occlusive plastic film.
After 16 hr the films and guards were removed and the presence or absence
of vasoconstriction was recorded; dramatic effects on skin pallor occurred
after occlusion. McKenzie (1962) then used the test to rank commercially
available steroids in order of potency.
     McKenzie and Atkinson (1964) used a refined bioassay to assess the
ability of betamethasone and 23 esters to induce skin pallor; this work led
to the introduction of betamethasone 17-valerate into dermatological therapy.
McKenzie (1966) emphasized that the test was most valuable for demon-
strating those compounds that blanched at high dilutions, which correlated
with the most effective clinical anti-inflammatory activity. However, Zaun
(1966) concluded that the test was not sufficiently sensitive to demonstrate
quantitatively differences between compounds—a conclusion amply disproved
by subsequent work.
     Further work with alcoholic solutions of steroids developed the test and
gave additional insight into the variables which affected the precision and

accuracy of the bioassay (Heseltine et al., 1964; Baker and Sattar, 1968; Stoughton, 1969; Place et al., 1970; Bickhardt, 1972; Stewart et al., 1973; Bagatell and Augustine, 1974; Harris, 1975; Moore-Robinson and Christie, 1970; Moore-Robinson, 1971; Garnier, 1971; Burdick, 1972a; Weirich and Lutz, 1974; Engel et al., 1974; Falconi and Rossi, 1972; Barry and Brace, 1975).

In the meantime, corticosteroids were being tested in solvents other than simple ethanol (Stoughton and Fritsch, 1964; Tissot and Osmundsen, 1966; Schlagel, 1972; Altmeyer and Zaun, 1974a; du Vivier and Stoughton, 1975).

In the clinic dermatologists seldom use ethanolic solutions or other single solvents, but they employ complex formulations. The remainder of this section will therefore discuss a suitable modification of the vasoconstriction assay using human volunteers—a bioassay which has been improved and extended from the original McKenzie-Stoughton assay. This bioassay may be employed both to screen new steroids for clinical efficacy and to determine the bioavailability of steroids from topical vehicles. The term "bioavailability" is taken here to mean the relative absorption efficiency for a medicament as determined by the release of the steroid from the formulation and its penetration through the stratum corneum and viable epidermis into the dermis to produce the characteristic vasoconstrictor effect (Barry, 1976). Thus we may measure the intensity and duration of the steroid-induced pallor to assess both the activity of a corticosteroid and its bioavailability from different vehicles, as determined by a pharmacological response (Barry and Woodford, 1978). We will consider the design, development, precision, and reproducibility of the modified vasoconstrictor test, together with some theoretical and practical aspects.

1. Development of a standard vasoconstrictor test

In the years since the vasoconstrictor test was introduced, many of its practitioners have proposed their own modifications of the test design. The most important variables have included such features as the method of application—occluded or nonoccluded; the duration of steroid application—from 1 hr to 20 hr; and the method for assessing the response—graded or present/absence, single or multiple readings with time. Table 5.1 is a chronological classification of some publications which report assays applied to topical formulations and which use the most common method of assessment—visual observation. The table cites many of the important references to this topic; for a more detailed treatment, the reader may consult Woodford (1977).

2. Design considerations for the vasoconstrictor test

To design a standard procedure using the arms of volunteers, many features must be considered. For example, blanching may be inconsistent for people with very short or very narrow forearms, for application sites

TABLE 5.1 Chronological Classification (1964–1982) of Human Vasoconstrictor Assays on Corticosteroid Formulations Using a Subjective Method of Measurement

Reference	Method of application	Duration of application time	Measurement of response	
			Method of assessment	Single or multiple measurement
Barrett et al. (1964)	Occlusion	Long (?)	Graded (?)	Single (?)
Sarkany et al. (1965)	Occlusion	Long	Graded (scale)	Single
Barrett et al. (1965)	Occlusion	Long	Graded (scale)	Single
Reid & Brookes (1968)	Occlusion	Long	Graded (area and pallor)	Single
Child et al. (1968)	Occlusion	Long	Presence or absence	Single
Busse et al. (1969)	Occlusion	Long	Graded (area)	Single
Christie & Moore–Robinson (1970)	Occlusion and nonocclusion	Short	Graded (scale)	Multiple
Burdick et al. (1970)	Occlusion	Short	Presence or absence	Multiple
Garnier (1971)	Occlusion	Short	Graded (scale)	Multiple
Pepler et al. (1971)	Occlusion	Short	Graded (scale)	Multiple
Ostrenga et al. (1971a)	Occlusion and nonocclusion	Short	Presence or absence	Multiple
Goldman et al. (1971a, b)	Nonocclusion	Short	Graded (scale)	Multiple
Reinstein et al. (1972)	Nonocclusion	Short	Presence or absence	Multiple
Burdick (1972a, b)	Occlusion and nonocclusion	Short	Presence or absence	Multiple
Stoughton (1972b)	Nonocclusion	Long	Graded (scale)	Single
Burdick et al. (1973)	Occlusion and nonocclusion	Short	Presence or absence	Multiple
Smith et al. (1973)	Occlusion	Short	Presence or absence	Single
Poulsen et al. (1974)	Occlusion and nonocclusion	Short	Presence or absence and graded (scale)	Multiple
Zaynoun & Kurban (1974)	Occlusion	Short	Graded (scale)	Single
Kaidbey & Kligman (1974)	Occlusion	Short	Graded (scale)	Single

Study	Condition	Duration	Scoring	Application
Woodford & Barry (1974)	Occlusion	Short	Graded (scale)	Multiple
Barry & Woodford (1974)	Occlusion and nonocclusion	Short	Graded (scale)	Multiple
Barry & Woodford (1975)	Occlusion and nonocclusion	Short	Graded (scale)	Multiple
Whitefield & McKenzie (1975)	Occlusion	Long	Presence or absence	Single
Fredriksson et al. (1975)	Occlusion	Long	Graded (scale)	Single
Barry & Woodford (1976)	Occlusion	Short	Graded (scale)	Multiple
Woodford & Barry (1977a)	Occlusion and nonocclusion	Short	Graded (scale)	Multiple
Woodford & Barry (1977b)	Occlusion	Short	Graded (scale)	Multiple
Barry and Woodford (1977)	Nonocclusion with multiple application	Multiple periods	Graded (scale)	Multiple
Barry and Woodford (1978)	Occlusion and nonocclusion	Short	Graded (scale)	Multiple
Poulsen et al. (1978)	Occlusion and nonocclusion	Short	Presence or absence and graded (scale)	Multiple
Girard et al. (1978)	Occlusion	Short	Graded (scale)	Multiple
Wallace et al. (1979)	Occlusion	Long	Graded (scale)	Single
Barbier et al. (1979)	Occlusion and nonocclusion	Short	Graded (scale)	Multiple
Woodford & Barry (1979)	Occlusion	Short	Graded (scale)	Multiple
Coleman et al. (1979)	Occlusion and nonocclusion	Short	Graded (scale)	Multiple
Poulsen & Rorsman (1980)	Occlusion and nonocclusion	Short	Graded (scale)	Multiple
Bengtsson (1980)	Occlusion and nonocclusion	Short and long	Graded (scale)	Multiple
Woodford (1981)	Occlusion	Short	Graded (scale)	Multiple
Woodford et al. (1981, 1982)	Nonocclusion with multiple application	Multiple periods	Graded (scale)	Multiple

Source: Barry and Woodford (1978).

nearer to the pulse or elbow than 4 cm, and for typists, i.e., persons exer-
cising the forearm muscles during the period of steroid application (Burdick,
1974; Barry and Woodford, 1978). Because of the differences between sites
on the same forearm (McKenzie and Atkinson, 1964; Kirsch et al., 1982),
preparations should be applied according to randomization charts. Lower
blanching scores and more inter- and intrasubject variation arise with
nonocclusion. A short steroid application time of 6 hr provides better differentiation between products than does 12 hr of occlusion. Variations in the
applied amount of a cream or ointment between 3 and 8 mg applied over
50 mm^2 of skin do not significantly affect the degree of pallor produced over
96 hr. After the application period of 6 hr, skin sites may be gently washed
with soap and water (30° to 40°C) and patted dry. Vigorous drying may produce erythema which obscures the immediate blanching response. Washing
with 70% aqueous ethanol confers no advantage and may produce occasional
transient pallor.

The blanching readings should be taken under standard lighting conditions
with the arms held horizontally or slightly upward; the blood vessels in some
volunteers enlarge when their arms hang downward, and this swelling may
obscure the pallor.

The pallor may be assessed against untreated skin on a 0 to 4 scale with
half-point ratings as follows: 0, normal skin; 1, slight pallor of indistinct
outline; 2, more intense pallor with at least two corners of the application
square outlined; 3, even pallor with a clear outline of the application area;
4, very intense pallor. Only the most potent formulations applied to very
sensitive volunteers produce a score of 4 at the peak time of 9 to 12 hr.
Pallor should be assessed by observing the response for a minute before
allocating scores, when the eye can seek out the less intense sites.

The main objection to tests of this type is the subjective nature of the
assessment, which makes training of the observer essential and interlaboratory comparisons difficult. It is advisable to include a standard steroid formulation in every trial so as to help to control the test. Over the years there
have been several attempts to replace a visual method of assessment by an
instrumental approach. Greeson et al. (1973) modified the xenon-133 gas
clearance technique of Sejrsen (1966) to measure cutaneous blood flow alterations caused by flurandrenolide, and they correlated decreased blood flow
and vasoconstriction. Tronnier (1970) reported the "thermal conductivity"
of areas blanched by steroid. Stüttgen (1976) reported that blanching was
accompanied by a decrease in IR radiation, although Kiraly and Soos (1976)
could not detect such differences with an IR camera. Gibson (1971) discussed
the disadvantages of visual standards and the limitations of normal photographic techniques.

Reflectometry and colorimetry have been used in anthropological studies
of different races, and these methods have received some attention in steroid
assessment studies. Simple reflectometry is suitable for measuring changes
in pigmentation and has been used to quantify erythema, but the technique

lacks sensitivity (Gibson, 1971). Heseltine et al. (1964) found that the procedure was no improvement over the visual assessment for pallor. Zaun
and Altmeyer (1973) and Altmeyer and Zaun (1974a,b, 1976a,b) used a
reflex-photometric technique to study the blanching activity of steroids but
found that the difference between blanched areas and normal skin was never
more than 6%. This disparity is too small to allow precise measurements
in biopharmaceutical studies.

Reid and Brookes (1968) assessed blanching with a reflectance spec-
trometer but found that differentiation between steroid products was difficult.
Tring (1973a,b) used a similar technique to assess the effects of various
treatments, including steroid application, on skin color in psoriasis. It is
possible that reflectance measurements are more satisfactory for determining skin color than for assessing blanching. Considerable success has
been achieved by workers determining the logarithm of the inverse of the
reflectance of the skin (Feather et al, 1981, 1982).

Kiraly and Soos (1976) used a tristimulus colorimeter to measure
blanching and claimed the same statistical differentiation between potent
steroids as were obtained by simultaneous subjective pallor assessments.
However, Woodford (1977) found that a Mark 3 Lovibond Flexible Optic
Tintometer was tedious to use, subject to operator error (for example, the
pressure of the measuring head changed the skin color), and the instrument
was not sufficiently sensitive to distinguish adequately among different degrees of pallor.

Aiache et al. (1980) used a thermographic method of analysis and concluded that there was no relation between the traditional blanching assay
and thermography.

For optimal value in biopharmaceutical studies, any instrumental
method for assessing the blanching response must meet certain criteria.
The instrument must not contribute to the response which it measures, nor
should it change the physiological or physicochemical condition of the skin.
Thus, methods which apply even a slight weight to the skin can cause a
spurious pallor, and occlusive methods may hydrate the skin and alter the
percutaneous absorption of the steroid. The determination must be rapid
compared with the time scale of the absorption process. The measurement
should be sensitive, reproducible, and accurate, and the technique must be
acceptable to the volunteers. The method has to allow for physiological
variables, such as the normal variation of skin temperature during the day
(Shahidullah et al., 1969; Durocher and Bielmann, 1975; Woodford and
Barry, 1973). Most importantly, any instrumental technique must not be
affected by—or must compensate for—skin imperfections which may alter,
for example, a reflectance measurement. Difficulties can arise with
freckles, moles, scars, and other skin discolorations, as well as prominent
blood vessels, hairs, excessive tanning, etc. At the present time, the only
really satisfactory technique employs the trained human eye, which is adept
at assessing subtle color differences and at making automatic allowances

for skin imperfections. In particular, the eye-brain combination can readily compare a steroid application site with the adjacent untreated skin; it is this comparison, rather than some arbitrary fixed standard of pallor, which is the cornerstone of a successful vasoconstrictor assay. Thus, Barry and Woodford (1978) found that a visual assessment method was more sensitive and precise than an objective, instrumental method such as reflectance spectroscopy.

The assessed response may be slightly higher than the true reading when, for example, the volunteer has been sedentary in cold weather. Scoring following 1 hr of normal activity indoors produces a result which fits smoothly on the blanching curve (Burdick, 1972a,b; Barry and Woodford, 1978).

The blanching response fades quickly and erratically if volunteers become hot or their arms become wet; panel members may need to change their life-style somewhat during a test period.

To use the vasoconstrictor assay as a biopharmaceutical technique, it is not essential to know precisely how steroids produce pallor. This is fortunate, as the exact mechanism by which topical corticosteroids blanch skin remains in doubt. Most workers agree that the pallor arises from a vasoconstrictor action and the terms "vasoconstriction," "blanching," and "pallor" are widely used as synonyms. Several studies suggest that the effect is caused indirectly by sensitization of the vascular musculature to norepinephrine (noradrenalin), while other experiments indicate a mechanism which does not implicate norepinephrine exclusively. For the interested reader, relevant discussions have been provided by Fritz and Levine (1951), Ashton and Cook (1952), Zweifach et al. (1953), Reis (1960), Juhlin (1964), Frank et al. (1964), Altura (1966), Solomon et al. (1965), Möller (1962), Kopin and Axelrod (1963), du Vivier and Stoughton (1975), Wolf et al. (1974), Snell (1976), and Woodford (1977). Attempts have been made to determine which skin blood vessels are involved in the blanching response (Frank et al., 1964; Zweifach et al., 1953; Thune, 1970a,b, 1971a,b, 1972, 1976; Stüttgen, 1976; Kramor, 1975).

3. The Barry-Woodford vasoconstrictor test:
occluded

Semisolid formulations are stored at room temperature, and the first gram of product from a tube is rejected. Caucasian volunteers are screened for a consistent response to a standard preparation [Betnovate Cream (Glaxo, United Kingdom), containing 0.1% betamethasone 17-valerate]. They are ranked as good, medium, or poor responders. Ten volunteers are selected to provide a team with a balance of such responders. In subsequent trials, any particular volunteer not available may be replaced by one with a similar sensitivity ranking. This procedure leads to greater consistency of results from trial to trial. No volunteer should have received topical application of a steroid for at least 2 months prior to an investigation.

Some 5 ± 1 mg of each product is applied to the washed flexor surface of both forearms (avoiding regions with skin blemishes or large blood vessels, and the wrist and elbow). Application sites are paired 7 × 7 mm areas punched out of double-sided adhesive Blenderm polyethylene tape (3M Medical Products, London); formulations are applied by reference to randomization tables. The sites are occluded with type S 12 μm Melinex film (I.C.I. Plastics Division, Welwyn Garden City, United Kingdom) for 6 hr. The sites are then washed with soap and water at skin temperature, dried, and the degree of pallor is estimated 10 min later under standard lighting conditions using the 0 to 4 scale.

Readings may then be taken as a function of time to provide data points for skin blanching at 6, 7, 8, 9, 12, 24, 32, 48, 72, 80, and 96 hr after application. A full blanching profile may then be drawn. All estimations of pallor are performed in a double-blind manner by an experienced investigator, without reference to application charts. During the test period, as far as possible, volunteers should avoid high temperatures and water.

4. The Barry-Woodford vasoconstrictor test: nonoccluded

The nonoccluded design is similar to the occluded tests, except that after application of samples to the skin the Blenderm tapes are removed and a perforated plastic screen is used for 6 hr instead of the polyester film. This design removes the occlusive, hydrating effect of the water-impervious film.

Unless otherwise specified, the remainder of this discussion will refer to the occluded test.

5. Precision and reproducibility of the Barry-Woodford vasoconstrictor test

For a test which depends on a pharmacological response in humans assessed subjectively, it is important to investigate how results may alter as the panel composition changes and how reproducible the test is from year to year. For this purpose, Betnovate Cream was selected as a suitable formulation, as this is our standard preparation which we use when assessing the activities and bioavailabilities of topical steroid products. Sixteen volunteers were employed, six being used throughout as members of every panel and the remainder being called upon as necessary to produce full panels of 10 volunteers.

The occluded blanching test was used, and the results for all volunteers were expressed in a standard manner as the percentage of the total possible score at each time period of assessment. A blanching profile could then be drawn from a plot of percentage total possible score as a function of time. Ten experiments at different seasons over a period of $3\frac{1}{2}$ years have provided the curves in Fig. 5.6. The graphs were similar, and the season of the year did not affect the results.

The areas under the blanching curves (from the 6-hr reading to the disappearance of pallor) were obtained by planimetry and were expressed in units of "percentage of the total possible score × hours." The mean value was 1,860 (range: 1,448 to 2,045), with a standard deviation of 187 (10% of mean value) and a standard error of the mean (n = 10) of 59. Figure 5.7 illustrates an alternative method of presenting the data—as a blanching profile of the mean ± standard error of the mean for the data

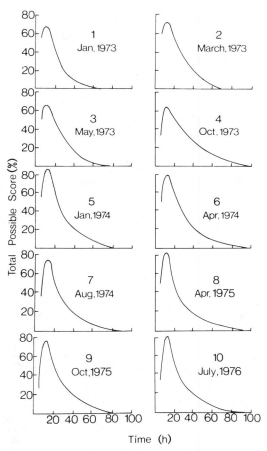

FIG. 5.6 Percentage total possible score as a function of time for Betnovate Cream: 10 experiments performed over $3\frac{1}{2}$ years. (From Barry and Woodford, 1978; reproduced with permission of Blackwell Scientific Publications Ltd.)

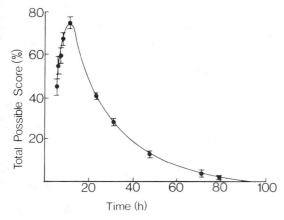

FIG. 5.7 Percentage total possible score as a function of time for Betnovate Cream: mean of 10 experiments ± standard error of the mean, n = 10. (From Barry and Woodford, 1978; reproduced with permission of Blackwell Scientific Publications Ltd.)

points determined at each time interval up to 96 hr. The area under this curve is 1,855% TPS (total possible score)-hour units.

For statistical treatment, the scores for each volunteer over all reading times for each experiment are summed and subjected to an analysis of variance. The computer program analyzes the data without transformation or in one of five transformations [x^{-1}, $x^{-1/2}$, $x^{1/2}$, log x, and x^2 (Tukey, 1975)]. Tests for nonadditivity (Harter and Lum, 1962) will then indicate a preferred order from which the variance analysis may be calculated. For most of our experiments, the square root values are used.

Alternative statistical treatments of blanching data have recently been reported by Poulsen and Rorsman (1980) and Clanachan et al. (1980).

The main conclusion from our work is that for experienced investigators adhering to a strict protocol and using a controlled panel of volunteers the bioassay is sensitive, accurate, and reproducible. The variability between individual volunteers is only of the order of 25% standard deviation.

6. Dose-response relationships in the vasoconstrictor test

To give confidence in the use of the vasoconstrictor test for biopharmaceutical assessments, it is important to establish dose-response relationships. Experiments were therefore performed to see if model preparations which contained different concentrations of steroid in the same base produced graded blanching responses. An essential criterion in this program is that the steroid in each formulation should be entirely in solution. There would then be no problem with suspended drug dissolving on dilution with

placebo vehicle and thus maintaining the thermodynamic activity of the
penetrant. Two commercial formulations were selected, Bebate Gel
(0.025% betamethasone 17-benzoate) and Topilar Cream (0.025% fluclorolone
acetonide). Five serial dilutions were made in their respective placebo
bases, and all preparations were tested for vasoconstrictor activity using
the occluded procedure with an additional pallor estimate at 56 hr (Barry
and Woodford, 1978).

The blanching profiles for the two series of preparations illustrated
in Fig. 5.8 show a satisfactory gradation of response with applied steroid
concentration. The curves were hand drawn, but the position of the maximum was determined by computer to obtain the peak maximum score, B_{max}.
The areas under the curve, peak times (t_{max}), and B_{max} are listed in
Table 5.2. The blanching profiles for each series of diluted preparations
were similar to that of the undiluted formulation, allowing for the difficulty
of precise assessment at low vasoconstriction scores (i.e., below 10-15%
total possible score).

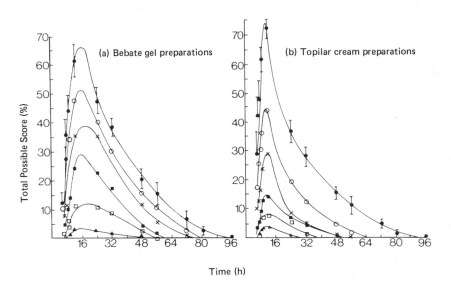

FIG. 5.8 Percentage total possible score as a function of time for Bebate
Gel and Topilar Cream and their respective dilutions in placebo bases.
(a) Bebate Gel: •, $2.5 \times 10^{-2}\%$; o, $1.5 \times 10^{-2}\%$; ×, $5 \times 10^{-3}\%$; ■, $3 \times 10^{-3}\%$;
□, $1 \times 10^{-3}\%$; ▲, $2 \times 10^{-4}\%$. (b) Topilar Cream: •, $2.5 \times 10^{-2}\%$; o, $5 \times$
$10^{-3}\%$; ×, $1 \times 10^{-3}\%$; ■, $5 \times 10^{-4}\%$; □, $2 \times 10^{-4}\%$; ▲, $4 \times 10^{-5}\%$. Undiluted
preparations ± SEM (n = 10) as example. (From Barry and Woodford, 1978;
reproduced with permission of Blackwell Scientific Publications Ltd.)

TABLE 5.2 Blanching Parameters for Bebate Gel and Topilar Cream
Dilutions in Their Respective Placebo Bases

Steroid preparation	Applied concentration (% w/w)	B_{max} [a] (% TPS)	t_{max} [b] (hr)	Area under the curve [c] (% TPS × hr)
Bebate Gel	2.5×10^{-2}	65.3	14.9	2150
	1.5×10^{-2}	51.0	15.5	1610
	5.0×10^{-3}	38.4	17.0	1240
	3.0×10^{-3}	29.5	16.1	740
	1.0×10^{-3}	10.3	22.0	337
	2.0×10^{-4}	3.1	14.1	86.2
Mean t_{max} = 16.7 hr (SD 2.77)				
Topilar Cream	2.5×10^{-2}	72.0	11.0	1790
	5×10^{-3}	43.8	12.5	873
	1×10^{-3}	28.7	11.0	466
	5×10^{-4}	14.3	10.6	282
	2×10^{-4}	8.2	15.3	141
	4×10^{-5}	4.4	12.4	58.7
Mean t_{max} = 12.1 hr (SD 1.74)				

[a] Peak response, i.e., maximum percentage possible score (TPS).
[b] Time of peak response.
[c] Obtained by planimetry of the blanching profile (three significant figures).
Source: From Barry and Woodford (1978).

Wagner (1968) suggested some empirical treatments to relate pharmacological responses to the dose of the drug employed. The data in Table
5.2 were used to see if these relationships were valid for the vasoconstrictor
response.

Figure 5.9 illustrates the data for the peak responses (B_{max}) expressed
as functions of the applied concentration. Similar plots were obtained using
the area-under-the-curve values as the ordinate. Figure 5.9a presents a
graph on Cartesian coordinates, illustrating two separate regions; thus the
response is not directly proportional to the applied steroid concentration.
The curve shapes may arise in part from decreased receptor availability
as the maximum response is approached (Ariens, 1966), or the plot could
reflect nonlinearity in the 0 to 4 scoring scale.

Figure 5.9b illustrates the traditional pharmacological method for
plotting data in the form of log dose (equated to applied steroid concentration)

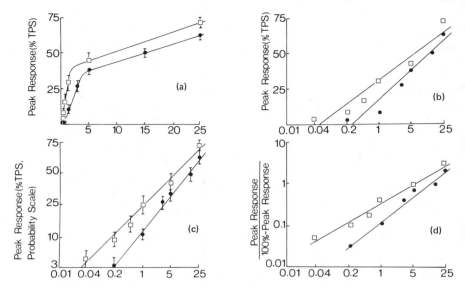

FIG. 5.9 Applied steroid concentration ($\% \times 10^{-3}$): a, linear scale;
b through d, log scale. Applied concentration versus peak response relationship for formulations and dilutions in placebo bases: ●, Bebate Gel;
□, Topilar Cream. (a) Cartesian; (b) semilog; (c) log-probability; (d) log-
logistic coordinates. SEM (n = 10) shown in (a) and (c) as examples; TPS,
total possible score. (From Barry and Woodford, 1978; reproduced with
permission of Blackwell Scientific Publications Ltd.)

against response. The results suggest partial sigmoid curves and straight
lines could be drawn through the approximate linear portions of the curves.
However, such selection of linear regions requires a subjective judgement
as to the onset of linearity. Instead, best straight lines were drawn through
all data points using least-squares linear regression. The extrapolation of
these plots to the dose axis produces the "minimum effective concentration"
(Wagner, 1968). In such semilog plots the response is expressed as a discontinuous function of concentration because the equations predict no real
maximum response (Wagner, 1975).

     Figure 5.9c illustrates the blanching data as log-normal probability
(probit) plots, in which the partial sigmoid shapes of Fig. 5.9b become
more linear. In fact, Finney (1952) stated that probit transformation is
simply a means for representing the sigmoid curve of response versus
concentration by a straight line.

     Blanching data are plotted in the form of the log-logistic function (or
log-log plot) in Fig. 5.9d. Berkson (1951, 1953) discussed the application
of a logistic function as an alternative to normal sigmoid and probit graphs.

In practice, log-normal probability and log-logistic plots have similar
shapes over a wide response range (Wagner, 1968). However, the function
of choice for presenting the blanching data is log-logistic, as proposed by
Wagner, because such plots (1) predict a zero response at zero concentration, (2) fully characterize a sigmoid curve over its entire range, (3) are
continuous over the entire concentration range, and (4) predict a maximum
response as the concentration increases indefinitely.

7. The steroid reservoir and the vasoconstrictor test

The use of the blanching test to assess the so-called steroid reservoir
has been dealt with in Chap. 3, Sec. III.

8. Additional pharmacokinetic and bio-availability considerations

Theoretically, we could extend the treatment discussed here to a full
pharmacokinetic analysis. For example, we could employ the peak response-
concentration curves of Fig. 5.9 as calibration curves to convert observed
blanching response versus time graphs into corresponding site of action
drug concentration plots. Then, we could use the dose–effect curve in an
analogous manner to a nonlinear Beer's law plot and we could apply nonlinear
pharmacokinetic methods. However, after full investigations which showed
that the process was applicable in principle, it was not proceeded with
further (Brace, 1977). Essentially, the problem is that in the majority of
instances the precision of a subjective visual method, although accurate
enough for most purposes, is not sufficiently precise to provide firm,
unequivocal conclusions in pharmacokinetic terms.

The development of a precise and sensitive in vivo test, demonstration
of a dose-related response, use of appropriate pharmacological effect–time
curves, and correlations of in vitro and in vivo data (Barry and Woodford,
1978) all comply with the FDA Bioequivalence Requirements and In Vivo
Bioavailability Procedures (Gardner, 1977). In fact, they far exceed these
requirements for topical steroid preparations.

9. Multiple application of topical steroids: tachyphylaxis of the vasoconstrictor response

An interesting feature of the vasoconstrictor response is the phenomenon
of tachyphylaxis to multiple application of topical steroids. Barry and Woodford (1977) applied commercial preparations of fluocinonide, fluocinolone
acetonide, betamethasone 17-valerate, hydrocortisone 17-butyrate, and
hydrocortisone according to a multiple dosage regimen. The blanching response first increased but then diminished with continued application over
a 5-day period. After 2 days of rest during which no steroid was applied,
the application sites recovered considerably but tachyphylaxis again
occurred from subsequent repeated applications. Even the hydrocortisone

formulations produced acute tolerance similar to that occurring with the more potent steroids. Woodford et al. (1981, 1982) developed this approach further to assess the bioavailabilities and activities of three amcinonide preparations and Betnovate Cream using three multiple dosage regimen blanching assays. This work assessed the clinical implications of the tachyphylactic response to topical steroids and suggested that the most advantageous dosage regimen is a once–daily application with no loading dose (du Vivier and Stoughton, 1975, 1976; Altmeyer and Zaun, 1976b).

10. Summary of the possible uses for the vasoconstrictor test

The vasoconstrictor bioassay is a very valuable technique with which to assess the combination of intrinsic activity at a receptor site and skin penetrability of a topical glucocorticoid. The test can also be exploited to scrutinize other drugs which blanch tissues (Stoughton, 1972a). Some possible applications for the assay include the following.

a. Screening of novel synthetic steroids   When medicinal chemists synthesize new topical steroids, they may acquire considerable information about structure-activity relationships by conducting the blanching test with the molecules dissolved in a simple solvent such as ethanol (e.g., see Schlagel, 1972; Barry and Brace, 1975). There are close correlations between the results of the vasoconstrictor test and anti-inflammatory potencies as judged in the clinic, both for alcoholic solutions of steroids and for developed, marketed formulations.

b. Development of topical formulations   When developing optimal formulations for a new steroid, it is uneconomical in time and money for the manufacturer to submit all possible formulation candidates to a full clinical trial. One of the most valuable features of the vasoconstrictor bioassay is that it allows the pharmaceutical scientist to select only the best formulations to go forward to a clinical trial. For example, Fig. 5.10 shows the blanching profiles of 0.025% betamethasone benzoate as presented in a quick-break aerosol foam, in the foam concentrate, and in a range of semisolid dosage forms. The superiority of the aerosol foam preparation is readily apparent, as is the inferiority of the cream.

c. Testing of marketed products and their ranking in terms of clinical efficacy   The activities and bioavailabilities of many proprietary corticosteroid formulations have been assessed by the single-application vasoconstrictor test of Barry and Woodford (1974, 1975, 1976). This work ranked the preparations in a classification which often demonstrated comparability between the blanching results and the conclusions of clinical trials (Portnoy, 1972; Baran, 1972; Rex, 1973; Goodwin et al., 1973; MacDonald and Fry, 1974; Sparks and Wilson, 1974; Whitefield and McKenzie, 1975; Corbett, 1976; Wilson, 1976). Even though we cannot

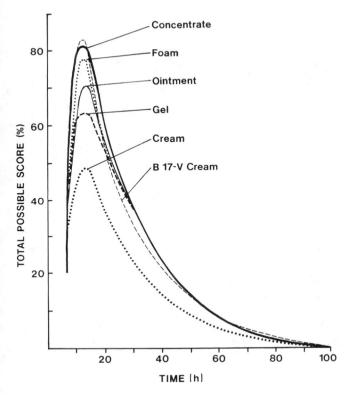

FIG. 5.10 Blanching response to betamethasone benzoate formulations containing 0.025% steroid and to 0.1% betamethasone 17-valerate (B 17-V) cream. (From Woodford and Barry, 1977a.)

prove conclusively that there is a correlation between the clinical efficacy of topical steroids and vasoconstriction in the bioassay, in the absence of comprehensive comparative clinical investigations we have good reason to base the classification of these preparations on vasoconstrictor studies (Poulsen and Rorsman, 1980; Place et al., 1970). Stoughton (1976) reported five different investigations in which two steroid preparations were compared with regard to vasoconstriction and clinical performance in psoriasis; there was close correlation in all studies. Maibach and Stoughton (1975) employed pallor assessment to classify steroids in order of potency. They maintained that because of the time and work required from highly qualified experts which are needed to make a thorough clinical comparison, there is no reasonable alternative to the vasoconstrictor assay for assessing steroid potency. There appear to be no examples of gross lack of correlation between clinical anti-inflammatory activities and vasoconstrictor bioassays competently performed.

Blanching tests can often expose quite subtle interactions, such as the modulating potential of an antimicrobial in a bioassay (Barry and Woodford, 1974, 1975). In one combination product the blanching response of the steroid decreased, and this reduction was traced to the irritant action of an ingredient which had been added to the formulation simply to aid in the chemical assay of the germicide. On another occasion a commercial steroid cream produced an unexpectedly high vasoconstrictor response. On investigation it was discovered that the chemical control procedures used in the industrial laboratory were at fault and that as a consequence the cream contained a greater steroid concentration than its label claimed.

d. Fundamental studies on percutaneous absorption   The vasoconstrictor assay furnishes a means for testing various aspects of fundamental theory, in vivo, and in humans. Examples of investigations which are currently in progress include work on the thermodynamic activity of steroids in topical formulations as well as the elucidation of the mode of action of penetration enhancers (Woodford and Barry, 1982).

e. Development of dosage regimens for topical steroids   Topical therapy differs from other routes of medication, such as oral or parenteral treatment, in that the drug regimen is seldom developed from and tested by fundamental pharmacokinetic/pharmacodynamic principles. However, we may use the multiple application of topical steroids, as modified by the tachyphylactic response, to design effective dosage regimens. This topic was discussed in Sec. IV.F.9.

REFERENCES

Aiache, J. M., Lafaye, C., Bouzat, J., and Rabier, R. (1980). J. Pharm. Belg. 35:187.
Ainsworth, M. (1960). J. Soc. Cosmetic Chemists 11:69.
Albery, W. J., and Hadgraft, J. (1979). J. Pharm. Pharmacol. 31:65.
Albery, W. J., Couper, A. M., Hadgraft, J., and Ryan, C. (1974). J. Chem. Soc. (Faraday I) 70:1124.
Albery, W. J., Burke, J. F., Leffler, E. B., and Hadgraft, J. (1976). J. Chem. Soc. (Faraday I) 72:1618.
Alexander, H., and Miller, D. L. (1979). J. Invest. Dermatol. 72:17.
Al-Khamis, K. I. (1981). Ph.D. Thesis, University of Nottingham, United Kingdom.
Altmeyer, P., and Zaun, H. (1974a). Arch. Dermatol. Forsch. 248:387.
Altmeyer, P., and Zaun, H. (1974b). Arch. Dermatol. Forsch. 250:381.
Altmeyer, P., and Zaun, H. (1976a). Arch. Dermatol. Res. 255:43.
Altmeyer, P., and Zaun, H. (1976b). Arch. Dermatol. Res. 255:51.

Altura, B. M. (1966). Am. J. Physiol. 211:1393.

Ariens, E. J. (1966). Adv. Drug Res. 3:1.

Asherson, G. L., and Ptak, W. (1968). Immunology 15:405.

Ashton, N., and Cook, C. (1952). Br. J. Exp. Pathol. 33:445.

Astley, J. P., and Levine, M. (1976). J. Pharm. Sci. 65:210.

Ayres, J. W., and Laskar, P. A. (1974). J. Pharm. Sci. 63:1402.

Bagatell, F. K., and Augustine, M. A. (1974). Curr. Ther. Res. 16:748.

Baker, B. L. (1951). Ann. N.Y. Acad. Sci. 53:690.

Baker, H., and Kligman, A. M. (1967a). Arch. Dermatol. 96:441.

Baker, H., and Kligman, A. M. (1967b). J. Invest. Dermatol. 30:315.

Baker, H., and Sattar, H. A. (1968). Br. J. Dermatol. 80:46.

Banfi, S., Cornelli, U., and Carpi, C. (1976). Curr. Ther. Res. 19:126.

Baran, R. (1972). Acta Derm. Venereol. (Stockh.) 52(Suppl. 67):79.

Barbier, A., Girard, J., Tardieu, J. C., and Lafille, C. (1979). Clin. Ther. 2:194.

Barnes, H., Gaylarde, P. M., Brock, A. P., and Sarkany, I. (1975). Br. J. Dermatol. 92:459.

Barrett, C. W., Hadgraft, J. W., and Sarkany, I. (1964). J. Pharm. Pharmac. 16 Suppl. 104T.

Barrett, C. W., Hadgraft, J. W., Caron, G. A., and Sarkany, I. (1965). Br. J. Dermatol. 77:576.

Barry, B. W. (1976). Dermatologica 152(Suppl. 1):47.

Barry, B. W., and Brace, A. R. (1975). J. Invest. Dermatol. 64:418.

Barry, B. W., and Brace, A. R. (1977). J. Pharm. Pharmacol. 29:397.

Barry, B. W., and El Eini, D. I. D. (1976). J. Pharm. Pharmacol. 28:219.

Barry, B. W., and Woodford, R. (1974). Br. J. Dermatol. 91:323.

Barry, B. W., and Woodford, R. (1975). Br. J. Dermatol. 93:563.

Barry, B. W., and Woodford, R. (1976). Br. J. Dermatol. 95:423.

Barry, B. W., and Woodford, R. (1977). Br. J. Dermatol. 97:555.

Barry, B. W., and Woodford, R. (1978). J. Clin. Pharm. 3:43.

Baxter, D. C., and Stoughton, R. B. (1970). J. Invest. Dermatol. 54:411.

Bengtsson, G. E. (1980). Drugs Exp. Clin. Res. 6:385.

Berenson, G. S., and Burch, G. E. (1951). Am. J. Trop. Med. Hyg. 31:842.

Berkson, J. (1951). Biometrics 7:327.

Berkson, J. (1953). J. Am. Statist. Anlz. 48:565.

Berliner, D. L. (1964). Ann. N.Y. Acad. Sci. 116:1078.

Berliner, D. L., and Nabors, C. J. (1967). J. Reticuloendothel. Soc. 4:284.

Berliner, D. L., and Ruhmann, A. G. (1966). Endocrinology 78:373.

Berliner, D. L., and Ruhmann, A. G. (1967). J. Invest. Dermatol. 49:117.

Berliner, D. L., Ruhmann, A. G., Berliner, M. L., and Dougherty, T. F. (1966). Excerpta Med. 111:180.

Berliner, D. L., Gallegos, A. J., and Schneebeli, G. L. (1967). J. Invest. Dermatol. 48:44.

Berliner, D. L. , Bartley, M. H. , Kenner, G. H. , and Jee, W. S. S. (1970). Br. J. Dermatol. 82(Suppl. 6):53.

Bettley, F. R. (1961). Br. J. Dermatol. 73:448.

Bettley, F. R. , and Grice, K. A. (1965). Br. J. Dermatol. 77:627.

Bickardt, R. (1972). Hautarzt 23:301.

Bielicky, T. , and Döring, H. F. (1974). Arch. Dermatol. Forsch. 250:369.

Billups, N. F. , and Patel, N. K. (1970). Am. J. Pharm. Educ. 34:190.

Blank, I. H. (1952). J. Invest. Dermatol. 18:443.

Blank, I. H. (1960a). J. Occup. Med. 2:6.

Blank, I. H. (1960b). J. Soc. Cosmetic Chemists 11:59.

Bottari, F. , Di Colo, G. , Nannipieri, E. , Saettone, M. F. , and Serafini, M. F. (1977). J. Pharm. Sci. 66:926.

Bowser, R. T. , and Baer, H. (1963). J. Immunol. 91:791.

Brace, A. R. (1977). Ph.D. Thesis, Council for National Academic Awards, Portsmouth Polytechnic, United Kingdom.

Bradshaw, M. (1961). Am. Perfumer 76:15.

Brogden, R. N. , Pinder, R. M. , Sawyer, P. R. , Speight, T. M. , and Avery, G. S. (1976). Drugs 12:249.

Bronaugh, R. L. , Congdon, E. R. , and Scheuplein, R. J. (1981). J. Invest. Dermatol. 76:94.

Brunner, M. J. , and Finkelstein, P. (1960). Arch. Dermatol. 81:453.

Burdick, K. H. (1972a). Acta Derm. Venereol. (Stockh.) 52(Suppl. 67):19.

Burdick, K. H. (1972b). Acta Derm. Venereol. (Stockh.) 52(Suppl. 67):24.

Burdick, K. H. (1974). Arch. Dermatol. 110:238.

Burdick, K. H. , Poulsen, B. , and Place, V. A. (1970). J. Am. Med. Assoc. 211:462.

Burdick, K. H. , Haleblian, J. K. , Poulsen, B. J. , and Cobner, S. E. (1973). Curr. Ther. Res. 15:233.

Burrows, W. M. , and Stoughton, R. B. (1976). Arch. Dermatol. 112:175.

Busse, M. J. , Hunt, P. , Lees, K. A. , Maggs, P. N. D. , and McCarthy, T. M. (1969). Br. J. Dermatol. 81(Suppl. 4):103.

Butler, J. A. (1966). Br. J. Dermatol. 78:665.

Calman, K. C. (1970). Br. J. Dermatol. 82(Suppl. 6):26.

Chase, M. W. (1969). Toxicol. Appl. Pharmacol. (Suppl. 3):45.

Chaudhury, A. P. , Halberg, F. , and Bittner, J. J. (1956). Proc. Soc. Exp. Biol. Med. 91:602.

Chayen, J. , Bitensky, L. , Butcher, R. G. , Poulter, L. W. , and Ubhi, G. S. (1970). Br. J. Dermatol. 82(Suppl. 6):62.

Child, K. J. , English, A. F. , Gilbert, H. G. , Hewitt, A. , and Woollett, E. A. (1968). Arch. Dermatol. 97:407.

Chimoskey, J. E. , Holloway, G. A. , and Flanagan, W. J. (1975). J. Invest. Dermatol. 65:241.

Choman, B. R. (1960). J. Soc. Cosmetic Chemists 11:138.

Christie, G. A. , and Moore-Robinson, M. (1970). Br. J. Dermatol. 82 (Suppl. 6):93.

Clanachan, I., Devitt, H. G., Foreman, M. I., and Kelly, I. P. (1980). J. Pharmacol. Methods 4:209.

Coldman, M. F., Poulsen, B. J., and Higuchi, T. (1969). J. Pharm. Sci. 58:1098.

Coldman, M. F., Lockerbie, L., and Laws, E. A. (1971a). Br. J. Dermatol. 85:381.

Coldman, M. F., Lockerbie, L., and Laws, E. A. (1971b). Br. J. Dermatol. 85:573.

Coleman, G. L., Magnus, A. D., Haigh, J. M., and Kanfer, I. (1979). S. Afr. Med. J. 56:447.

Cooper, E. R. (1982). Personal communication.

Corbett, M. F. (1976). Br. J. Dermatol. 94(Suppl. 12):89.

Crank, J. (1975). The Mathematics of Diffusion, 2nd ed. Oxford Univ. Press (Clarendon), New York.

Cyr, G., Skauen, D., Christian, J. E., and Lee, C. (1959). J. Pharm. Sci. 38:615.

Davis, S. S., and Khanderia, M. S. (1977). Proc. 1st Int. Conf. Pharm. Technol., Paris, Vol. 3, p. 30.

Delforno, C., Holt, P. J. A., and Marks, R. (1978). Br. J. Dermatol. 98:619.

Devitt, H., Clark, M. A., Marks, R., and Picton, W. (1978). Br. J. Dermatol. 98:315.

Di Colo, G., Carelli, V., Giannaccini, B., Serafini, M. F., and Bottari, F. (1980). J. Pharm. Sci. 69:387.

Dietrich, F. M., and Hess, R. (1970). International Archives of Allergy 38:246.

DiPasquale, G., Rassaert, C. L., and McDougall, E. (1970). J. Pharm. Sci. 59:267.

DiPolo, R., Sha'afi, R. I., and Solomon, A. K. (1970). J. Gen. Physiol. 55:63.

Dorfman, R. I. (1970). Br. J. Dermatol. 82(Suppl. 6):45.

Dougherty, T. F., and Schneebeli, G. L. (1955). Ann. N.Y. Acad. Sci. 61:328.

Draize, J. H. (1959). Dermal toxicity. In Appraisal of the Safety of Chemicals in Foods, Drugs and Cosmetics. The Association of Food and Drug Officials of the United States, Austin, Texas.

Duemling, W. W. (1941). Arch. Dermatol. Syphilol. 43:264.

Dürrheim, H., Flynn, G. L., Higuchi, W. I., and Behl, C. R. (1980). J. Pharm. Sci. 69:781.

Dumas, K. J., and Scholtz, J. R. (1972). Acta Derm. Venereol. (Stockh.) 52:43.

Durocher, L. P., and Bielmann, P. (1975). Dermatologica 151:168.

du Vivier, A., and Stoughton, R. B. (1975). Arch. Dermatol. 111:581.

du Vivier, A., and Stoughton, R. B. (1976). Br. J. Dermatol. 94(Suppl. 12): 25.

Dyer, A., Hayes, G. G., Wilson, J. G., and Catterall, R. (1979). Int. J. Cosmet. Sci. 1:91.

Dykes, P. J., and Marks, R. (1979). Br. J. Dermatol. 101:599.

Eaglstein, W. H., and Mertz, P. M. (1978). J. Invest. Dermatol. 71:382.

Elias, P. M. (1981). Arch. Dermatol. Res. 270:95.

Elias, P. M., Mittermayer, H., Tappeiner, G., Fritsch, P., and Wolff, K. (1974a). J. Invest. Dermatol. 63:467.

Elias, P. M., Mittermayer, H., Fritsch, P., Tappeiner, G., and Wolff, K. (1974b). J. Lab. Clin. Med. 84:414.

Elias, P. M., Goerke, J., and Friend, D. S. (1977). J. Invest. Dermatol. 69:535.

Elias, P. M., Brown, B. E., and Ziboh, V. A. (1980). J. Invest. Dermatol. 74:230.

Elias, P. M., Cooper, E. R., Korc, A., and Brown, B. E. (1981). J. Invest. Dermatol. 76:297.

Engel, D. J. C., Marx, A. F., Rekker, R. F., and Van Wijk, L. (1974). Arch. Dermatol. 109:863.

Evans, D. P., Hossak, M., and Thomson, D. S. (1971). Br. J. Pharmacol. 43:403.

Everall, J., and Fisher, L. (1952). J. Invest. Dermatol. 19:97.

Falconi, G., and Rossi, G. L. (1972). Arch. Dermatol. 105:856.

Feather, J. W., Dawson, J. B., Barker, D. J., and Cotterill, J. A. (1981). In Bioengineering and the Skin, R. Marks and P. A. Payne (Eds.). M.T.P. Press, Boston, p. 275.

Feather, J. W., Ryatt, K. S., Dawson, J. B., Cotterill, J. A., Barker, D. J., and Ellis, D. J. (1982). Br. J. Dermatol. 106:437.

Feldmann, R. J., and Maibach, H. I. (1965). Arch. Dermatol. 91:661.

Feldmann, R. J., and Maibach, H. I. (1966). Arch. Dermatol. 94:649.

Feldmann, R. J., and Maibach, H. I. (1967). J. Invest. Dermatol. 48:181.

Feldmann, R. J., and Maibach, H. I. (1968). J. Invest. Dermatol. 50:351.

Feldmann, R. J., and Maibach, H. I. (1969). J. Invest. Dermatol. 52:89.

Feldmann, R. J., and Maibach, H. I. (1970). J. Invest. Dermatol. 54:399.

Finney, D. (1952). Probit Analysis: A Statistical Treatment of the Sigmoid Response Curve, 2nd ed. Cambridge Univ. Press, New York.

Fisher, L. B., and Maibach, H. I. (1971). Arch. Dermatol. 103:39.

Flynn, G. L., and Roseman, T. J. (1971). J. Pharm. Sci. 60:1788.

Flynn, G. L., and Smith, E. W. (1971). J. Pharm. Sci. 60:1713.

Flynn, G. L., and Smith, R. W. (1972). J. Pharm. Sci. 61:61.

Foreman, M. I., Clanachan, I., and Kelly, I. P. (1977). J. Pharm. Pharmacol. 30:152.

Foreman, M. I., Picton, W., Lukowiecki, G. A., and Clark, C. (1979). Br. J. Dermatol. 100:707.

Francis, G. S., and Hagen, A. D. (1977). Angiology 28:873.

Frank, L., Stritzler, C., and Kaufman, J. (1955). Arch. Dermatol. 71:117.

Frank, L., Rapp, Y., and Bird, L. (1964). Arch. Dermatol. 89:55.

Franz, T. J. (1975). J. Invest. Dermatol. 64:190.

Franz, T. J. (1978). Curr. Probl. Dermatol. 7:58.

Fredriksson, T., Gip, L., and Hamfelt, A. (1975). Curr. Ther. Res. 18: 324.

Fregnan, G. B., and Torsello, A.L. (1975). Curr. Ther. Res. 17:375.

Frewin, D. B. (1969). Aust. J. Derm. 10:61.

Fritz, I., and Levine, R. (1951). Am. J. Physiol. 165:456.

Frosch, P. J., Behrenbeck, E.-M., Frosch, K., and Macher, E. (1981). Br. J. Dermatol. 104:57.

Fry, L., and McMinn, R. M. H. (1968). Br. J. Dermatol. 80:373.

Fukuyama, K., and Baker, B. L. (1958). J. Invest. Dermatol. 31:327.

Gardner, I. S. (1977). Fed. Register 42(5):1624.

Garnier, J. P. (1971). Clin. Trials J. 8:55.

Garrett, E. R. (1973). J. Pharmacokin. Biopharm. 1:341.

Garrett, E. R., and Chemburkar, P. B. (1968a). J. Pharm. Sci. 57:944, 949.

Garrett, E. R., and Chemburkar, P. B. (1968b). J. Pharm. Sci. 57:1401.

Gary-Bobo, C. M., DiPolo, R., and Solomon, A. K. (1969). J. Gen. Physiol. 54:369.

Gazith, J., Schalla, W., Bauer, E., and Schaeffer, H. (1978). J. Invest. Dermatol. 71:126.

Gellin, G. A. (1975). In Animal Models in Dermatology, H. Maibach (Ed.). Churchill Livingstone, Edinburgh and London, p. 267.

Gemmell, D. H. O., and Morrison, J. C. (1957). J. Pharm. Pharmacol. 9:641.

Gemmell, D. H. O., and Morrison, J. C. (1958a). J. Pharm. Pharmacol. 10:167.

Gemmell, D. H. O., and Morrison, J. C. (1958b). J. Pharm. Pharmacol. 10:553.

Gibson, I. M. (1971). J. Soc. Cosmetic Chemists 22:725.

Girard, J., Sagon, J., Barbier, A., Tardieu, J. C., and Lafille, C. (1978). J. Pharm. Belg. 33:341.

Go, M. (1969). Arzneim. Forsch. 19:1801.

Goldlust, M. B., Palmer, D. M., and Augustine, M. A. (1976). J. Invest. Dermatol. 66:157.

Goldzieher, J. W. (1949). J. Gerontol. 4:104.

Goldzieher, J. W., Roberts, I. S., Rawls, W. B., and Goldzieher, M. A. (1952). Arch. Dermatol. Syphilol. 66:304.

Goldzieher, M. A. (1946). J. Gerontol. 1:196.

Gomez, E. C., and Frost, P. (1975). In Animal Models in Dermatology, H. Maibach (Ed.). Churchill Livingstone, Edinburgh and London, p. 190.

Goodwin, P. G., Hamilton, S., and Fry, L. (1973). Br. J. Dermatol. 86: 61.

Gray, H. R., Wolf, R. L., and Doneff, R. H. (1961). Arch. Dermatol. 84: 18.

Greeson, T. P., Levan, N. E., Freedman, R. I., and Wong, W. H. (1973). J. Invest. Dermatol. 61:242.

Griesemer, R. D., Blank, I. H., and Gould, E. (1958). J. Invest. Dermatol. 31:255.

Gupta, N., and Levy, L. (1973). Br. J. Dermatol. 47:240.

Guy, R. H., and Fleming, R. (1979). Int. J. Pharm. 3:143.

Haleblian, J. K. (1976). J. Pharm. Sci. 65:1417.

Haleblian, J., Runkel, R., Mueller, N., Christopherson, J., and Ng, K. (1971). J. Pharm. Sci. 60:541.

Haleblian, J. K., Poulsen, B. J., and Burdick, K. H. (1977). Curr. Ther. Res. 22:713.

Harman, R. R. M., Mathews, C. N. A., Jensen, N. E., MacConnell, L. E. S., and Milne, J. A. (1971). Clin Trials J. 8:51.

Harris, D. M. (1975). J. Steroid Biochem. 6:711.

Harter, H. L., and Lum, M. D. (1962). Aeronautical Research Laboratory, U.S. Air Force ARL 62-313, p. 1.

Haxthausen, H. (1955). J. Invest. Dermatol. 24:111.

Haxthausen, H. (1956). Acta Derm. Venereol. (Stockh.) 36:381.

Heite, von H.-J., Kalkoff, K. W., and Kohler, H. (1964). Arzneim. Forsch. 14:222.

Hennings, H., and Elgjo, K. (1971). Virchows Arch. [Zellpathol.] 8:42.

Hershberger, L. G., and Calhoun, D. W. (1957). Endocrinology 60:153.

Heseltine, W. W., McGilchrist, J. M., and Gartside, R. (1962). Nature 196:486.

Heseltine, W. W., McGilchrist, J. M., and Gartside, R. (1964). Br. J. Dermatol. 76:71.

Hollander, J. L., Stoner, E. K., Brown, E. M., and De Moor, P. (1950). Ann. Rheum. Dis. 9:401.

Homburger, F., Tregier, A., Baker, J. R., and Crooker, C. M. (1961). Proc. Sci. Sect. Toilet Goods Assoc. 35:5.

Horhota, S. T., and Fung, H.-L. (1978). J. Pharm. Sci. 67:1345.

Hosler, J. H., Tschanz, C., Hignite, C. E., and Azarnoff, D. L. (1979). J. Invest. Dermatol. 74:51.

Howze, J. M., and Billups, N. F. (1960). Am. J. Pharm. 138:193.

Hunke, W. A., and Matheson, L. E. (1982). J. Pharm. Sci. 70:1313.

Idson, B. (1968). J. Pharm. Sci. 57:1.

Idson, B. (1971). In Absorption Phenomena (Topics in Medicinal Chemistry, Vol. 4), J. L. Rabinowitz and R. M. Myerson (Eds.). Wiley (Interscience), New York, p. 181.

Idson, B. (1975). J. Pharm. Sci. 64:901.

Iizuka, Y., Endo, Y., Misawa, Y., and Misaka, E. (1981). Agents Actions 11:254.

Inman, P. M., Gordon, B., and Trinder, P. (1956). Br. Med. J. 2:1202.

Jablonska, S., Groniowska, M., and Dabrowski, J. (1979). Br. J. Dermatol. 100:193.

Jarvinen, K. A. (1951). Br. Med. J. 2:1377.

Jones, H. E. (1975). In Animal Models in Dermatology, H. Maibach (Ed.). Churchill Livingstone, Edinburgh and London, p. 168.

Juhlin, L. (1964). Acta Derm. Venereol. (Stockh.) 44:322.

Kaidbey, K. H., and Kligman, A. M. (1974). J. Invest. Dermatol. 63:292.

Kaidbey, K. H., and Kligman, A. M. (1978). J. Invest. Dermatol. 72:253.

Kaidbey, K. H., and Kligman, A. M. (1981). J. Invest. Dermatol. 76:352.

Kaidbey, K. H., and Kurban, A. K. (1976). J. Invest. Dermatol. 66:153.

Kalkoff, K. W., Born, W., and Reinhard, W. (1966). Arch. Klin. Exp. Dermatol. 227:857.

Kalz, F., and Scott, A. (1956). J. Invest. Dermatol. 26:165.

Kammerau, B., Klebe, U., and Zesch, H. (1976). Arch. Dermatol. Res. 255:31.

Kanof, N. B. (1955). J. Invest. Dermatol. 25:329.

Katz, M., and Poulsen, B. J. (1971). In Handbook of Experimental Pharmacology, B. B. Brodie and J. Gillette (Eds.), Vol. 28, Pt. 1. Springer-Verlag, New York, p. 103.

Kepel, E., Rooks, W. H., Rodolfo, M. S., Ferraresi, W., and Scott, L. D. (1974). J. Invest. Dermatol. 62:595.

Kincl, F. A., Benagiano, G., and Angee, I. (1968). Steroids 11:673.

Kiraly, K., and Soos, Gy. (1976). Dermatologica 152(Suppl. 1):133.

Kirby, J. D., and Munro, D. D. (1976). Br. J. Dermatol. 94(Suppl. 12): 111.

Kirsch, J., Gibson, J. R., Darley, C. R., Barth, J., and Burke, C. A. (1982). Br. J. Dermatol. 106:495.

Kligman, A. M., and Christophers, E. (1963). Arch. Dermatol. 88:702.

Kligman, A. M., and Wong, T. (1979). Br. J. Dermatol. 100:699.

Kopin, I. J., and Axelrod, J. (1963). Ann. N.Y. Acad. Sci. 107:848.

Kotwas, J., von, Schaeffer, H., and Zesch, A. (1979). Arzneim. Forsch. 29(1), 3:562.

Kramar, J. (1975). Int. Arch. Allergy Appl. Immunol. 39:341.

Krawczyk, W. S., and Wilgram, G. E. (1975). J. Invest. Dermatol. 64: 263.

Lamke, L. O., Nilsson, G. E., and Reithner, H. L. (1977). Scand. J. Clin. Lab. Invest. 37:325.

Laug, E. P., Vos, E. A., Kunze, F. M., and Umberger, E. J. (1947a). J. Pharmacol. Exp. Ther. 89:52.

Laug, E. P., Vos, E. A., Umberger, E. J., and Kunze, F. M. (1947b). J. Pharmacol. Exp. Ther. 89:42.

Lee, P. I. (1980). In Controlled Release of Bioactive Materials. R. Baker (Ed.). Academic Press, New York, p. 135.

Lerner, L. J., Bianchi, A., Turkheimer, A. R., Singer, F. M., and Borman, A. (1964a). Ann. N.Y. Acad. Sci. 116:1071.

Lerner, L. J., Turkheimer, A. R., Bianchi, A., Singer, F. M., and Borman, A. (1964b). Proc. Soc. Exp. Biol. Med. 116:385.

Lewis, A. J. (1976). Br. J. Dermatol. 56:385P.
Lewis, A. J., and Fox, P. K. (1976). J. Pharm. Pharmacol. 28(Suppl):
    82P.
Leyden, J. J., Stewart, R., and Kligman, A. M. (1979). J. Invest. Derma-
    tol. 72:165.
Liebsohn, E., and Bagatell, F. K. (1974). Br. J. Dermatol. 90:435.
Ljunggren, B., and Möller, H. (1973). Arch. Dermatol. Forsch. 248:1.
Lorenzetti, O. J. (1975). In Animal Models in Dermatology, H. Maibach
    (Ed.). Churchill Livingstone, Edinburgh and London, p. 212.
Lorenzetti, O. J. (1979). Curr. Ther. Res. 25:92.
Lovering, E. G., and Black, D. B. (1974). J. Pharm. Sci. 63:1399.
Lovering, E. G., Black, D. B., and Rowe, M. L. (1974). J. Pharm. Sci.
    63:1224.
Lyman, D. J., Loo, B. H., and Crawford, R. W. (1964). Biochemistry 3:
    985.
MacDonald, A., and Fry, L. (1974). Br. J. Dermatol. 90:470.
MacKee, G. M., Sulzberger, M. B., Hermann, F., and Baer, R. L.
    (1945). J. Invest. Dermatol. 6:43.
McKenzie, A. W. (1962). Arch. Dermatol. 86:611.
McKenzie, A. W. (1966). Br. J. Dermatol. 78:182.
McKenzie, A. W., and Atkinson, R. M. (1964). Arch. Dermatol. 89:741.
McKenzie, A. W., and Stoughton, R. B. (1962). Arch. Dermatol. 86:608.
Magnus, I. (1976). Dermatological Photobiology: Clinical and Experimental
    Aspects. Blackwell Sci. Publns., Oxford, England, p. 164.
Maibach, H. (1975). Animals Models in Dermatology. Churchill Livingstone,
    Edinburgh and London.
Maibach, H. (1976). Ann. Rev. Pharmacol. Toxicol. 16:401.
Maibach, H. I., and Stoughton, R. B. (1975). Steroid Therapy. Saunders,
    Philadelphia, p. 174.
Maili, J. W. H. (1956). J. Invest. Dermatol. 27:451.
Malkinson, F. D. (1956). J. Soc. Cosmetic Chemists 7:109.
Malkinson, F. D. (1958). J. Invest. Dermatol. 31:19.
Malkinson, F. D. (1964). In The Epidermis, W. Montagna (Ed.), Academic
    Press, New York.
Malkinson, F. D., and Kirschenbaum, M. B. (1963). Arch. Dermatol. 88:
    427.
Malone, T., Haleblian, J. K., Poulsen, B. J., and Burdick, K. H. (1974).
    Br. J. Dermatol. 90:187.
Manna, V., Bem, J., and Marks, R. (1982). Br. J. Dermatol. 106:169.
Marks, R. (1976). Dermatologica 152(Suppl. 1):117.
Marks, R. (1978). J. Soc. Cosmetic Chemists 29:433.
Marks, R., and Payne, P. A. (1981). Bioengineering and the Skin. M.T.P.
    Press, Boston.
Marks, R., Halprin, K., Fukui, K., and Graff, D. (1971). J. Invest.
    Dermatol. 56:470.

Marks, R., Pongsehirun, D., and Saylan, T. (1973). Br. J. Dermatol. 88:69.

Marks, R., Dykes, P., and Roberts, E. (1975). Arch. Dermatol. Res. 253:93.

Marzulli, F. N. (1962). J. Invest. Dermatol. 39:387.

Marzulli, F. N., Brown, D. W. C., and Maibach, H. I. (1969). Toxicol. Appl. Pharmacol. Suppl. 3:76.

Mériaux-Brochu, A., and Paiement, J. (1975). J. Pharm. Sci. 64:1055.

Meyer, F. (1966). Arch. Exp. Pathol. Pharmakol. 255:47.

Miller, O. B., and Selle, W. A. (1949). J. Invest. Dermatol. 12:19.

Mills, O. H., and Kligman, A. M. (1975). In Animal Models in Dermatology, H. Maibach (Ed.). Churchill Livingstone, Edinburgh and London, p. 176.

Möller, H. (1962). Acta Derm. Venereol. (Stockh.) 42:386.

Möller, H., and Rorsman, H. (1960). Acta Derm. Venereol. (Stockh.) 40: 381.

Montagna, W. (1954). Proc. Soc. Exp. Biol. Med. 86:668.

Moore-Robinson, M. (1971). Clin. Trials J. 8:45.

Moore-Robinson, M., and Christie, G. A. (1970). Br. J. Dermatol. 82 (Suppl. 6):86.

Most, C. F. (1970). J. Appl. Polym. Sci. 11:1019.

Muller, G. H., and Kirk, R. W. (1969). Small Animal Dermatology. Saunders, Philadelphia.

Nakano, M., and Patel, N. K. (1970). J. Pharm. Sci. 59:985.

Nakano, M., Kuchiki, A., and Arita, T. (1976). Chem. Pharm. Bull. (Tokyo) 24:2345.

Nambu, N., Nagai, T., and Nogami, H. (1971). Chem. Pharm. Bull. (Tokyo) 19:808.

Nambu, N., Sakurae, S., and Nagai, T. (1975). Chem. Pharm. Bull. (Tokyo) 23:1404.

Neild, V. S., and Scott, L. V. (1982). Br. J. Dermatol. 106:199.

Newcomer, V. D., and Landau, J. W. (1964). The current role of animals in the development of topically applied preparations. In The Evaluation of Therapeutic Agents and Cosmetics, T. H. Sternberg and W. D. Newcomer (Eds.). McGraw-Hill, New York.

Nguyen, T. T., Ziboh, V. A., Uematsu, S., McCullough, J., and Weinstein, G. (1981). J. Invest. Dermatol. 76:384.

Nilsson, G. E. (1977). Linköping University (Sweden) Medical Dissertation No. 48.

Novak, M. (1972). Cs. Dermatol. 47:28.

Novak, M., and Bartak, P. (1971). Cs. Dermatol. 46:147.

Nugent, F. J., and Wood, J. A. (1980). Can. J. Pharm. Sci. 15:1.

Örsmark, K., Wilson, D., and Maibach, H. (1980). Acta Derm. Venereol. (Stockh.) 60:403.

Oishi, H., Ushio, Y., Narahara, K., and Takehara, M. (1976). Chem. Pharm. Bull. (Tokyo) 24:1765.

O'Neill, W. P. (1980). In Controlled Release Technologies: Methods, The-
ory, and Applications, A. F. Kydonieus (Ed.), Vol. 1. CRC Press,
Boca Raton, Fla., p. 129.
Onken, H. D., and Moyer, C. A. (1963). Arch. Dermatol. 87:584.
Ortega, E., Rodriguez, C., Burdick, K. H., Place, V. A., and Gonzales,
L. (1972). Acta Derm. Venereol. (Stockh.) 52(Suppl. 67):95.
Ostrenga, J., Haleblian, J., Poulsen, B., Ferrell, B., Mueller, N., and
Shastri, S. (1971a). J. Invest. Dermatol. 56:392.
Pang, S. C., Daniels, W. H., and Buck, R. C. (1978). Am. J. Anat. 153:
177.
Parrish, J. A., Anderson, R. R., Urbach, F., and Pitts, D. (1978).
UV-A: Biological Effects of Ultraviolet Radiation with Emphasis on
Human Response to Longwave Ultraviolet. Plenum Press, New York.
Parrish, J. A., Zaynoun, S., and Anderson, R. R. (1981). J. Invest.
Dermatol. 76:356.
Patel, N. K., and Foss, N. E. (1964). J. Pharm. Sci. 53: 94.
Pepler, A. F., Woodford, R., and Morrison, J. C. (1971). Br. J. Derma-
tol. 85:171.
Pitman, I. H., and Rostas, S. J. (1981). J. Pharm. Sci. 70:1181.
Pitman, I. H., and Rostas, S. J. (1982). J. Pharm. Sci. 71: in press.
Place, V. A., Velazquez, J. G., and Burdick, K. H. (1970). Arch.
Dermatol. 101:531.
Platt, W. B. (1978). J. Invest. Dermatol. 71:24.
Pochi, P. E. (1975). In Animal Models in Dermatology, H. Maibach (Ed.).
Churchill Livingstone, Edinburgh and London, p. 184.
Ponec, M., de Haas, C., Bachra, B. N., and Polano, M. K. (1977a).
Arch. Dermatol. Res. 259:117.
Ponec, M., Hasper, I., Vianden, G. D. N. E., and Bachra, B. N.
(1977b). Arch. Dermatol. Res. 259:125.
Ponec, M., de Kloet, E. R., and Kempenaar, J. A. (1980). J. Invest.
Dermatol. 75:293.
Portnoy, B. (1972). Acta Derm. Venereol. (Stockh.) 52(Suppl. 67):72.
Poulsen, B. J. (1970). Br. J. Dermatol. 82(Suppl. 6):49.
Poulsen, B. J., and Rorsman, H. (1980). Acta Derm. Venereol. (Stockh.)
60:57.
Poulsen, B. J., Young, E., Coquilla, V., and Katz, M. (1968). J. Pharm.
Sci. 57:928.
Poulsen, B. J., Burdick, K., and Bessler, S. (1974). Arch. Dermatol.
109:367.
Poulsen, B. J., Chowhan, Z. T., Pritchard, R., and Katz, M. (1978).
Curr. Probl. Dermatol. 7:107.
Priestley, G. C. (1978). Br. J. Dermatol. 99:253.
Priestley, G. C., and Brown, J. C. (1980). Br. J. Dermatol. 102:35.
Quattrone, A. J., and Laden, K. (1976). J. Soc. Cosmetic Chemists 27:
607.

Ragan, C., Howes, E. L., and Platz, C. M. (1949). Proc. Soc. Exp. Biol. Med. 72:718.

Reaven, E. P., and Cox, A. J. (1968). J. Invest. Dermatol. 50:118.

Reddy, B. S. N., and Singh, G. (1976). Br. J. Dermatol. 94:191.

Reid, J., and Brookes, D. B. (1968). Br. J. Dermatol. 80:328.

Reinstein, J., Ostrenga, J., Haleblian, J., Shastri, S., Poulsen, B., and Katz, M. (1972). Acta Derm. Venereol. (Stockh.) 52(Suppl. 67):13.

Reis, D. J. (1960). J. Clin. Endocrinol. 20:446.

Rex, I. H. (1973). Curr. Ther. Res. 15:833.

Riddiford, A. C. (1966). Adv. Electrochem. Electrochem. Eng. 4:47.

Rietschel, R. L., and Akers, W. A. (1978). J. Soc. Cosmetic Chemists 29:778.

Ringler, I. (1964). In Methods in Hormone Research, R. I. Dorfman (Ed.), Vol. 3. Academic Press, New York, p. 227.

Roberts, M. S., Shorey, C. D., Arnold, R., and Anderson, R. A. (1974). Aust. J. Pharm. Sci. [NS] 3:81.

Roger, S. (1967). Techniques of Autoradiography. Elsevier, New York.

Roseman, T. J., and Higuchi, W. I. (1970). J. Pharm. Sci. 59:353.

Rosenberg, E. W., Blank, H. I., and Resnik, S. (1962). J. Am. Med. Assoc. 179:809.

Roth, L. J. (1971). In Handbook of Experimental Pharmacology, B. B. Brodie and J. Gillette (Eds.), Vol. 27, Pt. 1. Springer-Verlag, New York, p. 286.

Ruhmann, A. G., and Berliner, D. L. (1965). Endocrinology 76:916.

Ruhmann, A. G., and Berliner, D. L. (1967). J. Invest. Dermatol. 49:123.

Runikis, J. O., McLean, D. I., and Stewart, W. D. (1978). J. Invest. Dermatol. 70:348.

Rutter, N., and Hull, D. (1979). Arch. Dis. Child. 54:858.

Saarni, H., Jalkanen, M., and Hopsu-Havu, V. K. (1980). Br. J. Dermatol. 103:167.

Samitz, M. H., Katz, S., and Shrager, J. D. (1967). J. Invest. Dermatol. 48:514.

Sarkany, I., and Gaylarde, P. M. (1973). Trans. St. John's Hosp. Dermatol. Soc. 59:241.

Sarkany, I., Hadgraft, J. W., Caron, G. A., and Barrett, C. W. (1965). Br. J. Dermatol. 77:569.

Schaaf, F., and Gross, F. (1953). Dermatologica 106:357.

Schaeffer, H., Stüttgen, G., Zesch, A., Schalla, W., and Gazith, J. (1978). Curr. Probl. Dermatol. 7:80.

Schalla, W., Schaeffer, H., Kammerau, B., and Zesch, A. (1976). J. Invest. Dermatol. 66:258.

Scheuplein, R. (1978). In The Physiology and Pathophysiology of the Skin, A. Jarrett (Ed.), Vol. 5. Academic Press, New York, p. 1693.

Scheuplein, R. J., and Blank, I. H. (1971). Physiol. Rev. 51:702.

Scheuplein, R. J., and Ross, L. W. (1974). J. Invest. Dermatol. 62:353.

Schlagel, C. A. (1965). J. Pharm. Sci. 54:335.

Schlagel, C. A. (1972). Adv. Biol. Skin. 12:339.

Schlagel, C. A. (1975). In Animal Models in Dermatology, H. Maibach (Ed.). Churchill Livingstone, Edinburgh and London, p. 203.

Schlagel, C. A., and Northam, J. I. (1959). Proc. Soc. Exp. Biol. Med. 101:629.

Scholtz, J. R., and Dumas, K. J. (1968). Proc. 13th Int. Cong. Dermatol., Vol. 2. Springer-Verlag, New York, p. 179.

Schutz, E. (1957). Arch. Exp. Pathol. Pharmakol. 232:237.

Scott, A. I. (1965). Br. J. Dermatol. 77:586.

Scott, A., and Kalz, F. (1956a). J. Invest. Dermatol. 26:149.

Scott, A., and Kalz, F. (1956b). J. Invest. Dermatol. 26:361.

Scott, R. C. (1982). Ph.D. Thesis, University of Bradford, United Kingdom.

Scott, R. C., and Dugard, P. H. (1981). J. Pharm. Pharmacol. 33(Suppl): 2P.

Sejrsen, P. (1966). Scand. J. Clin. Lab. Invest. 99(Suppl):52.

Selye, H. (1953). Proc. Soc. Exp. Biol. Med. 82:329.

Shahidullah, M., Raffle, E. J., Frain-Bell, W., and Rimmer, A. R. (1969). Br. J. Dermatol. 81:866.

Shelmire, J. B. (1958). Arch. Dermatol. 78:191.

Shima, K., Matsusaka, C., Hirose, M., Noguchi, T., Noguchi, T., and Yamahira, Y. (1981). Chem. Pharm. Bull. (Tokyo) 29:2338.

Sidi, E., and Bourgeois-Gavardin, J. (1953). Press Med. 61:1760.

Smith, E. B., Gregory, J. F., and Bartruff, J. K. (1973). South. Med. J. 66:325.

Snell, E. S. (1976). In Mechanisms of Topical Corticosteroid Activity, a Glaxo Symposium, L. Wilson and R. Marks (Eds.). Churchill Livingstone, Edinburgh and London, p. 136.

Snyder, D. S. (1975). J. Invest. Dermatol. 64:322.

Snyder, D. S., and May, M. (1975). J. Invest. Dermatol. 65:543.

Sobel, A. E., Parnell, J. P., Sherman, B. S., and Bradley, D. K. (1958). J. Invest. Dermatol. 30:315.

Solomon, L. M., Wentzec, E., and Greenberg, M. S. (1965). J. Invest. Dermatol. 44:129.

Southwell, D., and Barry, B. W. (1982). In preparation.

Sparkes, C. G., and Wilson, L. (1974). Br. J. Dermatol. 90:197.

Spearman, R. I. C., and Jarrett, A. (1975). Br. J. Dermatol. 92:581.

Stelzer, J. M., Colaizzi, J. L., and Wurdack, P. J. (1968). J. Pharm. Sci. 57:1732.

Stevanovic, D. V. (1976). In Mechanisms of Topical Corticosteroid Activity: A Glaxo Symposium, L. Wilson and R. Marks (Eds.). Churchill Livingstone, Edinburgh and London, p. 97.

Stewart, W. D., Runikis, J. O., Verma, S. C., and Wallace, S. (1973). Can. Med. Assoc. J. 108:33.

Stolar, M. E., Rossi, G.V., and Barr, M. (1960). J. Pharm. Sci. 49:144.

Stoughton, R. B. (1964). In Progress in the Biological Sciences in Relation to Dermatology, A. Rook and R. H. Champion (Eds.). Cambridge Univ. Press, New York.

Stoughton, R. B. (1969). Arch. Dermatol. 99:753.

Stoughton, R. B. (1970). Arch. Dermatol. 101:160.

Stoughton, R. B. (1971). In Proceedings of the International Symposium on Psoriasis, Stanford University, E. M. Farber and A. J. Cox (Eds.). Stanford Univ. Press, Stanford, Cal., p. 367.

Stoughton, R. B. (1972a). Adv. Biol. Skin. 12:535.

Stoughton, R. B. (1972b). Arch. Dermatol. 106:825.

Stoughton, R. B. (1975). In Animal Models in Dermatology, H. Maibach (Ed.). Churchill Livingstone, Edinburgh and London, p. 121.

Stoughton, R. B. (1976). Dermatologica 152(Suppl. 1):27.

Stoughton, R. B., and Fritsch, W. (1964). Arch. Dermatol. 90:512.

Strakosch, E. A. (1943). Arch. Dermatol. Syphilol. 48:384.

Strakosch, E. A. (1944). Arch. Dermatol. Syphilol. 49:1.

Stüttgen, G. (1961). Klin. Wochenschrift 39:267.

Stüttgen, G. (1976). Dermatologica 152(Suppl. 1):91.

Sved, S., McLean, W. M., and McGilveray, I. J. (1982). J. Pharm. Sci. 70:1368.

Swarbrick, J., Lee, G., and Brom, J. (1982). J. Invest. Dermatol. 78: 63.

Täuber, U. (1976). Arzneim. Forsch. 26:1479.

Täuber, U., Amin, M., Fuchs, P., and Speck, U. (1976). Arnzneim. Forsch. 26:1493.

Takehara, M., and Koike, M. (1977a). Yakugaku Zasshi 97:770.

Takehara, M., and Koike, M. (1977b). Yakugaku Zasshi 97:780.

Takehara, M., and Koike, M. (1979a). Yakugaku Zasshi 99:1122.

Takehara, M., and Koike, M. (1979b). Yakugaku Zasshi 99:302.

Tan, C. Y., Marks, R., and Payne, P. (1981a). J. Invest. Dermatol. 76:126.

Tan, C. Y., Marks, R., Roberts, E., and Guibarrer, K. (1981b). In Bioengineering and the Skin, R. Marks and P. A. Payne (Eds.). M.T.P. Press, Boston, p. 215.

Tanaka, M., Fukuda, H., and Nagai, T. (1978). Chem. Pharm. Bull. (Tokyo) 26:9.

Tas, J., and Feige, Y. (1958). J. Invest. Dermatol. 30:193.

Thune, P. (1970a). Acta Derm. Venereol. (Stockh.) 50:27.

Thune, P. (1970b). Acta Derm. Venereol. (Stockh.) 50:263.

Thune, P. (1971a). Acta Derm. Venereol. (Stockh.) 51:183.

Thune, P. (1971b). Acta Derm. Venereol. (Stockh.) 51:261.
Thune, P. (1972). Acta Derm. Venereol. (Stockh.) 52:303.
Thune, P. (1976). In Mechanisms of Corticosteroid Activity: A Glaxo Symposium, L. Wilson and R. Marks (Eds.). Churchill Livingstone, Edinburgh and New York, p. 25.
Tissot, J., and Osmundsen, P. E. (1966). Acta Derm. Venereol. (Stockh.) 46:447.
Tonelli, G., Thibault, L., and Ringler, I. (1965). Endocrinology 77:625.
Tree, S., and Marks, R. (1975). Br. J. Dermatol. 92:195.
Tregear, R. T. (1966). Physical Functions of Skin. Academic Press, New York.
Tring, F. C. (1973a). Acta Derm. Venereol. (Stockh.) 53:199.
Tring, F. C. (1973b). Dermatologica 147:309.
Tronnier, H. (1970). Arch. Klin. Exp. Dermatol. 237:769.
Tukey, J. W. (1957). Ann. Math. Stat. 28:602.
Urbach, F., Forbes, P. D., Davies, R. E., and Berger, D. (1976). J. Invest. Dermatol. 67:209.
Van Scott, E. J. (1972). Adv. Biol. Skin 12:523.
Wagner, J. G. (1968). J. Theoret. Biol. 20:173.
Wagner, J. G. (1975). Fundamentals of Clinical Pharmacokinetics. Drug Intelligence Publns., Hamilton, Ill.
Wahlberg, J. E. (1965). Acta Derm. Venereol. (Stockh.) 45:397.
Wallace, S. H., Falkenberg, H. M., Runikis, J. O., and Stewart, W. D. (1979). Arch. Dermatol. 115:440.
Walters, K. A., Flynn, G. L., and Marvel, J. R. (1981). J. Invest. Dermatol. 76:76.
Warin, A. P. (1978). Br. J. Dermatol. 98:473.
Washitake, M., Takashima, Y., Tanaka, S., Anmo, T., and Tanaka, I. (1980). Chem. Pharm. Bull. (Tokyo) 20:2855.
Watson, B., Rhodes, E. L., and Majewski, B. B. J. (1979). Br. J. Dermatol. 101:553.
Weirich, E. G., and Longauer, J. (1974). Z. Exp. Med. Exp. Chir. 163: 229.
Weirich, E. G., and Lutz, U. (1974). Arch. Dermatol. Forsch. 250:359.
Wells, G. C. (1957). Br. J. Dermatol. 69:11.
Wendt, H., and Reckers, R. (1976). Arzneim. Forsch. 26:1495.
Wester, R. C., and Noonan, P. K. (1978). J. Invest. Dermatol. 70:92.
Whitaker, W. L., and Baker, B. L. (1948). Science 108:207.
Whitaker, W. L., and Baker, B. L. (1951). Univ. Mich. Med. Bull. 17: 384.
Whitefield, M., and McKenzie, A. W. (1975). Br. J. Dermatol. 92:585.
Wickrema Sinha, A. J., Shaw, S. R., and Weber, D. J. (1978). J. Invest. Dermatol. 71:372.

Wilkes, G. L., Brown, I. A., and Wildnaur, R. H. (1973). CRC Crit. Rev. Bioeng., p. 453.
Wilson, L. (1976). Br. J. Dermatol. 94(Suppl. 12):33.
Wilson Jones, E. (1976). Dermatologica 152(Suppl. 1):107.
Winder, C. V., Wax, J., Burr, V., Been, M., and Rosiere, C. E. (1958). Arch. Int. Pharmacodyn. Ther. 116:261.
Winter, G. D., and Burton, J. C. (1976). Br. J. Dermatol. 94(Suppl. 12): 107.
Winter, G. D., and Wilson, L. (1976a). In Mechanisms of Topical Corticosteroid Activity: A Glaxo Symposium, L. Wilson and R. Marks (Eds.). Churchill Livingstone, Edinburgh and London, p. 77.
Winter, G. D., and Wilson, L. (1976b). Br. J. Dermatol. 94:545.
Witkowski, G. D., and Kligman, A. (1956). J. Invest. Dermatol. 26:111.
Witkowski, J., and Kligman, A. (1959). J. Invest. Dermatol. 32:481.
Wolf, J. (1939). Z. Mikrosk.-Anat. Forsch. 46:170.
Wolf, J. E., Hubler, W. R., and Guznick, N. D. (1974). Paper presented at Society for Investigative Dermatology Meeting, Chicago; cited in du Vivier and Stoughton (1975), vide supra.
Woodford, R. (1977). Ph.D. thesis, Council for National Academic Awards, Portsmouth Polytechnic, United Kingdom, p. 32.
Woodford, R. (1981). Curr. Ther. Res. 29:17.
Woodford, R., and Barry, B. W. (1973). Br. J. Dermatol. 89:53.
Woodford, R., and Barry, B. W. (1974). Curr. Ther. Res. 16:338.
Woodford, R., and Barry, B. W. (1977a). J. Pharm. Sci. 66:99.
Woodford, R., and Barry, B. W. (1977b). Curr. Ther. Res. 21:877.
Woodford, R., and Barry, B. W. (1979). Curr. Ther. Res. 26:601.
Woodford, R., and Barry, B. W. (1982). J. Invest. Dermatol. (in press).
Woodford, R., Haigh, J. M., and Barry, B. W. (1981). J. Pharm. Pharmacol. 33(Suppl):4P.
Woodford, R., Haigh, J. M., and Barry, B. W. (1982). Dermatologica (in press).
Wuepper, K. D., Harber, L. C., Malkinson, F. D., and Parrish, J. A. (1981). J. Invest. Dermatol. (Spec. Issue) 77(1).
Wurster, D. E., and Kramer, S. F. (1961). J. Pharm. Sci. 50:288.
Young, J. M., Wagner, B. M., and Fisk, R. A. (1978a). Br. J. Dermatol. 99:665.
Young, J. M., Yoxall, B. K., and Wagner, B. M. (1978b). Br. J. Dermatol. 99:655.
Zacarian, S. A., and Adham, M. I. (1967). J. Invest. Dermatol. 48:7.
Zaun, H. (1966). Arch. Klin. Exper. Dermatol. 226:359.
Zaun, H., and Altmeyer, P. (1973). Arch. Dermatol. Forsch. 247:379.
Zaynoun, S. T., and Kurban, A. K. (1974). Br. J. Dermatol. 90:85.
Zweifach, B. W., Shorr, E., and Black, M. M. (1953). Ann. N.Y. Acad. Sci. 56:626.

— 6 —

FORMULATION OF DERMATOLOGICAL VEHICLES

I. INTRODUCTION

Cosmetic consumers and dermatology patients apply many preparations to the skin, ranging in their physicochemical nature from powders through semisolids to liquids. In the past, formulators developed such preparations in terms of the stability, compatibility, and patient or consumer acceptability of the vehicle, rather than considering the influence which components of the topical product may have on the bioavailability of a drug. It is only relatively recently that investigators have shown with any precision that the type of vehicle can affect the percutaneous absorption of a drug (Schutz, 1957; Poulsen et al., 1968; Busse et al., 1969; Coldman et al., 1969; Poulsen, 1970, 1973; Burdick, 1972; Christie and Moore-Robinson, 1970; Katz and Shaikh, 1965; Dempski et al., 1969; Sarkany et al., 1965).

Barr (1962) and Rothman (1954) discussed the early work on topical vehicles; reviews of more recent work include those of Malkinson (1964), Vickers (1966), Malkinson and Rothman (1963), Barrett et al. (1964a), Barrett (1969), Munro (1969), Sarkany and Hadgraft (1969), Hadgraft (1972), Katz and Poulsen (1971, 1972), Katz (1973), Poulsen (1973), and Idson (1971, 1975). Because topical steroids are so important in current dermatological therapy, studies on the percutaneous absorption of corticosteroids have yielded much information on vehicle effects. Relevant references, additional to those already listed, include Feldmann and Maibach (1969), Stoughton and Frisch (1964), Munro and Stoughton (1965), Barrett et al. (1964b), Barrett et al. (1965), Portnoy (1965), Caldwell et al. (1968), Tissot and Osmundsen (1966), and Brode (1968). We can use the vasoconstrictor test for topical steroids to monitor the release of a steroid from a preparation and its penetration into man. This assay is thus a valuable procedure not only for assessing the activity of a steroid but also for determining how the vehicle affects steroid bioavailability. Such information, directly relevant to marketed corticosteroid preparations, has been provided by Woodford and Barry (1974a, 1977a,b, 1979), Barry and Woodford (1974, 1975, 1976, 1977), and Barry (1976); see Barry and Woodford (1978) for references to other relevant work.

The literature which discusses the influence which a vehicle may impose on the skin penetration of a drug is often confusing and occasionally contradictory. A variety of factors combine to make interpretation complex. Workers have used different experimental animals and test techniques and have not always been aware of possible drug-vehicle interactions, the functions of different vehicles, or the importance of a correct interpretation of thermodynamic parameters. Ideally, the best method of approach that we can use to design a vehicle which will provide optimum bioavailability of a topical drug is to employ those fundamental permeation theories outlined in Chaps. 2, 3, and 4. We must also take into account that in the clinic the treatment regime and the diseased skin usually violate the constraints of simple diffusion theory (see Chap. 4, Sec. III.E.5). However, in our present state of knowledge, such a formal approach tends to limit the investigator to manipulating the components of a simple vehicle which is only a single-phase system, such as a polar gel; multiphase systems usually provide intractable theoretical problems. But dermatologists usually insist that a topical application must provide several therapeutic effects in addition to the requirement that the vehicle should readily release the drug for optimum absorption. We may list those major aims or effects as (Lorincz, 1964):

1. Anti-inflammatory effects in acute inflammation—vasoconstriction, cooling, astringent and antiexudative effects
2. Symptomatic relief of pain and itch—analgesic and antipuritic effects
3. Protection—from mechanical, microbiological, thermal, actinic, and chemical irritation
4. Cleansing—removal of dirt, exudates, crust, scales, and previous applications
5. Lubricant and emollient effects—smoothing of the skin surface, replacement of deficient surface lipids, alleviation of dry, chapped skin

A single-phase vehicle cannot readily achieve such multifarious effects; we need complex, multicomponent bases to treat many dermatological conditions.

The remainder of this chapter therefore will consider the science and near art of formulating such bases, mainly in terms of unmedicated preparations. When we design a base to be suitable for a specific dermatological treatment, we must ensure that it fosters the remarkable recuperative capability of the skin. It is often as important to select a vehicle which promotes healing and which does no further damage as it is to apply a therapeutic agent (Heisel, 1967). In the past, dermatologists have accepted as an axiom the rule that, if the lesion is wet, they should prescribe an aqueous dressing and, if the skin is dry, a lipophilic salve is the base of choice. Thus, in acute eczema, the treatment should be mainly aqueous, providing cooling preparations which also cleanse the skin of its exudates. In contrast, chronic dermatoses require oily preparations to conserve body fluids and temperature, to protect and to lubricate, and to help to restore normal keratinization. However, some modern practitioners consider that the classic rule is outdated which requires steroid creams to be used in preference to an ointment when treating weeping dermatoses (Ive and Comaish, 1980). Pharmaceutically, the selected preparation should meet the esthetic criteria of satisfactory appearance and ease of application, and also must be odorless, nonstaining, and homogeneous.

When we apply formulation science to design topical bases, one approach among many is to consider that most vehicles are blended from one or more of the three main classes of component—aqueous, powder, and oil. If we permutate and combine members of these classes in the presence of auxiliary thickening agents, emulsifying agents, buffers, antioxidants, preservatives, colors, propellants, etc., we can formulate a wide range of topical medications (Fig. 6.1). An exhaustive survey of topical pharmaceutical formulation and compounding would produce an encyclopedic presentation. Instead, we shall consider here only typical examples of the main types of preparation available for skin treatment. However we can use some space to expand the discussion for those specific delivery systems that are widely used and exemplify fundamental principles (hydrocarbons, Carbopol gels)

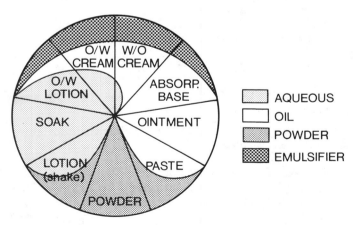

FIG. 6.1 Diagrammatic representation of how aqueous, oil, powder, and emulsifier materials combine to supply a variety of topical products. (From Katz, 1973.)

or for which the theory is not well developed in standard texts (self-bodied creams).

As a guide to further study the following references are valuable: Jenkins et al. (1957), Lerner and Lerner (1960), Sprowls (1963), Bennett et al. (1968), Ansel (1969), Zografi (1970), Cooper and Lazarus (1970), Katz and Poulsen (1971), Katz (1973), Carter (1975), Swinyard (1975), Blaug (1975), Rawlins (1977a), Wilkinson (1979a), and Flynn (1979). In addition there are the pharmacopoeias, codexes, and formularies of various countries. The literature of the cosmetic industry also offers elegant, sophisticated approaches to formulation and evaluation techniques and a wide range of raw ingredients (Sagarin, 1957; De Navarre, 1962; Hibbott, 1963; Wells and Lubowe, 1964; Sternberg and Newcomer, 1964; Jellinek, 1970; Wilkinson, 1973).

II. DERMATOLOGICAL FORMULATIONS

A. Liquid Preparations

Liquid preparations for external application to the skin include simple soaks or baths, applications, liniments, lotions, paints, varnishes, tinctures, and eardrops. External preparations such as gargles, mouthwashes, nasal drops, spray solutions, and inhalations do not concern us here.

A simple soak or bath provides an active ingredient in an aqueous solution or suspension, which water-miscible solvents may modify. A wide range of gums and gelling agents, either natural and synthetic carbohydrates or clays or synthetic polymers, may vary the consistency from a mobile liquid to a stiff, ringing gel. Bath additives such as Oilatum Emollient (Stiefel) deposit a layer of liquid paraffin on the skin in an attempt to maintain the moisture content of the stratum corneum.

Applications, be they liquid or viscous preparations, often incorporate parasiticides, e.g., dicophane, benzyl benzoate, gamma benzene hexachloride, and malathion.

Patients may apply liniments with or without friction, but they should not treat broken skin with them. Liniments may be alcoholic solutions (Aconite Liniment BPC), oily solutions (Methyl Salicylate Liniment BPC), or emulsions (Turpentine Liniment BP).

Lotions are aqueous solutions or suspensions (shake lotions). After application, the water evaporates to leave a large area of the body covered with a thin uniform coating of powder. Evaporation cools and soothes the skin, so lotions are valuable in treating acutely inflamed areas. Alcohol enhances the cooling effect, and glycerol sticks the powder to the skin. Suspending agents such as bentonite or sodium carboxymethylcellulose disperse insoluble powders in shake lotions (Calamine Lotion BP). Lotions may also be dilute emulsions, usually of the oil-in-water type stabilized

by emulsifying wax at a concentration which does not form a continuous
matrix in the continuous phase (see Sec. II.E for a discussion on how
emulsifying waxes stabilize emulsions).

Paints, varnishes, and tinctures present solutions of active ingredients
in volatile solvents such as water (Crystal Violet Paint BPC), industrial
methylated spirits (Brilliant Green and Crystal Violet Paint BPC), acetone
(Cantharidin Wart Paint), or ether (Flexible Collodion BP).

Eardrops are often aqueous solutions, although glycerol and alcohol
may also be used. Typical examples include Hydrogen Peroxide Eardrops
BPC and Phenol Eardrops BPC.

B. Gels (Jellies)

Alexander and Johnson (1949) defined a gel as a two-component system of
a semisolid nature, rich in liquid. Although different authors emphasize
various properties within their definitions, the one common feature which
they identify as characteristic of a gel is the presence of some form of
continuous structure which provides solid-like properties. In a typical polar
gel, a natural or synthetic polymer at a relatively low concentration (usually
much less than 10%) builds a three-dimensional matrix throughout a hydrophilic liquid. The system may be clear or turbid, because the gelling agent
does not fully dissolve or because it froms aggregates which disperse the
light. Typical polymers include the natural gums tragacanth, carrageen,
pectin, agar, and alginic acid; semisynthetic materials such as methyl-
cellulose, hydroxyethylcellulose, hydroxypropylmethylcellulose, and
carboxymethylcellulose; and the synthetic polymer Carbopol. We may also
use certain clays.

The cellulose derivatives form colloidal solutions in water which gel
at relatively high concentrations. These celluloses resemble the natural
gums in many respects but are not as vulnerable to bacterial or fungal
attack. Sodium carboxymethylcellulose, an anionic compound, stabilizes
and thickens suspensions, lubricating jellies, and topical emulsions.

Sodium alginate, which consists mainly of the sodium salt of alginic
acid, produces aqueous solutions that gel firmly on the addition of small
amounts of soluble calcium salts, e.g., gluconate, tartrate, or citrate.
For example, in the presence of calcium citrate a 3% solution yields a
stable water-soluble jelly base (Blaug, 1975).

Bentonite, a colloidal hydrated aluminum silicate, is insoluble in
water but swells when mixed with 8 to 10 parts of water to generate a
slightly alkaline gel resembling petrolatum. Veegum (colloidal magnesium
aluminum silicate) and Laponite (a synthetic hectorite) behave somewhat
similarly.

Pharmaceutical and cosmetic manufacturers now extensively employ
the synthetic polymer Carbopol to formulate gels; for example, the U.S.

preparation Topsyn Gel and the U.K. preparation Synalar Gel both use this polymer to gel a propylene glycol/water solution of a topical steroid.

The Carbopols (carbomers), a group of carboxyvinyl polymers cross-linked with allyl sucrose, are hydrophilic colloidal materials which thicken better than the natural gums. They disperse in water to form cloudy acidic solutions which are neutralized by strong bases such as sodium hydroxide, by amines (e.g., triethanolamine), or by weak inorganic bases (e.g., ammonium hydroxide), thereby increasing the consistency and decreasing the turbidity.

Several mechanisms may be responsible for gelation and it seems likely that a combination of processes occurs. Under acid conditions a small proportion of the carboxyl groups on the polymer chain dissociates to promote a flexible coil. Base addition dissociates more groups and electrostatic repulsion between the charged regions extends the molecule, making it more rigid and so augmenting the gel. However, further base thins the gel because the cations screen the carboxy groups and so reduce the electrostatic repulsion (Dittmar, 1957). If we add excess amine to a Carbopol dispersion the consistency does not decrease, possibly because steric effects prevent screening of the charged carboxyls. The theory which accounts for the thickening of hydrophilic, organic solvents without neutralization proposes that solvent molecules hydrogen bond to the carboxyl groups on the carbomer. Thus the solvent molecules orient along the polymer chain to enhance the rigid structure (Lang, 1972). Of course, in aqueous systems hydrogen bonds must also form, but because water molecules are small such binding only marginally affects the flexibility of the polymer. A third mechanism takes into account the cross-links in the polymer. The carbomer absorbs water to form a gel from macroscopic, swollen particles (Taylor and Bagley, 1974, 1975; Bagley and Taylor, 1974). Shear stresses can deform the close-packed arrangement of the particles, and under extreme conditions the aggregates may disrupt to decrease permanently the gel strength.

Different grades of Carbopol thicken over slightly different pH ranges: Carbopol 934, pH 5.5 to 11.0; Carbopol 940, pH 4.5 to 11.0; and Carbopol 941, pH 3.5 to 11.0. Over these ranges and at equal concentrations the consistencies of the gels remain almost constant and in general the firmness is greater than that of a gel of a traditional gum such as sodium alginate or tragacanth. Carbopol gels provide good "freeze thaw" stability, and they can withstand autoclaving without serious loss of consistency. Dispersions of carbomer should contain a suitable antimicrobial preservative such as chlorocresol 0.1% or thiomersal 0.01%.

Soluble salts such as sodium chloride reduce Carbopol gel consistency (Testa and Etter, 1973) and basic salts employed as neutralizers (e.g., sodium carbonate) promote gels only over a restricted pH range of 2.0 to 3.0. The metal cations screen the charged carboxyl groups, preventing the formation of a rigid matrix (Dittmar, 1957; Cohen, 1956). Divalent metal compounds such as zinc oxide precipitate metal-polymer complexes (Misek et al., 1956; Ory, 1962). If we increase the pH with an inorganic base so that a soluble salt forms, this disruptive interaction is reduced (Lee and Nobles, 1959).

Carbopols thicken many hydrophilic organic solvents such as alcohols and glycols provided that we neutralize the solution with amines; otherwise metal-polymer salts precipitate. In dispersions of carbomer in high-molecular-weight polyethylene glycols, amines precipitate polymer complexes. Insoluble complexes also form with nonionic surfactants of the polyoxyethylene ether type (Saito and Taniguchi, 1973). However, we can gel many of these apparently incompatible organic solvents without neutralization (Lang, 1972). Hydrophobic organic solvents gel provided that we incorporate sufficient of a hydrophilic solvent to dissolve the polymer.

In light, Carbopol gels gradually decrease in consistency but antioxidants minimize the reaction; gamma radiation breaks down the structure completely (Shwarz and Levy, 1958; Adams and Davis, 1973). This consistency loss is a depolymerization reaction catalyzed by trace metals and arises from side-group scission (Morimoto and Suzuki, 1972). Alcohol, glycerol, and chelating agents stabilize the gel.

The synthetic nature of the Carbopols permits strict quality control during their production and batches vary little. This close control, together with the exceptional gelling abilities of the polymer, have led to its extensive use in the pharmaceutical and cosmetic industries. Several authors reported on the use of Carbopol 934 and its sodium salt in topical formulations (Swafford and Nobles, 1955; Lee et al., 1957; Caver et al., 1957). Preparations were either suspensions (e.g., ammoniated mercury), emulsions (e.g., coal tar) or clear gels (e.g., boric acid). In general, the products were stable with only a few instances of incompatibility (e.g., phenol, resorcinol, and mercuric oxide). In a comparison of the in vitro diffusion rates of iodine, salicylic/benzoic acids, and sulfathiazole contained in Carbopol and standard formulations, only the Carbopol-sulfathiazole formulation showed a reduced rate (Streeter et al., 1955). Saski (1960) neutralized Carbopol 934 gels with the physiologically active amines ephedrine and atropine. The investigation of these and other similar amine preparations, using both Carbopol 934 and 940, showed that Carbopol 940 gels were more stable (Schrenzel, 1964).

Giroux and Schrenzel (1964) studied the percutaneous and ocular tolerances of Carbopol 934 and 940 gels, together with the in vivo release of medicaments; Dolan et al. (1960) and Van Oudtshoorn and Potgeiter (1971) investigated oral formulations. These authors concluded that Carbopols are neither toxic nor sensitizers and do not affect the biological activities of specific drugs.

Steroids release well from propylene glycol/water gels, in vivo and in vitro (Poulsen et al., 1968; Ostrenga et al., 1971a, b; Woodford and Barry, 1974a, b; Barry and Woodford, 1978). The pores in the gel allow relatively free diffusion of compatible molecules provided that they are not excessively large. Thus, many of the fundamental studies on drug release considered in Chap. 4, Sec. III. D used Carbopol as the gelling agent.

General reviews on the pharmaceutical applications of the Carbopols appear in the works of Nobles (1955), Secard (1962), and Meyer (1978). Investigations of specific carbomer formulations include those by Levy and Schwartz (1957), Heyd (1971), Newton et al. (1973), and Testa and Etter (1975a,b). The cosmetic industry uses Carbopols to formulate shampoos, lotions, after-shaves, and deodorants (see B.F. Goodrich, Manufacturer, n.d.; Lang, 1972). Lang (1974) has suggested that gels neutralized with amino acids can be used as moisturizing lotions. Other reviews on the cosmetic applications of carbomers are those of Nobles (1955), Hynniman and Lamy (1969), and Courtney (1972).

Chapter 7 emphasizes the importance of a full rheological characterization of a topical semisolid. At very low Carbopol concentration, the gels are pseudoplastic, becoming plastic at higher concentrations; their flow curves reveal little or no hysteresis (Dodge and Metzner, 1959; Cohen, 1956; Fischer et al., 1961; Barry and Meyer, 1979a). Taylor and Bagley (1974, 1975) and Bagley and Taylor (1974) observed a similar flow behavior. They also found that low-strain, low-frequency oscillatory pretreatment of Carbopol 941 gels built up the matrix structure, which was observed as maxima in torque and normal stress values on subsequent testing of a sample in steady shear. The combination of yield value and high consistency accounts for the good suspending properties of Carbopol gels. Meyer and Cohen (1959) made permanent sand suspensions (particle size: 0.06 cm) with gels containing as little as 0.25% Carbopol. The same stability with gums such as tragcanth requires a polymer concentration of ca. 3%. Carbopols also stabilize emulsions either by thickening the continuous phase, which reduces creaming and coalescence, or by their action as emulsifiers. In the latter role a fatty amine neutralizes the carbomer and provides a lipophilic portion for the emulsifier molecule. The polymer then concentrates at the oil/water interface and develops a network around the dispersed phase (Wolff and Meyer, 1961; Weiner et al., 1969).

It is important that a topical semisolid should maintain its consistency under the influence of the varied processes which it is likely to encounter during a production cycle. In this respect, the continuous shear properties of neutralized Carbopol 940 gels are not greatly affected by centrifuging, milling, temperature cycling, or aging; milling of neutralized Carbopol 941 preparations, however, breaks down some structure and the apparent viscosity decreases (Barry and Meyer, 1979a). For both types of unneutralized carbomer gels the apparent viscosity reduces much more than for the neutralized forms. This difference is consistent with the theory that the unneutralized gel develops its structure primarily via hydrogen bonding—which shear easily disrupts.

The apparent viscosities of gels vary exponentially with carbomer concentration; increasing temperature only gradually decreases the consistency. Solvents such as water, ethylene glycol, propylene glycol, and glycerol affect the apparent viscosity in a manner unrelated to solvent viscosity or molecular weight. The apparent viscosities of gels neutralized with monoethanolamine, diethanolamine, triethanolamine, and sodium hydroxide are independent of the type of base employed.

We can use techniques of small strain testing to evaluate the fundamental rheological properties of Carbopol gels and also to determine the effects of polymer concentration, temperature, neutralization, and different solvents and neutralizers (Barry and Meyer, 1979a,b). Carbopol gels of a consistency sufficient to maintain their form unsupported are linear viscoelastic systems. To a first approximation, they behave as elastic solids. The creep compliance decreases exponentially with concentration, and the compliance is uncorrelated with solvent or neutralizer type. Oscillatory data confirm the dominant elastic nature of carbomer gels, and the results indicate that the polymer is strongly entangled. If we transform creep data into dynamic functions and combine the results with oscillatory data, the rheological trends suggest that Carbopols are high-molecular-weight amorphous polymers with long side chains.

Barry and Meyer (1973) employed Carbopol gels to derive Master Curves with which to assess the spreadability of hydrophilic topical preparations. Section II.C.2 of Chap. 7 discusses this work.

The cosmetic industry produces gels formulated with high concentrations of surfactants. Dermatological therapy does not use them, and so we will not consider them here.

C. Powders

We may formulate dusting powders for application to skin folds by mixing together several finely divided insoluble powders. Such medicaments function as drying, protective, and lubricant agents. Examples include talc, zinc oxide, starch, and kaolin; dusting powders should no longer contain boric acid since abraded skin may absorb it in toxic amounts.

In all systems which incorporate powders, including shake lotions and pastes, the individual powder particles should be impalpable, i.e., incapable of being perceived as individual particles by touch. The palpability of a powder is a function of its hardness, shape, and size; particles smaller than 20 μm in their longest dimension are impalpable. A coarser powder makes the preparation gritty to the skin.

D. Ointments

Ointments are greasy, semisolid preparations which are often anhydrous and which contain the medicament either dissolved or dispersed in the vehicle. We can classify ointment bases into hydrocarbons, fats and fixed oils, silicones, absorption bases, emulsifying bases, and water-soluble bases.

1. Hydrocarbon bases

These usually consists of soft paraffin (Vaseline petroleum jelly or petrolatum) or a mixture of soft paraffin with hard paraffin to produce a suitable consistency. Paraffins deposit a greasy film on the skin surface that retards moisture loss. This occlusive property improves the hydration of the horny layer in dry, scaly conditions. Although practitioners usually assume that petrolatum is pharmacologically inert, its wide spectrum of usage in dermatology raises the suspicion that petrolatum may contain traces of compounds which act at some cell receptors. For example, Woodford and Barry (1973, 1974b) showed that white soft paraffin produced a response in the skin blanching test used to assess topical steroid activity.

Yellow and white soft paraffin differ only in color, since the latter is bleached. Hard paraffin and microcrystalline waxes are chemically similar to white soft paraffin but contain no fluid components. Schindler (1961) has reviewed the history of soft paraffin since the first patent relating to this material appeared in 1872. Franks (1964) has reviewed the chemistry and the properties of petrolatum and mineral oil, and Grace (1971) and Barry and Grace (1971a) have discussed the structural, rheological, and textural properties of soft paraffins.

Petrolatum contains n-paraffins, isoparaffins, and cyclic paraffins (Presting and Keil, 1956; Longworth and French, 1969; Gstirner and Meisenberg, 1970; Gstirner, 1970); it may also contain unsaturated and aromatic hydrocarbons (Schindler, 1961). The properties of the various paraffins vary considerably between different batches and grades of petrolatum, and this complexity can lead to difficulties with quality control. The reasons for the variation in the constituents of petrolatum, and therefore in its physical properties, include the diverse sources of the crude material, different types and extents of refining, and alternative bleaching processes.

Microscopically, petrolatum appears as a two-phase colloidal system containing liquid, microcrystalline, and crystalline paraffins (Schulte and Kassem, 1963; Franks, 1964; Meyer, 1968; Münzel, 1968). The microcrystalline fraction is mainly iso- and cyclic paraffins. On production, after the molten material cools, the liquid paraffin may be supersaturated with respect to solid paraffins (Nelson and Stewart, 1949). The stiffening wax phase develops a three-dimensional matrix which forms a compact network with voids of molecular dimensions. Sorption phenomena tightly bind the supersaturated liquid phase to this matrix (Franks, 1964; Erdi et al., 1968).

Optical microscopy provides direct information about the structure of petrolatum. Meyer (1968) and Van der Have and Verver (1957) used polarized light to identify anisotropic crystals. Barry and Grace (1971b) employed a

polarizing microscope fitted with a Kofler hot stage to determine the
melting point range of large acicular crystals (mainly n-paraffins) in
petrolatum. Birdwell and Jesson (1966) discussed the crystal habits of
n- and isoparaffins.

A finer scale of scrutiny reveals detail of the filamentous structure of
the material. The electron microscope shows that the crystals consist of
fiber-like bundles of colloidal dimensions linked at numerous points of
contact (Pajor et al., 1967; Kato and Saito, 1967; Christov et al., 1970).

Thermal methods can investigate the crystalline state of petrolatum.
Kato and Saito (1967) used specific heat and differential thermal analysis
techniques to show that a component of petrolatum passes through a phase
transition to a more stable configuration within 2 weeks of preparation.

Workers have exploited many procedures to investigate and to
standardize the flow properties of petrolatum. Semiempirical tests such
as cone penetrometry are popular because the analysis is unsophisticated
and the apparatus is simple and inexpensive. Mottram (1961) correlated
yield values derived by penetrometry with low shear rate viscosity data
for pseudoplastic materials. Van Ooteghem (1965) derived yield values for
petrolatum, and Delonca et al. (1967) determined the thixotropy of the
material with a modified penetrometer. Berneis et al. (1964) correlated
penetration data with the dilution of petrolatum by liquid paraffin, and
Cerezo and Sune (1970) evaluated semisolid preparations for topical application with a penetrometer. Mutimer et al. (1956) investigated the relationship between temperature and penetration depth in petrolatum. Barry and
Grace (1971a) distinguished various grades of petrolatum with a Boucher
Electronic Jelly Tester, using both conical and spherical penetration heads.

Other empirical methods can provide a limited insight into the rheological characteristics of petrolatum (Gretsky and Blagovidova, 1969) and
the extrusion properties of semisolids in general (Marriot, 1961; Wood
et al., 1964). For fundamental work such empirical test methods are best
avoided since the techniques and the experimental results do not lend themselves to mathematical analysis and interlaboratory comparisons are difficult. However, in limited circumstances such methods may be valuable
because they are easy to use and can assess, however approximately, complex parameters such as extrudability.

Investigators have used continuous shear viscometry extensively to
study soft paraffin and its formulations (Mutimer et al., 1956; Fabian et al.,
1965; Boylan, 1966, 1967; Christov, 1967; Erös and Kedvessy, 1969;
Tsagareishvili et al., 1969; Davis, 1969; Barry and Grace, 1970, 1971a,b).
However, the method has several disadvantages (discussed in detail in
Chap. 7). In general, petrolatum yields a hysteresis loop because its flow
properties arise from a combination of true thixotropy and irreversible
shear breakdown. The yield stress relates linearly to the absolute temperature for petrolatum and related materials (Berneis and Münzel, 1964;
Barry and Grace, 1970, 1971a). Barry and Grace (1970) investigated the

grade variation of petrolatum using six samples; apparent viscosities varied by a factor of 8, yield stresses varied by a factor of 3, and activation energies for viscous flow (as determined from Arrhenius-type plots) increased from 59 to 106 kJ mol^{-1}.

In oscillation, one can approximate petrolatum to a Hookean solid (Warburton and Davis, 1969) or to a linear viscoelastic material of very small phase angle, between 0° and 3° (Barry and Grace, 1971a).

In creep, Davis (1969) reported that at low stresses petrolatum was elastic, but not viscoelastic, and that it yielded at higher stresses, becoming nonlinear viscoelastic without residual flow. Creddle (1965) found lubricating greases to be linear viscoelastic for strains approaching ultimate yield strain. Barry and Grace (1971a, b) experimented with samples of petrolatum over a 45° temperature range to find that the material was linearly viscoelastic up to 45°C and nonlinear at 50°C. The residual viscosity data in Arrhenius-type plots yielded graphs with inflections at 30° to 35°C. Plots of infrared transmittance at 720 and 730 cm^{-1} versus temperature likewise showed inflections within this temperature range. We do not completely understand the cause of the discontinuity in these physical properties of petrolatum, but it could arise from solid state transitions which the normal paraffin fraction undergoes (Kato and Saito, 1967; Piper et al., 1931; Müller, 1930, 1932; Kolvoort, 1938; Seyer et al., 1944; Smith, 1953; Nielsen and Hathaway, 1963; Gray, 1943; Mnyukh, 1963; Stein and Sutherland, 1954). However, large amounts of iso- and cyclic paraffins alter the crystalline form of n-paraffins and eutectic mixtures may develop; different crystal types of isoparaffins exist (Birdwell and Jesson, 1966).

Work softening may be important in the pharmaceutical industry, where material may soften on mixing, milling, and pumping. A topical vehicle may also work soften when a patient rubs it into the skin. Petrolatum decreases in consistency on shearing because its three-dimensional crystalline matrix breaks down. However, if left undisturbed the material partially recovers its original structure and rheological properties (Barry and Grace, 1971c; Gstirner, 1970; Longworth and French, 1969; Mandak et al., 1969a).

As different petrolatums vary so much, pharmacopoeial and other standards are necessarily wide and there is a variety of miscellaneous methods for quality assessment. These techniques assess variables such as "melting point," drop point (or congealing point), color, odor, taste, acidity or alkalinity, foreign organic matter, and sulfated ash. Longworth and French (1969) suggested two additional methods for inclusion in the British Pharmacopoeia—measurement of bleeding tendency and lump-forming tendency. Formulators usually subjectively assess ductility, i.e., the ability of a material to form filaments on extension, although they can also use instruments (Kinsel and Schindler, 1948; Charm, 1964; Barry and Grace, 1970). Casparis and Meyer (1935) suggested a water index, which is the maximum quantity of water which 100 g of the anhydrous excipient

retains in a relatively stable manner at approximately 20 °C. One can also
use the index to determine how hydrophilic an ointment base such as petrolatum is when mixed with cetyl alcohol or lanolin (Castillo and Sune, 1968).

To alter the consistency of soft paraffin, a manufacturer may incorporate a polymer such as a relatively low-molecular-weight polyisobutylene.
If we clap a sample between our hands we may detect the additive as it falls
out in the form of fine, fibrous particles.

Petrolatum for cosmetic and pharmaceutical use should be free from
pathogenic organisms and preferably be sterile. Myers (1969) found pathogenic organisms of <u>Bacillus</u>, <u>Pseudomonas</u>, and <u>Clostridium</u> species sur-
viving for more than 3 years in pharmaceutical oils. Myers and Leslie
(1969) reported a new species of microorganism, <u>Mycobacterium rhodo-</u>
<u>chrons</u>, which used liquid petrolatum as its sole carbon source.

The effect of diluting petrolatum with liquid paraffin has been considered
by Berneis et al. (1964), Berneis and Münzel (1964), Kostenbauder and
Martin (1954), and Barry and Grace (1971d). In general, rheological
parameters change linearly with the extent of dilution. The effects have
been investigated of added oil or wax, lanolin, complex emulsifiers, simple
surfactants, emulsified water, and other ingredients (Van Ooteghem, 1968;
Erös and Kedvessy, 1969; Mandak et al., 1969a; Christov, 1967; Mutimer
et al., 1956; Regdon and Kovacs, 1969; Füller and Münzel, 1962; Gruntova
et al., 1967a,b).

Since topical applications so often incorporate petrolatum and similar
materials, scientists have attempted to correlate rheological measurements
with sensory parameters as assessed by the user. The complete texture
profile of a product also involves nonrheological considerations such as
visual appearance (Sherman, 1970, 1971). Barry and Grace (1971c, 1972)
developed a Master Curve method to assess the shear stress/shear rate
relationship which operates when we spread on the skin a topical lipophilic
material such as petrolatum. Section II.C.2 of Chap. 7 discusses this
approach; the same chapter also contains further information on the rheological properties of petrolatum.

Mandak et al. (1969b) and Olszewski and Kubis (1969) have compiled
information on the effect which petrolatum has on the release rate of drugs
to the skin.

Hydrocarbon bases may contain ingredients additional to petrolatum;
for instance, Paraffin Ointment BP is a blend of white beeswax, hard paraffin, cetostearyl alcohol, and soft paraffin. Ozokerite is a mined wax consisting mainly of C_{35} to C_{55} saturated hydrocarbons. Ceresin is a mixture
of ozokerite and paraffin wax (hard paraffin). Ozokerite and ceresin can
retain oils within their matrix structure without bleeding or oozing.

The Plastibases provide a series of hydrocarbon vehicles in which the
manufacturing process incorporates polyethylene into mineral oil at high
temperature, followed by rapid cooling. The polyethylene, a large hydro-

carbon polymer, forms the structural matrix in a system which is fluid at
the molecular or diffusant scale but is a typical dermatological semisolid
at the macroscopic level. This feature suggests that drug release should
be favored from these vehicles compared to petrolatum systems (Foster
et al., 1951).

Plastibases are soft, smooth, homogeneous, neutral, colorless, odorless, nonirritating, nonsensitizing, extremely stable vehicles, as one
would expect from their formula. They are compatible with a wide range
of medicaments and maintain their consistency even at high concentrations
of solids and under extremes of temperature. The base applies easily and
spreads readily, adheres to the skin at body temperature, imparts a
velvety, nongreasy feel to the skin, and can readily be removed. Mutimer
et al. (1965) have discussed the properties of the Plastibases in some
detail.

For many experimental purposes, these mineral oil-polyethylene gels
would appear to provide near-ideal systems. Section III of Chap. 7 discusses the role which Plastibases have played in experiments designed to
correlate the rheological properties of topical vehicles with drug bioavailability.

Soap-base greases may be exemplified by preparations produced by
incorporating aluminum stearate in a heavy mineral oil. A random arrangement of metallic soap fibers weave throughout the oil in the form of rods,
ribbons, or twisted strands. The fibers produce a product which changes
its consistency only slightly over the temperature range 8° to 45°C (Singiser
and Beal, 1958). The base readily incorporates drugs, and the addition of
lanolin permits the absorption of a small amount of water.

2. Fats and fixed oil bases

Topical vehicles have frequently contained fixed oils of vegetable origin,
which consist essentially of the mono-, di-, and triglycerides of mixtures
of saturated and unsaturated fatty acids. The most common oils include
peanut, sesame, olive, cottonseed, almond, arachis, maize, and persic
oils. Such oils are prone to decompose on exposure to light, air, and high
temperatures, and they may become rancid. Trace metal contaminants in
the oils catalyze oxidative reactions which the formulator minimizes with
antioxidants such as butylated hydroxytoluene, butylated hydroxyanisole,
or propyl gallate or with chelating agents such as the salts of ethylene-
diaminetetraacetic acid (EDTA). However, antioxidants may themselves
introduce problems with respect to drug compatibility or may sensitize
some patients.

Lard, the purified internal fat of the abdomen of the hog, and lard-
containing vehicles are now only of historical interest since we rarely use
them in modern dermatological therapy.

3. Silicones

Silicones provide formulations with similar properties to hydrocarbon bases. The silicones are a family of polymers with a structure consisting of alternate atoms of silicon and oxygen, with organic groups such as methyl or phenyl bonded to the silicon atom. The most important are the dimethicones, or dimethyl polysiloxanes. They are fluid polymers with the general formula $CH_3[Si(CH_3)_2O]Si(CH_3)_3$; in each unit two methyl groups and an oxygen atom attach to a silicon atom in the chain. Silicones are water repellent, with a low surface tension; they are used in barrier creams to protect the skin against water-soluble irritants. Creams, lotions, and ointments containing 10 to 30% of a dimethicone can prevent diaper rash and bedsores and protect the skin against the trauma associated with colostomy discharge or incontinence (Roberts, 1960; McEwan, 1968).

4. Absorption bases

Absorption bases possess hydrophilic (water-absorbing) properties so that they can soak up water to form water-in-oil emulsions yet retain their semisolid consistencies. In general they are anhydrous vehicles composed of a hydrocarbon base and a substance that is miscible with the hydrocarbon but also carries polar groups and therefore functions as a water-in-oil emulsifier. These polar groups may be hydroxyl, sulfate, sulfonate, carboxyl, or an ether linkage. Typical materials include lanolin, lanolin isolates, cholesterol, lanosterol and other sterols, acetylated sterols, or the partial esters of polyhydric alcohols such as sorbitan monostearate or monooleate.

Anhydrous lanolin (wool fat) is the purified anhydrous fat-like substance derived from the wool of the sheep. It consists mainly of the fatty acid esters of cholesterol, lanosterol, and fatty alcohols and has the remarkable ability of taking up at least twice its own weight of water to form water-in-oil emulsions. It is probable that its emulsifying properties depend on the presence of high-molecular-weight diesters of hydroxyacids, although some workers claim that lanolin needs its complex mixture of alcohols to retain its excellent water-absorbing properties.

Several derivatives and modifications of wool fat exhibit the fundamental properties of this material together with certain other advantages. Liquid lanolin, a mixture of liquid esters derived from the fractionation of wool fat, is less tacky on the skin. Reaction of wool fat with ethylene oxide yields liquid and solid polyoxyethylene derivatives, i.e., the water-soluble lanolins. Hydrogenated wool fat is free from stickiness, and its water-absorbing capacity is 50% greater than that of wool fat (Barnett, 1957, 1958; Lowek and Cressey, 1957; Conrad, 1958). Hydrous wool fat (lanolin) is a mixture of seven parts of wool fat and three parts of water (Breit and Bandmann, 1973; Cronin, 1966).

The preparation known as wool alcohols (wool wax alcohols) consists of the alcoholic fraction of the product we obtain by saponifying the wool grease of the sheep. It contains not less than 30% cholesterol, together with 10 to 13% isocholesterol and other steroid and triterpene alcohols; 500 to 1,000 ppm butylated hydroxyanisole or butylated hydroxytoluene provide antioxidant protection. Wool alcohols is a useful emulsifier since its water-in-oil emulsions do not darken on storage or develop an objectionable odor in hot weather. The addition of only 5% of wool alcohols allows soft paraffin to absorb three times more water and weak acids do not crack the resulting emulsion; cetostearyl alcohol further stabilizes the dispersion (Clark, 1968).

Simple Ointment BP, a mixture of wool fat, hard paraffin, cetostearyl alcohol, and white or yellow soft paraffin, absorbs about 15% of its weight of water to yield a water-in-oil emulsion.

Wool Alcohols Ointment BP contains wool alcohols, hard paraffin, liquid paraffin, and white or yellow soft paraffin; it takes up an equal weight of water.

Absorption bases such as Wool Alcohols Ointment and Simple Ointment deposit a greasy film on the skin in a similar manner to that of a hydrocarbon base, but they suppress less the transepidermal water loss (Baker, 1968). However, they may assist the stratum corneum to hydrate by applying a water-in-oil emulsion to the skin and thus prolonging the time during which the horny layer may absorb moisture.

Some individuals are sensitive to lanolin (Baer, 1955; Calnan, 1962; Everall and Truiter, 1954; Newcomb, 1966). However, as judged in terms of its extensive usage by the general population, we may consider lanolin to be an infrequent sensitizer (Wilkinson, 1979b). For example, Clark (1975) calculated that the incidence of specific allergy to hydrous wool fat in the general population is less than 10 per million. Nevertheless, lanolin sensitization is important in dermatology because it occurs unexpectedly and physicians frequently overlook it, especially in atopic patients who may apply large quantities of lanolin-containing emollients for protracted periods. The availability of so many proprietary preparations, including cosmetics, which contain lanolin, further compounds the problem: nearly 200 were listed in the United Kingdom in 1966 (Conrad, 1966; Cronin, 1966; Evans, 1970). Patients with leg ulcers are particularly prone to a reaction (Breit and Bandsmann, 1973; Wilkinson, 1972). Over recent years, many proprietary corticosteroid formulations have had their lanolin deleted.

The offending agents in the lanolin are probably the alcohol constituents (Cronin, 1966; Clark, 1977; Sugai and Higaski, 1975).

5. Emulsifying bases

These essentially anhydrous bases contain oil-in-water emulsifying agents which make them miscible with water and so washable or "self-emulsifying." Often, the preparation incorporates the emulsifying agents in the form of a wax—a granular material which a formulator can more easily handle and weigh, and which he can also use separately to produce a semisolid emulsion (a cream). Depending on the ionic nature of the surface active portion of the water-soluble emulsifying agent, we can classify emulsifying bases into three main types—anionic, cationic, or nonionic.

Emulsifying Ointment BP, an anionic base, contains emulsifying wax, white soft paraffin, and liquid paraffin. Emulsifying Wax BP is a mixture of sodium lauryl sulfate (an anionic oil-in-water emulsifier) and ceto-stearyl alcohol (a water-in-oil emulsifier); it is incompatible with cationic organic medicaments and the salts of barium and heavy metals.

An example of a cationic emulsifying base is Cetrimide Emulsifying Ointment BP. It is a blend of cetrimide (a cationic oil-in-water emulsifier), cetostearyl alcohol, white soft paraffin, and liquid paraffin. The analogous wax is Cetrimide Emulsifying Wax BPC, a combination of cetrimide with cetostearyl alcohol which is compatible with cationic medicaments and incompatible with anionics.

An official model for a nonionic emulsifying ointment is Cetomacrogol Emulsifying Ointment BPC, a mixture of cetomacrogol emulsifying wax, white soft paraffin, and liquid paraffin. Cetomacrogol Emulsifying Wax BP comprises cetostearyl alcohol and cetomacrogol 1000 (the nonionic oil-in-water emulsifier, a polyethylene glycol ether of cetostearyl alcohol); it is compatible with most ionic medicaments and fairly high concentrations of electrolytes, but the cetomacrogol is incompatible with phenols.

A recurrent feature of these bases is that they contain a mixture of emulsifiers of the opposite type. The water-in-oil emulsifier is ceto-stearyl alcohol; it combines with the oil-in-water emulsifier, which may be ionic or nonionic. Formulators employ such or similar blends to stabilize oil-in-water emulsions, particularly dermatological and cosmetic creams. Section II.E.2 considers their mechanism of action in more detail.

Because they contain surfactants, emulsifying bases may help to bring the medicament into more intimate contact with the skin. They mix with aqueous skin secretions and may be readily washed off the skin; they are therefore useful for treating the scalp.

6. Water-soluble bases

Formulators prepare water-soluble bases from mixtures of high- and low-molecular-weight polyethylene glycols (macrogols, Carbowaxes) with the general formula $CH_2OH(CH_2OCH_2)_mCH_2OH$. These condensation polymers of ethylene oxide and water are liquid when the average molecular weight lies between 200 and 700; those with a molecular weight greater than 1,000 increase in consistency with size, changing from soft unctuous materials to hard wax-like solids. The number in their name denotes the molecular weight. The liquid and semisolid members of the series are hygroscopic, but this attribute decreases with increasing molecular weight.

Suitable combinations of macrogols provide products of an ointment-like consistency which soften or melt on application to the skin. They are nonocclusive, mix readily with skin exudates, and do not stain bed linen or clothing; washing quickly removes any residue from the skin. The macrogols do not hydrolyze, deteriorate, support mold growth, or irritate the skin.

Macrogol Ointment BPC is a blend of macrogol 300 and macrogol 4000; it is similar to Polyethylene Glycol Ointment USP (macrogol 400 plus macrogol 4000). Because their components are water soluble, such preparations will not take up more than 8% of an aqueous solution before losing their desirable physicochemical characteristics. To enable the base to incorporate larger amounts of aqueous solution, we can substitute stearyl alcohol for some of the macrogol 4000.

Macrogol bases are used with local anesthetics such as lignocaine but are incompatible with a range of chemicals including phenols, iodine, potassium iodide, sorbitol, tannic acid, and the salts of silver, mercury, and bismuth. The bases reduce the antimicrobial activity of quaternary ammonium compounds and methyl and propyl p-hydroxybenzoates; the macrogols rapidly inactivate penicillin and bacitracin (Neuald and Adam, 1954; Patel and Foss, 1964).

E. Creams

The term "cream" as used in pharmacy, medicine, and cosmetics denotes an emulsion of semisolid consistency, formulated for application externally to the skin or mucous membranes. Essentially, an emulsion is a heterogeneous system containing two immiscible phases—an aqueous or polar liquid phase and a lipid or oil phase. If the mixture consists of polar droplets dispersed in oil, we refer to it as a water-in-oil (w/o) emulsion, even when the polar liquid is not water. An oil-in-water (o/w) emulsion has a nonpolar liquid dispersed in the aqueous phase; we use the term "oil" to include all lipid materials even when they are not true oils in the chemical sense, e.g., hydrocarbons. Emulsion droplet diameters generally lie in the range 0.1 to 100 μm. We may formulate more complicated systems as multiple emulsions in which, for example, individual oil droplets enclose several small water droplets, so forming a w/o/w emulsion; the analogous system of oil droplets enclosed in globules of water stabilized in an oily continuous phase provides an o/w/o emulsion. Such systems can occur at an emulsion inversion point or be deliberately formulated (Mulley and Marland, 1970). However, dermatological therapy does not often use multiple emulsions and so we will not consider them further.

The major outlet for pharmaceutical emulsions today is to function as emulsion basis in skin therapy: o/w emulsions are most useful as water-washable bases, whereas w/o emulsions provide emolliecy and a cleansing action.

1. Water-in-oil creams

Water-in-oil emulsions develop a wide range of consistencies depending on the components in the oil and the aqueous phase and in the emulsifier blend. The relative proportions of each phase and the properties of the various auxiliary agents also have a marked effect. Oily creams contain w/o emulsifying agents which typically may be wool fat, wool alcohols, a fatty acid ester of sorbitan, or the salt of a fatty acid with a divalent metal such as calcium. Patients often prefer a w/o cream to an ointment because the cream spreads more readily and is less greasy and because, as the water evaporates from the skin, the process soothes the inflamed tissue.

Oily Cream BP consists of a mixture of equal parts of wool alcohols ointment (see Sec. II.D.4) and water; it is incompatible with ichthammol, phenolics, and coal tar solution (Ashley, 1955). The preparation still leaves a somewhat greasy film on the skin, and when this is unacceptable a satisfactory w/o cream may be dispensed according to the formula wool fat, stearyl alcohol, isopropyl myristate (16:16:16), cetrimide 0.04, and water to 100% (Groves, 1964).

Zinc Cream BP contains zinc oxide suspended in a w/o emulsion of arachis oil stabilized by calcium oleate (formed in situ) and wool fat. Zinc oxide is a mild astringent for the skin and has a soothing and protective action on slight abrasions and in eczema.

The invention of the cold cream type of formulation is credited to Galen, a physician in second century Rome who may have obtained the recipe from Hippocrates. Originally the formula used beeswax as the emulsifier, whereas nowadays various recipes utilize a beeswax-borax combination as the stabilizer with a vegetable or mineral oil as the continuous phase. Beeswax is a complex mixture of fatty esters, acids, alcohols, and hydrocarbons. Its composition can vary considerably from batch to batch, depending on the place of collection. When the molten beeswax mixes with a borax solution, sodium salts of the wax acids lower the interfacial tension so as to favor the formation of an emulsion.

The beeswax-borax system is anomalous in that it produces both w/o and o/w creams without the aid of so-called secondary emulsifiers. The factors influencing the type of emulsion which forms in any particular circumstance include the phase ratio of oil to water, the proportion of beeswax which saponifies, the other constituents of the cream, and the temperature (Salisbury et al., 1954; Pickthall, 1954).

2. Oil-in-water creams

Oil-in-water creams ("vanishing" creams) rub into the skin and disappear with little or no trace of their former presence.

To prepare topical o/w creams, we often use mixed emulsifiers of the surfactant/fatty amphiphile type, in which the amphiphile is usually a long-chain alcohol although, particularly in cosmetic preparations, fatty acids

are popular. The recipe may list these mixed emulsifiers as separate
ingredients or as preformulated blends, such as Emulsifying Wax BP,
Lanette Wax (a partially sulfated mixture of cetyl and stearyl alcohols),
Cetrimide Emulsifying Wax BPC, and Cetomacrogol Emulsifying Wax BP
(see Sec. II. D. 5). Such mixed emulsifiers are used widely, mainly because
of their ability not only to stabilize the emulsion but also to impart "body"
and so turn a fluid into a semisolid cream. The amphiphiles are usually
higher fatty alcohols (of chain length C_{14} to C_{18}) or fatty acids such as
palmitic and stearic; on their own, they are weak emulsifiers of the w/o
type. The companion water-soluble surfactant may be anionic (e.g., sodium
lauryl sulfate), cationic (e.g., cetrimide), or nonionic (e.g., cetomacrogol,
Tweens); alone they are strong o/w emulsifiers, but their resultant emulsions are fluid and they tend to be unstable. Combining a surfactant with a
fatty amphiphile in the correct ratio produces a powerful emulsifying blend
of the o/w type, with superior stabilizing and thickening properties. Formulators may then prepare stable emulsions of nearly any desired consistency,
ranging from pourable mobile lotions to stiffer adhering creams, simply
by altering the concentration of the mixed emulsifier. We can refer to the
self-bodying action, a process by which a mixed emulsifier not only stabilizes an emulsion but also controls its consistency between wide limits. An
essential feature of this exercise is that the mixed emulsifier introduces a
significant elastic component into the rheological behavior of the dispersion
(Barry, 1969; see also Chap. 7 of the present book for a further discussion
of the relevant rheological considerations).

When we assess the literature on emulsion stabilization, it is apparent
that workers agree that mixed emulsifiers of the surfactant/fatty alcohol
type stabilize o/w emulsions by forming complex, condensed monomolecular
films at the oil/water interface, as Schulman and Cockbain (1940) described
in their classic paper. However, in time a rather misleading concept developed, and investigators often referred to the water-soluble surfactant as
the primary emulsifier and the fatty alcohol as the auxiliary, secondary, or
coemulsifier. In addition, it was often assumed that, by some unexplained
mechanism, the solid nature of the interfacial monomolecular film (i.e.,
solid within the plane of the monolayer) was sufficient to make the bulk
emulsion semisolid. However, this simple concept cannot be true because
we can readily make emulsions which range in consistency from fluid to
semisolid, yet the mixed emulsifier concentration within every formulation
is in excess of that required to form a condensed monomolecular film at
the droplet interface (Barry, 1968; Barry and Saunders, 1970a, 1971a,
1972a; Barry and Eccleston, 1973; Eccleston, 1976, 1977a,b). Thus, interfacial film rheology does not control bulk consistency. Because most formulations have more fatty amphiphile than surfactant, many texts refer to
such amphiphiles as bodying agents or consistency improvers. However,
as we will see later, the simple presence of excess fatty amphiphile in a
cream cannot account for the elastic nature of the preparation. It is theo-

retically more correct to consider the surfactant and the amphiphile as equally important, with their combination fulfilling the dual function of stabilization and ensuring optimum flow properties.

The critical feature is that mixed emulsifiers control the consistency of a cream by developing a viscoelastic network throughout the continuous phase of the emulsion, thus linking droplets together. Such networks form when the mixed emulsifier interacts with water in a specific manner so as to assemble a liquid crystal phase. To understand the overall process, it is best to consider first the nature and the properties of the ternary systems which develop when the mixed emulsifier, or its components, disperse in water, and then to examine the emulsion obtained by adding an oil phase. The thesis which evolves—the gel network theory—allows us to explain and to control many of the colloidal phenomena which occur in o/w emulsions, and so to avoid stability problems. For example, the theory explains: how fatty alcohols and acids act as consistency improvers; why some creams thicken during manufacture; why, with a nonionic surfactant, the cream often increases in consistency on storage, changing from a mobile liquid to a semisolid; how some creams, which are semisolid initially, become unstable and thin during storage; why droplet sizes are generally larger in emulsions prepared with nonionic surfactants than those which incorporate ionic emulsifiers; and why many semisolid creams, particularly cosmetic preparations, exhibit a pearly or lustrous sheen.

We can gain valuable preliminary information about ternary system networks and how the surfactant and the amphiphile interact in water by doing a penetration experiment. In this technique we observe microscopically how an aqueous solution of the surfactant penetrates the amphiphile surface. Two types of reaction are important: the reaction that proceeds at ambient storage temperature (the low-temperature interaction), and the molecular penetration occurring at the higher temperature used in the initial stages of manufacture of these creams (the high-temperature interaction).

If we melt a few milligrams of the amphiphile (e.g., cetostearyl alcohol) on a cavity slide, allow it to cool and to recrystallize, flood the cavity with an aqueous surfactant solution such as cetrimide, and seal on a cover slip, we can detect microscopically, in normal and in polarized light, any subsequent interactions. For low-temperature investigations, we periodically examine the slide, maintained at 25°C, over 24 to 48 hr. As the ionic surfactant solution contacts the crystalline cetostearyl alcohol, the sharp edges blur and, as the interaction progresses, the penetrated alcohol mass disrupts, spreading over the field of view. Within 24 hr a gel network forms (Barry and Eccleston, 1973; Eccleston, 1977b).

A nonionic surfactant solution, such as cetomacrogol 1000, penetrates similarly into cetostearyl alcohol, although slower than an ionic surfactant. In contrast, if we apply a cetrimide solution to pure stearyl alcohol (i.e., a simple homolog), although the components interact at the alcohol surface the penetration product fails to link together successfully to form a continuous network (Eccleston, 1976).

In a high-temperature experiment, we heat the microscope slide on a Kofler hot stage and observe events. Any interaction other than the low-temperature interaction is ill defined until a specific temperature, the penetration temperature (T_{pen}). At T_{pen} mobile liquid crystals appear and a mesomorphous membrane develops at the surface of the crystalline alcohol. As the surfactant and water infiltrate the alcohol, myelin-like protruberances extrude into the aqueous solution and disintegrate into liquid crystal spherulites as surface tension forces act. The spherulites often dissolve into isotropic solution. Lawrence (1959, 1961a, b) published photomicrographs of the results of diffusion processes occurring at and above T_{pen}.

The value of T_{pen} increases with ionic surfactant chain length and decreases with surfactant concentration (Barry and Shotton, 1968; Barry and Saunders, 1970b, 1971b). However, we were unable to obtain T_{pen} values for aqueous nonionic cetomacrogol/cetostearyl alcohol systems. Although there is a temperature at which penetration accelerates and mobile liquid crystals form, the microscopic structures by which this temperature may be identified are too small to be easily visible (Barry and Saunders, 1972a, b).

These penetration experiments provide clues as to the diffusional processes which operate during the first few hours of interaction. To examine the quasi-equilibrium structures that form, we need to prepare bulk ternary systems in a way which corresponds to the industrial manufacturing process for self-bodied creams.

We can prepare ternary system gels by mixing molten alcohol with aqueous surfactant solution at 70 °C and then cooling rapidly to a storage temperature of 25 °C while still mixing vigorously. Under hot conditions penetration processes (similar to those we observe during high-temperature penetration experiments) form liquid crystal phases. We do not try to equilibrate the mesomorphous phase with the isotropic phase, as this may take a protracted time—much longer than that for which a manufacturing process would maintain a cream hot. On cooling to below T_{pen}, molecular interactions slow down and the smectic phase precipitates to yield a low-temperature surfactant/amphiphile/water ternary phase. Thus, at this stage in the preparative process, the system forms an intimate mixture of low-temperature ternary phase impregnated with isotropic solution and unreacted amphiphile. During storage, excess surfactant solution continues to permeate slowly into the crystalline alcohol, thus forming additional gel structure. The eventual quasi-equilibrium ternary phase may form a gel-like dispersion, or the system may be mobile, depending on the nature and the concentration of the reactants. Ternary systems consisting of water and cetostearyl alcohol reacted with cetrimide, sodium lauryl sulfate, or cetomacrogol 1000 appear as white shiny semisolids. Under the microscope we see scattered anisotropic globules, some of which contain small spherical structures at their centers. The small spheres are unreacted alcohol, enclosed

by ternary phase. Photomicrographs have been published of ternary systems
with sodium dodecyl sulfate, cetrimide, or cetomacrogol as the surfactant
(Barry and Shotton, 1967; Barry and Saunders, 1970a, 1972a,b; Eccleston,
1977b). Electron micrographs of the sodium dodecyl sulfate/cetostearyl
alcohol/water ternary system illustrate that the gel consists of straight
chains of submicroscopic particles interlinked to form a three-dimensional
network (Gstirner et al., 1969). Investigators have not yet fully elucidated
the exact structure of the network, although microscopic, rheological,
x-ray, and differential scanning calorimetry techniques indicate that the
matrix is stable only over a specific temperature range (Barry and Eccleston,
1973; Lawrence, 1959; Eccleston, 1975, 1980; Barry, 1975). The molecular
arrangement of the components probably parallels the conformation in semicrystalline gels and cogels, with the hydrocarbon chains in the same configuration as in a smectic phase but rigid (Vincent and Skoulios, 1966).

Under suitable conditions, molecular association at low temperature
leads to an alternative structure which is a crystalline adduct of surfactant
and alcohol (Lawrence, 1958; Epstein et al., 1956; Kung and Goddard,
1963, 1964, 1965; Goddard and Kung, 1965; Barry and Shotton, 1967). If
this molecular packing is stable, then the bulk system becomes mobile as
it degenerates into a simple dispersion of crystals in an aqueous phase.
This process tends to prevail when the alcohol is a single homolog instead
of a mixture; the resulting ternary systems thin rapidly as the adducts
precipitate and thus disrupt the gel network. This adjustment correlates
with the penetration behavior of cetrimide into pure stearyl alcohol (mentioned previously) when the alcohol masses failed to produce a continuous
network.

We prepare emulsions in a similar way to ternary systems. We dissolve the amphiphile (e.g., cetostearyl alcohol) in the hot "oil" phase
(typically liquid paraffin, mineral oil), mix the solution with hot aqueous
surfactant, and rapidly cool the mixture while agitating.

For most emulsion formulations, the concentration of the mixed emulsifier is greater than that required to form a complex, condensed monomolecular film at the oil droplet/water interface. At elevated temperatures,
therefore, an interfacial alcohol-surfactant complex stabilizes the newly
formed emulsion. Surfactant additional to that required to build the monolayer micellizes throughout the continuous phase. As the heterogeneous
system cools, the fatty alcohol becomes less soluble in the oil phase and
some alkanol partitions into the aqueous micellar phase to provide either
spherical mixed micelles or lamellar liquid crystals. A small amount of
the oil also solubilizes within these colloidal structures. The probability
that inverse mixed micelles solubilize a little water within each oil droplet
need not concern us, as the precise chemical constitution of the oil droplet
in a semisolid cream has little effect on the overall rheological properties.
When the temperature decreases to below T_{pen} (which may be depressed by
the solubilized oil), the smectic structure precipitates to form the low-

temperature gel network. We can detect at what temperature this matrix
forms by the manner in which many creams suddenly increase in consistency
at a particular moment of the cooling cycle. Thus, at room temperature, a
typical self-bodied cream consists essentially of a ternary surfactant/
amphiphile/water gel (containing a little solubilized oil), but with the majority of the oil dispersed and held in place within the gel. This ternary gel
assists the complex monomolecular film to stabilize the emulsion, and the
network contributes most to the overall consistency of the cream.

We can most easily see this gel network in a cream if we dilute a
sample and examine it microscopically. Remnants of the anisotropic phase
appear surrounding the larger globules and the aggregates of smaller droplets. Some formulations may contain such a high concentration of the long-
chain alcohol that crystals precipitate within the oil and so distort the
droplets (Barry, 1968). Gstirner et al. (1969) have published electron
photomicrographs of an ionic emulsion that show a three-dimensional network permeating the continuous phase.

With stable networks, surfactant solution continues to penetrate slowly
during storage into any remaining crystalline amphiphile so as to form
additional matrix structure, in a fashion analogous to that of the ternary
system. We can sometimes see this happening as unreacted beads of alcohol originally present in the fresh emulsion slowly disappear as the emulsion ages and thickens. Such gradual changes taking place over several
days are most noticeable with nonionic creams, such as cetomacrogol/
cetostearyl alcohol formulations (Barry and Eccleston, 1973; Barry and
Saunders, 1972c). Thus, in equilibrated nonionic emulsions, the droplet
particle sizes are often larger than in comparable ionic preparations. This
is because the droplets have more time to coalesce and thus to grow before
the gel network consolidates, holding them fixed, separate from their
neighbors, and with Brownian motion suppressed. With an ionic surfactant
such as cetrimide, networks develop so rapidly (mainly during the high-
temperature part of the preparative cycle) that we rarely see unreacted
alcohol and the consistency reaches almost its equilibrium value within a
few hours after manufacture. (Chapter 7 discusses some of the rheological
data which support the gel network theory.)

Nonetheless, just as for the ternary system preparations, if the gel
network which forms in a freshly prepared emulsion is unstable at the
storage and use temperatures, then slow phase transitions lead to an alternative phase. Thus, if the formulation uses pure cetyl or pure stearyl alcohol (i.e., a single homolog), the cream often thins on storage and may,
for example, produce a "watery" product in a tube. This is because the
viscoelastic continuous phase changes to a mobile liquid as the matrix
precipitates as crystalline adducts. The droplets, released from the mesh-
work, cream and eventually coalesce. These phase transitions may be
very slow; the system may reach a metastable state in which the emulsion
is still semisolid but contains well-dispersed crystalline adducts of the

mixed emulsifier. These adducts, reflecting light, may give the cream a sheen or pearly luster; in cosmetic preparations such an appearance provides consumer appeal.

In light of the basic theory of this rather complicated class of dermatological formulations, we can devise a logical program to select suitable combinations of surfactants and amphiphiles and so formulate stable creams (Eccleston, 1977b).

The formulator must first ensure that a proposed mixed emulsifier blend does form a coherent, viscoelastic gel in the continuous phase while also stabilizing the oil/water interfacial film. If the emulsifier combination precipitates crystalline adducts at ambient temperatures, there is a considerable risk that the cream will become unstable and mobile. Thus, the type of molecular association is critical; it depends on many factors including the nature, size, and physicochemical state of the polar and nonpolar regions of the mixed emulsifier molecules, the presence and nature of any drug and other adjuvants in the cream (buffers, antioxidants, preservatives, etc.), and the temperature.

In general, the formulation risks developing adducts if it employs pure amphiphiles and surfactants (i.e., single homologs) with small polar groups and straight hydrocarbon chains of a comparable length. These conditions favor close packing of the surfactant and amphiphile molecule, which can lead to crystallization. Alternatively, if the molecular structures prevent too close a packing in the continuous phase, then the temperature range over which the gel network is stable expands. Thus, bulky components of mixed homolog composition with different hydrocarbon chain lengths yield the most stable semisolid creams.

These general concepts can settle the controversies which sometimes arise as to the suitability of certain fatty alcohols for use as components of mixed emulsifiers (see, for example, Mapstone, 1974, and the discussion by Eccleston, 1977b). Many formulations and experimental investigations do not distinguish between the use of pure and commercial grades of cetyl and stearyl alcohol, or of these and cetostearyl alcohol. However, the choice of a specific grade can markedly affect the stability and the properties of the resulting emulsion. For example, cetrimide or sodium dodecyl sulfate creams prepared with pure cetyl or pure stearyl alcohol are unstable and break down on storage, whereas similar creams compounded with commercial cetyl alcohol or cetostearyl alcohol are stable (Barry, 1970; Eccleston, 1976). This difference in behavior arises because commercial grades of cetyl alcohol may contain up to 30% of homologs other than the C_{16} and because cetostearyl alcohol is also a mixture of straight-chain homologs. Even a small proportion of homologous impurity can lower and extend the temperature range over which a satisfactory network can form. The large polar head group (the polyoxyethylene chain) of cetomacrogol 1000 tends to loosen its alignment with an amphiphile, so that even cetomacrogol/pure alcohol networks do not break down as readily as might have been predicted from a knowledge of the alcohol composition alone.

Once the formulator has selected a suitable mixed emulsifier blend according to the foregoing considerations, taking into account any specific incompatibilities between the blend and other ingredients of the formulation, he can confirm his selection using the following protocol:

1. The formulator can perform penetration experiments over the range of temperature which it is reasonable to expect that the product will experience in use. In such investigations the surfactant solution should also contain any other water-soluble components in the formula, at the appropriate concentration. These determinations provide guidance as to whether gel networks or crystalline adducts will predominate in the continuous phase of the emulsion. If the formulator cannot readily detect an interaction between the amphiphile and the surfactant solution, even over a long time interval, it is unlikely that suitable gel networks will develop in the emulsion. Therefore the prospective emulsifier blend is unsuitable.

2. The formulator can then prepare a bulk ternary system at a composition and a concentration which relates to those to be used in the final cream (ratios of amphiphile to surfactant of from 4:1 up to 9:1 are suitable, with the overall mixed emulsifier concentration ranging up to 16%). He can use a normal heating and cooling cycle which mimics the usual manufacturing process for a cream. However, it is important to confirm that one can also prepare a ternary system of a suitable consistency by vigorously dispersing finely powdered amphiphile in surfactant solution at room temperature. This procedure checks whether or not low-temperature penetration occurs, as this can be important for stability on storage. If a satisfactory semisolid gel forms with both the high- and low-temperature procedures, then the formula should produce a satisfactory semisolid cream. If the gel develops only when the components are heated and cooled, and not when they are mixed at room temperature, then the cream will probably be unstable and it will thin on storage. Suitable ionic ternary systems become semisolid rapidly, independent of which method is used to prepare them, because the polar head group is small. Nonionics have bulky polar regions which slow down penetration processes so that most of the matrix structure forms during storage, even under the high-temperature regime of preparation.

3. The formulator can then prepare samples of the proposed cream by incorporating in the recipe an appropriate oil, together with any medicaments, colors, perfumes, preservatives, antioxidants, etc. Usually he need only make minor modifications, if any, to the mixed emulsifier composition and concentration used in the ternary gel. In general, the macroscopic appearance and the rheological properties of ternary systems are remarkably similar to their corresponding emulsions (Barry and Eccleston, 1973). This emphasizes the fact that the volume of oil in a self-bodied emulsion effects the consistency little, between wide limits. The adjuvants may improve stability by lowering transition temperatures (hence the suggestion to include all water soluble ingredients in stages 1 and 2, above).

A troublesome industrial problem with multiphase systems in general and emulsions in particular is that it is difficult to devise satisfactory accelerated stability testing procedures. The manufacturer may have to depend simply on storage tests, and faults in a formulation may show up only after months or years "on the shelf." It may well be that the above protocol will prove to be a satisfactory substitute for an accelerated stability test for assessing colloidal stability. (The protocol does not attempt, of course, to determine the chemical stability of either the medicament or any adjuvant, or to measure any interactions which are unrelated to the self-bodying action.)

This chapter has dealt with the theory of self-bodied creams at some length because in both the pharmaceutical and the cosmetic industries problems can arise with respect to the stability of such preparations. For example, a manufacturer may change his source of supply of a long-chain alcohol. The homolog composition of the amphiphile in his cream then alters, and stability becomes a problem. Patients start to complain that creams which they have found satisfactory for years now dribble from the tube instead of extruding as a smooth, shiny ribbon.

Typical pharmaceutical creams stabilized with mixed emulsifiers include anionic Aqueous Cream BP (sodium lauryl sulfate/cetostearyl alcohol), cationic Cetrimide Cream BPC and Dimethicone Cream BPC (cetrimide/cetostearyl alcohol), and nonionic Cetomacrogol Cream BPC (cetomacrogol 1000/cetostearyl alcohol). Such o/w creams may be diluted with water and are therefore washable and nonstaining. On application to the skin, much of the continuous phase evaporates and increases the concentration of a water-soluble drug in the adhering film. The concentration gradient for drug across the stratum corneum should therefore increase and promote percutaneous absorption. To minimize drug precipitation and to promote drug bioavailability, the formulation may include a nonvolatile water-miscible cosolvent such as propylene glycol. An o/w cream is nonocclusive because it does not deposit a continuous film of water-impervious lipid. However, a correctly formulated cream can deposit lipids and other moisturizers on and in the stratum corneum and so restore the tissues' ability to hydrate, i.e., the preparation has emollient properties. Self-bodied creams also serve as suitable diluents for therapeutic creams, provided that specific incompatibilities are avoided.

F. Pastes

Essentially, pastes are ointments which contain a high proportion of powder (as much as 50%) dispersed in a fatty base. Typical powder ingredients include zinc oxide, starch, calcium carbonate, talc, salicylic acid, and dithranol. Pastes are stiffer than the parent ointment as the powder contributes its own particle matrix to that of the base. They were originally formulated with the concept that the high solid content would absorb skin exudates, but it seems unlikely that a powder coated with a hydrocarbon could take up significant amounts of an aqueous liquid. However, pastes may be more successful in absorbing noxious chemicals such as the ammonia which bacteria liberate from urine.

Because of their consistency, pastes are useful for localizing the action of an irritant or staining materials, such as dithranol and coal tar, to circumscribed areas of the skin. They are less greasy than ointments because the powder absorbs some of the fluid hydrocarbons.

Pastes lay down a thick, unbroken, relatively impermeable film on the skin that can be opaque and act as an efficient sun filter. Skiers use such formulations on the face to minimize windburn (excessive dehydration) and to block out the sun's rays.

G. FAPG Base

A rather specialized formulation is FAPG base, which consists mainly of stearyl alcohol and propylene glycol, together with polyethylene glycol and glycerol (the initials stand for fatty alcohol/propylene glycol). The preparation is a smooth, white, soft, nonaqueous hydrophilic semisolid with a slightly pearly sheen. The originators claim that the base has possible significant advantages over traditional ointments and creams (Garner, 1971a,b; Rhodes, 1971). Its main use is as a vehicle for the topical steroid fluocinonide, as in the U.K. preparation Metosyn and the U.S. formulation Lidex. Problems can arise in the manufacture of the base; if overheated, the matrix structure alters from the microscopical appearance of an anisotropic flocculated suspension to a mosaic of thin, flat, anisotropic polyhedral crystals (Barry, 1973). The rheological behavior is that of a viscoelastic semisolid; continuous shear behavior develops from a mixture of thixotropy and irreversible shear breakdown. The material spreads readily on the skin and adheres there. The combination of rheological and sensory properties makes the formulation suitable as a topical vehicle.

H. Aerosols

Aerosols may function as drug delivery systems for solutions, suspensions, powders, semisolids, and emulsions (Sciarra, 1974, 1975a,b).

Solution aerosols are simple products, consisting of an active ingredient dissolved in a propellant or a mixture of a propellant and a miscible solvent. Suitable cosolvents include ethanol, acetone, hexadecyl alcohol, glycol ethers, and polyglycols; and typical dermatological agents are steroids, antibiotics, and astringents.

Powder aerosols (dispersions or suspensions) are similar to solution aerosols but contain solids dispersed throughout the propellant/solvent phase. Such systems encounter problems in respect of particle size growth, agglomeration and caking, and clogging of valves. The formulation may contain oily ingredients such as isopropyl myristate and light liquid paraffin to lubricate the valve and to promote slippage between the particles. Surfactants act as dispersing agents to minimize aggregation and caking. The powder aerosol methodology is useful for difficult soluble compounds such as steroids and antibiotics.

Semisolid preparations, such as ointments and creams, may be dispensed in a flexible bag type of arrangement which uses compressed nitrogen to expel the contents instead of a volatile propellant.

Emulsion systems provide a variety of products, producing foams which may be aqueous or nonaqueous, and stable or quick breaking (Richman and Shangraw, 1966; Lemlich, 1972). Medicinal stable foams are aqueous formulations which are employed for preoperative shaving, for contraception (Sobrero, 1960; Mears, 1962; Bushnell, 1965), and as adjuncts for the treatment of ulcerative colitis (Scherl and Scherl, 1973). The stable foam, which is similar to a shaving cream preparation but into which the formulator incorporates medicaments, varies in stability depending on the selection of surfactant, solvent, and propellant.

The basic aerosol quick-break foam contains a foaming agent (i.e., a surfactant), a solvent system, and a propellant. Polawax (an ethoxylated stearyl alcohol with auxiliary emulsifying agents) produces a satisfactory product (Chester, 1967); cetyl/stearyl combinations are less suitable (Sanders, 1966). When the patient actuates the valve, the propellant vaporizes, expelling and cooling the contents. This chilling, together with the loss of volatile cosolvent, crystallizes the foaming agent to form a lattice which initially stabilizes the bubbles of foam. The patient breaks the lattice by rubbing it, with his body heat redissolving the surfactant. The concept, then, is of a system which discharges from the container as a foam but which readily breaks on the skin. Although formulators usually base quick-break foams on ethanol, they may incorporate other solvents, such as propylene glycol (Sanders, 1970).

Woodford and Barry (1977b) formulated quick-break aerosol foams to deliver a variety of topical steroids (betamethasone valerate and benzoate, clobetasol propionate, triamcinolone acetonide, desonide, flumethasone pivalate, and hydrocortisone butyrate); activities and bioavailabilities as assessed using the vasoconstrictor assay were high. The authors concluded that such formulations offer a number of advantages over other dosage forms, including the stable aerosol foam: the quick-break foam presents the steroid to the skin in solution and is easy to apply; the patient can control the dosage via a metering valve—a feature unavailable in other topical medications; the preparation is economical in use and suitable for smooth

or hairy skin; there is less possibility of inhaling potent corticosteroids
with such foams as compared to aerosol sprays; and the delivery system
may be made sterile and remain so during use. One possible disadvantage
is the expulsion of halogenated hydrocarbons, because of their suggested
effects on the ozone layer (Anon, 1975). A suitable mixture of hydrocarbons
is a possible alternative propellant for a quick-break foam.

III. NONTHERAPEUTIC INGREDIENTS
OF DERMATOLOGICAL FORMULATIONS

Pharmaceutical and cosmetic topical formulations use a wide variety of
materials, ranging from pure chemicals through mixtures to natural
products. For example, a catalog of the surfactants available in the United
Kingdom includes details of 3,500 products, many of which are potential
topical ingredients (Hollis, 1980). It is neither practical nor desirable to
present here an encyclopedic treatment of dermatological ingredients, yet
investigators need to be familiar with at least the principal substances
employed in topical preparations, together with their main functions. In
Table 6.1 we attempt to condense into a manageable form information
relating to common topical constituents.

To develop a new topical preparation the formulator needs to understand not only the principles of colloid science and biopharmaceutics but
also to have an extensive knowledge of the available materials and considerable experience in formulation science. In practice, the formulator does
not usually start from scratch but begins with a published recipe which he
has found in a pharmaceutical or cosmetic book, in the patent literature,
or in a trade brochure. Occasionally, a novice formulator adopts a "me
too" approach and attempts simply to copy a product which is already well
established in the market, e.g., the brand leader. However, he should
bear in mind the dangers inherent in this approach. Many published recipes
have not been fully tested for long-term stability, and minor modifications
to component specifications may lead to additional stability problems (see,
for example, the discussion on self-bodied creams in Sec. II.E). Often the
principal aim of the originator of a model formulation was to achieve
cosmetic elegance. The pharmacist who incorporates a drug into this model
base must ensure additionally that the vehicle does not hinder the bioavailability of the medicament. For example, simply because a specific steroid
cream is successful in the clinic does not mean that the same complex
vehicle may be borrowed for use with a different steroid; this approach may
lead to therapeutic failure. The crucial requirement is that the manufacturer
should tailor each vehicle to fit a specific medicament in light of the unique
physicochemical characteristics of that drug.

TABLE 6.1 Common Nontherapeutic Ingredients of Topical Preparations and their Formulation Functions

Key to formulation functions:

1. Hydrophobic (lipid) vehicle
2. Water-miscible vehicle, cosolvent
3. Structural matrix agent
   (3a) Hydrophobic   (3b) Hydrophilic
   (3c) Oil-in-water self-bodied cream   (3d) Carbopol gel
4. Suspending, jelling or consistency promoting agent
5. Water-in-oil emulsifier
6. Oil-in-water emulsifier
7. Preservative/disinfectant
8. Buffer
9. Humectant—may withdraw moisture from skin
10. Antioxidant
11. Sequestering antioxidant
12. Penetration enhancer
13. Skin moisturizer
    (13a) By occlusion   (13b) Specific action
14. Drying, protective, lubricant

Ingredient	Principal functions
1. Hydrocarbons:	
Liquid petrolatum (liquid paraffin, mineral oil)	1, 13a
White/yellow petrolatum (soft paraffin, Vaseline petroleum jelly)	1, 3a, 13a
Paraffin (hard paraffin, paraffin wax)	1, 3a, 13a
Microcrystalline wax	3a
Ceresin (mineral wax, purified ozokerite)	3a
Polyethylene	3a
Squalane	1, 13a
Squalene	10
2. Silicones/silicates:	
Dimethicone (dimethylpolysiloxane, polydimethyl-siloxane)	1, 13a, 14
Colloidal silicon dioxide (Cab-O-Sil, Aerosil)	3a, 4
Bentonite (colloidal hydrated aluminum silicate)	3b, 4
Veegum (colloidal hydrated aluminum magnesium silicate)	3b, 4

TABLE 6.1 (Continued)

Ingredient	Principal functions
[2. Silicones/silicates]	
Hectorite (montmorillonite)	3a, 4
Laponite (synthetic hectorite)	3b, 4
Bentone (organically substituted montmorillonite)	3a, 4
3. Alcohols:	
Ethanol	2, 12?
Isopropyl alcohol	7
Lauryl (dodecanol, dodecyl)	1
Myristyl (tetradecanol, tetradecyl)	1
Cetyl (hexadecanol, hexadecyl, palmityl)	1, 3a, 3c, 5
Stearyl (octadecyl)	1, 3a, 3c, 5
Cetostearyl (cetyl plus stearyl)	1, 3a, 3c, 5
Oleyl	1, 5, 12
Benzyl	7
β-Phenoxyethyl	7
4. Polyols/polyglycols:	
Propylene glycol (propane-1,2-diol)	2, 12?
Glycerol (glycerin, propane-1,2,3-triol)	2, 9
Polyethylene glycol (liquid macrogol)	2, 9
Polyethylene glycol (hard macrogol)	2, 3b
Hexane-1,2,6-triol	2
Sorbitol solution, 70%	2, 9
p-Chlorphenyl propanediol	7
Bromonitropropanediol (Bronopol)	7
Polyvinyl alcohol	3, 4, 6
5. Sterols/sterol esters:	
Cholesterol	3a, 3c, 5
Lanolin (hydrous wool fat)	1, 5
Anhydrous lanolin (wool fat)	1, 5
Lanolin derivatives	1, 5
6. Phenolics:	
Phenol, cresol, thymol, halogenated derivatives	7
Parabens (methyl, ethyl, propyl, butyl p-hydroxy-benzoates)	7
BHA (butylated hydroxyanisole)	10
BHT (butylated hydroxytoluene)	10

TABLE 6.1 (Continued)

Ingredient	Principal functions
[6. Phenolics]	
Propyl gallate	10
Pyrogallol	10
7. Carboxylic acids and their salts:	
Lauric (dodecanoic)	1
Myristic (tetradecanoic)	1
Palmitic (hexadecanoic)	1, 3c, 5
Stearic (octadecanoic)	1, 3c, 5
Oleic (9-octadecenoic)	1, 5, 12
Salts of above acids (Na, K, amine, etc.)	6
Sorbic, benzoic, dehydroacetic, propionic	7
Citric acid and salts	8, 11
Sodium pyrrolidone carboxylate	13b?
Sodium or potassium salts of lactic acid	13b?
8. Esters/polyesters:	
Esters of pyrrolidone carboxylic acid	13b?
Beeswax (white and yellow)	3, 5, 6
Carnauba wax	3a
Spermaceti and synthetic spermaceti	3a
Cholesterol esters—long chain	1, 3a
Ethylene, propylene glycol monoesters—long chain	1, 5
Glyceryl monoesters—long chain	1, 5
Self-emulsifying monostearin (complex mixture)	1, 6
Sorbitol esters—long chain	1, 5
Sorbitan esters—long chain (Spans, Arlacels)	1, 5
Polyoxyethylene sorbitan esters—long chain (Tweens)	6
Polyoxyethylene esters—long chain (Myrj)	6
Oils (almond, corn, castor, cottonseed, olive, soybean, sesame, maize, peanut, persic; hydrogenated)	1
Sulfated oils	1, 5
Isopropyl myristate, palmitate	1
Essential oils (anethol, citronellol, eugenol, vanillates)	7
9. Ethers/polyethers:	
Macrogol ethers (polyoxyethylene fatty alcohol or alkyl phenol condensates—cetomacrogol, lauro-macrogol, nonoxynol)	6

TABLE 6.1 (Continued)

Ingredient	Principal functions
[9. Ethers/polyethers]	
Poloxamers (polyoxyethylene-polyoxypropylene copolymers)	5, 6
10. Gums/semisynthetic derivatives/synthetics:	
Agar, carrageen, tragacanth, pectin, alginic acid	4
Alginates, methylcellulose, carboxymethylcellulose, hydroxyethylcellulose, sodium carboxymethylcellulose	4
Microcrystalline cellulose (Avicel)	4
Carbopol (carbomer, carboxyvinyl polymer)	4
11. Powders:	
Talc	14
Zinc oxide	14
Starch	14
12. Miscellaneous:	
Anionic surfactants (monovalent ion)	6
Anionic surfactants (multivalent ion)	5
Cationic surfactants (e.g., cetrimide)	6, 7
Nonionic surfactants	5, 6
Borax (with beeswax)	5, 6
Ethanolamine, triethanolamine (with Carbopol)	4
Ethanolamine, triethanolamine (with stearic acid)	6
Ethylenediaminetetraacetic acid (EDTA)	11
Phosphoric acid and salts	8
Urea	12, 13b
Dimethyl sulfoxide (DMSO)	2, 12
Alkyl sulfoxides	2, 12
Dimethylacetamide (DMA)	2, 12
Dimethylformamide (DMF)	2, 12
Phosphine oxides	12?
Sugar esters	12?
Pyrrolidones	12
Azocycloalkan-2-ones	12
Tetrahydrofurfuryl alcohol	12
Quaternary ammonium compounds (benzalkonium chloride, cetyl pyridinium chloride)	7
Quinones (hydroxyquinone, hydroxycoumarins, tocopherols)	10

Source: Modified from Flynn (1979).

IV. COSMETIC OR ESTHETIC CRITERIA
FOR DERMATOLOGICAL FORMULATIONS

However well we may design a topical vehicle to maximize drug bioavailability, it is still important to ensure that the preparation is esthetically
acceptable to the patient. A poor product may mean that the treatment risks
patient noncompliance or the transfer of allegiance to an alternative, com-
petitor's product. Although a consumer may apply less stringent acceptability criteria to a dermatological than to, say, a cosmetic cream, patients
still generally prefer a preparation which is easy to remove from the container and which spreads readily and smoothly yet adheres to the treated
area while being neither tacky nor difficult to remove (Kostenbauder and
Martin, 1954).

   For cosmetic emulsions, Clark (1963) summarized the possible interrelationships between such properties as the appearance, feel, ease of
use, and consistency in terms of consumer requirements. Sherman (1971)
developed a consistency profile for dermatologicals which takes into account
product assessment prior to use, initial perception on the treatment area,
application to the skin site, and residual impression. Chapter 7 discusses
rheological experiments which assess the spreadability of topicals in terms
of preferred shearing conditions for maximum patient acceptability (Barry
and Grace, 1972; Barry, 1973; Barry and Meyer, 1973, 1975).

   In simple terms, the general objective is to formulate a product that
rubs into the skin to leave a residue which is undetectable to the eye and is
neither tacky nor greasy. Stiff pastes may be difficult to rub into the skin
or to apply as an even film; application to damaged skin may be painful.
However, it is often an advantage to leave a relatively thick layer of material on the skin to occlude the tissue or to protect it from mechanical,
chemical, or light damage. Ointments and pastes do this, and the viscous
drag imposed on application may provide further benefits. The application
procedure may loosen and dislodge scales, dead tissue, and remnants of
previous doses, so that the medicament comes into more intimate contact
with the diseased site; the stiff preparation also makes it easier to control
the area of treatment. The recipe usually controls the consistency of an
ointment by variation in the ratio of waxy components (structural matrix
agents) to the fluid fraction. For emulsions, the phase volume ratio is
important; for self-bodied creams, the mixed emulsifier concentration is
crucial. In gels, consistency control lies mainly in the concentration of the
polymer or clay.

   The tactile sensations of greasiness and tackiness arise from the
properties of these vehicle constituents which form the film left on the skin.
Particularly for creams, stearic acid and cetyl alcohol produce nontacky
films; hence the popularity of cosmetic vanishing creams composed of a
suspension of stearic acid dispersed in a stearate soap gel. In such preparations the "oil" phase is wax-like and the microcrystals spread well on

TABLE 6.2 Some Cosmetic and Usage Criteria for Topical Vehicles

1. Visual appearance of product

2. Odor: (a) development of pungent odor; (b) loss of fragrance

3. Sampling characteristics of product, e.g., ease of removal from container

4. Application properties: (a) hard, soft; (b) spreads easily or with difficulty; (c) softens when applied; (d) creamy, watery (e.g., runs off skin), adheres, viscous; (e) sticky, tacky, oily; (f) pasty, lumpy, gritty, smooth, powdery; (g) forms coherent film

5. Residual impression after application: (a) oily, greasy, or sticky residue on treatment area; (b) appearance of treatment area (e.g., dull, shiny, matt); (c) irritation; (d) odor on skin; (e) ease of removal of residue

Source: Modified from Sherman (1971).

the skin without rolling. Formulations which employ synthetic or natural gums as suspending agents should use the minimum amount, as these polymers tend to leave a tacky film on the skin.

Insoluble solids in a dermatological formulation leave the resultant film opaque, often with a powdery or crusty appearance. However, as the therapeutic treatment requires the presence of such solids in lotions and pastes, the formulator can do little to vary the nature of the film residue and patients accept the residue as an integral part of the treatment.

Table 6.2 is a summary of some of the more important cosmetic and usage criteria relevant to the formulation of a dermatological product.

V. PHYSICOCHEMICAL CRITERIA FOR DERMATOLOGICAL FORMULATIONS

The developer of a topical dosage form, as for any other drug delivery system, must be aware of the physical and chemical behavior of the drug and the dosage form during preformulation studies; throughout bench-scale work, pilot studies, and batch processing; at the manufacturing level including filling; and during storage and use of the product. Many of the criteria which he uses to assess the dosage form are common to several types of pharmaceutical, but some standards are particularly relevant to a topical semisolid. Table 6.3 presents a list of the general factors which a pharmacist evaluates for a new semisolid, both during developmental studies and as a function of time on storage. The assessment procedure for the stability

TABLE 6.3 Some Physicochemical Criteria for Pharmaceutical Semisolids

---

1. Stability of the active ingredients

2. Stability of the adjuvants

3. Rheological properties—consistency, extrudability

4. Loss of water and other volatile components

5. Phase changes—homogeneity/phase separation, bleeding

6. Particle size and particle size distribution of dispersed phase

7. Apparent pH

8. Particulate contamination

Source: From Flynn (1979).

of a pharmaceutical product examines the capability of a particular formulation, in a specific container, to remain within its physical, chemical, therapeutic, and toxicological specifications (Lintner, 1975).

The first difficulty arises in attempts to assess the chemical stability of the drug in its complex vehicle, together with the stability of any potentially labile adjuvants. A general methodology for predicting chemical stability uses an accelerated stability test which subjects the material to elevated temperatures and uses the Arrhenius relationship to establish a shelf life (Rawlins, 1977b; Lachman and DeLuca, 1970; Martin et al., 1969). However, in a multiphase system such as a cream, heat may alter the phase distribution and may even crack the emulsion. Thus, we may be limited to assessing the preparation over a long time at the storage temperature. A related problem is that, because of the complexity of the vehicle, it may be difficult to separate the drug or labile adjuvant from the base so as to analyze it.

In addition to performing specific analytical tests, the pharmacist should note any qualitative changes in the produce during storage; these changes are often apparent on inspection. The color may change, e.g., natural fats, oils, and lanolin brown with age as they oxidize, becoming rancid with a disagreeable odor. The texture may alter as phase relationships vary.

One method which readily quantifies changes in the structure of a colloidal system uses a rheological assessment, preferably by developing multipoint rheograms. Chapter 7 deals in some detail with the rheological analysis of pharmaceutical vehicles.

Many dermatologicals contain water or other volatile solvents, and batches may lose a proportion of the solvent either through the walls of unsuitable plastic containers or through faulty seams or ill-fitting caps.

The product may lose weight and may shrink away from the container wall, becoming puffy and stiff so that its application properties suffer.

Dermatological formulations are often heterogeneous systems which are susceptible to various phase changes when stored incorrectly. Emulsions may cream and crack, suspensions can agglomerate and cake, and ointments and gels may "bleed" as their matrices contract to squeeze out mobile constituents. High temperatures can produce or accelerate such adjustments.

For suspensions and emulsions, a stability protocol should monitor the particle size distribution and note any changes on storage. A particle size analysis may often detect a potentially unstable formulation long before any other parameter changes markedly. Emulsion globules may grow as a gel network breaks down on storage, thus allowing Brownian motion to bring droplets into contact so that they coalesce. Crystals may enlarge, or change their habit, or revert to a more stable, less active, polymorphic form. Such alterations in crystal form may affect the therapeutic activity of the formulation.

The apparent pH of a topical product may alter on storage as chemicals change. Although we cannot assign a fundamental meaning to a pH measurement in a complex dermatological vehicle, we can sometimes use a pH electrode as a tool to monitor variations in a formulation as it ages.

On the manufacturing scale, even with the most modern equipment and facilities, it can be difficult to produce creams and ointments completely free from foreign particles. Tin and aluminum tubes may contaminate a topical with "flashings"—metal slivers and shavings formed during the manufacture of the containers. Their presence is particularly undesirable in ophthalmic ointments, and various pharmacopoeial tests limit the extent of such contamination.

VI. MICROBIAL CONTAMINATION AND PRESERVATION OF DERMATOLOGICAL FORMULATIONS

Dermatological vehicles often contain aqueous and oily phases, together with carbohydrates and even proteins, and thus these bases are prone to attack by bacteria and fungi. Microbial growth not only spoils the formulation but is a potential toxicity hazard and a source of infection. Conditions which lower immunity, such as bodily injury, debilitating diseases, or drug therapy, may encourage organisms that are usually not highly infectious to infect a host, i.e., to become opportunistic pathogens (Bruch, 1971a,b). In 1969, a survey of 169 cosmetics and topical drugs revealed that 33 samples were microbially contaminated, half with gram-negative organisms which were a health hazard (Katz, 1973). In the mid-1960s, the source of an outbreak of serious eye infections in Scandinavia was an antibiotic ophthalmic ointment contaminated with Pseudomonas (Killings et al., 1966).

It is thought that contaminated topical formulations were responsible for hospital infections with gram-negative organisms (Bruch, 1971b; Dunnigan, 1968).

Of course, microbial growth is usually less likely to be dangerous when it occurs in a topical preparation than in injections or in eyedrops. However, it is desirable that all medicines should be free of pathogenic organisms such as Pseudomonas aeruginosa, Salmonella spp., Escherichia coli, Staphylococcus aureus, Candida albicans, and Aspergillus niger. It is especially important to preserve topicals which the patient may apply to broken or inflamed skin. The preservative concentration should be lethal to microorganisms rather than simply inhibitory.

The potential sources of microbial contamination are many and varied. Such contamination can occur: in raw materials (particularly those of natural origin) and water used in manufacture; in processing and filling equipment; in packing material such as drums, sacks, and cartons and final containers; if there is an unclean environment or poor plant hygiene; and if plant operatives fail to comply with good manufacturing procedures (Wedderburn, 1964).

Microorganisms depend on water to multiply, and in creams they proliferate in the aqueous phase where nutrients provide a favorable environment for growth. The constituents and properties of the polar phase, such as osmotic pressure, oxygen tension, pH, and surface tension determine whether the microorganisms are inhibited or survive in a quiescent state or thrive and multiply.

The most widely used methods of preservation include sterilization by moist heat (immersion in boiling water or using steam under pressure as in an autoclave; heating the material at 80°C for 1 hr, or at 100°C for less, on three successive days; heating with a bactericide), dry heat at 150° to 180°C for 1 or 2 hr, filtration, gaseous sterilization (ethylene oxide, β-propiolactone, formaldehyde, propylene oxide) and UV or ionizing radiation. However, most of these procedures are unsatisfactory for dermatologicals because of their multiphase physicochemical natures and because the moment the patient opens the container microorganisms contaminate the contents. In addition, killed bacteria may liberate endotoxins which may be potent sensitizers (Katz, 1973).

Chemical methods of preservation employ agents which inhibit microbial growth and thus constrain the subsequent decomposition of the product. Ideally, a suitable preservative should not only destroy potential pathogens but should extend the shelf life of the product and minimize the deleterious consequences of microbial contamination arising during use of the product. No single agent is appropriate for exploitation under all conditions for every class of topical vehicle.

Preservatives impede microbial metabolism, growth, and multiplication by a combination of mechanisms. They may oxidize, reduce, or hydrolyze cellular constituents, act on enzymes or other proteins, interfere with essential metabolites, or modify membrane permeability. By whatever route a particular preservative functions, there is a complex scheme of interaction between those factors which influence the growth of the microbe and the elements which modify the efficiency of the preservative. De Navarre (1962) outlined the basic concepts of microbial spoilage, and Wedderburn (1964) dealt with the control of microorganisms in emulsions. A convenient way to discuss this topic is to consider first some basic principles which Katz (1973) has summarized. Then we can deal in turn with the aqueous phase, the interfacial region, the lipid region, and the container, and within each of these sections we can note typical factors which influence microbial growth and facets which affect preservative efficiency.

Microbes grow readily in an aqueous phase; yeasts and molds prefer an acid pH, whereas bacteria thrive in a faintly alkaline medium. To be effective, a sufficient amount of preservative must dissolve in the aqueous phase and therefore the partition or distribution coefficient should favor the polar phase. The dissociation constant of the preservative, the intrinsic distribution constant of the undissociated species between the phases, and the pH all affect the partition coefficient of the preservative. In general, only the nonionized portion of the preservative is active, as the ionized part does not easily penetrate the microorganism; thus weak acids are potent at a pH below their pK_a, and weak bases kill on the alkaline side of their pK_a. Few microorganisms grow at extremes of pH, i.e., below pH 3 or above pH 9, but dermatological products buffered under such drastic conditions would damage skin. Preservatives differ in the chemical nature of their attack, in the part of the cell which they assault, and in the ease with which they penetrate the cell. Preservatives which contain an active hydrogen may bond or complex with dosage form adjuvants such as polymers, macromolecules, and ethoxylated compounds, and so be inactivated.

The aqueous phase of a topical cream may contain hydrocolloids, humectants, electrolytes, proteins, carbohydrates, particulate matter, and surfactants, in addition to water and polar solvents. In general, organisms require water to survive—and the more water present, the greater the growth. Cellulose derivatives and natural gums may be heavily contaminated, and the macromolecules may be rapidly metabolized. Propylene and hexylene glycols inhibit growth, provided that their concentrations are over 10%. Polyethylene glycol, polyvinylpyrrolidone, and cellulose derivatives may complex with some preservatives and so reduce their efficiency. Coates (1973) reviewed the interaction of preservatives with suspending agents, and Murray and Smith (1968) evaluated the incompatibilities of preservatives.

Glycols may increase the partition coefficient of the preservative so as to favor its concentration in the polar phase. Humectants such as glycerol and sorbitol inhibit growth when they are present above some 40 or 50% concentration, but microorganisms can metabolize them below this level.

Electrolytes influence the pH (and growth is favored at pH 5.0 to 7.5) and
thereby affect the dissociation of the preservative, depending on its pK_a.
Electrolytes also modify the critical micelle concentrations of surfactants.
Microorganisms can metabolize proteins, which also complex cationic
germicides strongly and other preservatives to a lesser extent. Similarly,
carbohydrates are liable to metabolism and complexation with some
preservatives.

Microorganisms may contaminate powders, and the solid particles may
adsorb the preservative. Nonionic and anionic surfactants may be metabolized, whereas cationics inhibit growth. Some surfactants can complex
with the preservative below the critical micelle concentration (CMC), and
the preservative may solubilize within the micelle and so become inactivated.
In general, nonionic surfactants reduce preservative efficiency markedly
and anionics to a lesser extent. At low concentrations (below the CMC) a
surfactant may promote a bactericidal action by lowering the interfacial
tension at the cell wall (Beckett and Robinson, 1958; Kostenbauder, 1959;
Garrett, 1966; Garrett and Woods, 1953; Bean et al., 1965; Bean et al.,
1969; Schwarz, 1971).

For a review and discussion of the interaction of nonionic surfactants
with preservatives, together with a survey of the physicochemical and
biological methods for determining such interactions, the articles of Parker
and Barnes (1967) and Coates (1973) may be consulted.

Microorganisms are attracted to the interfacial regions in an emulsion,
and preservatives may concentrate there.

The lipid phase may contain perfumes and particulate matter; essential
oils inhibit growth when present at high concentrations. As in the aqueous
phase, powders may be contaminated with microorganisms and the particles
may adsorb preservatives. The oil phase can dissolve nonpolar materials
and may therefore reduce the amount of some preservatives in the aqueous
phase.

Containers are frequently contaminated, particularly the closures.
Some types of containers may complex with preservatives or absorb them
(McCarthy, 1972).

From the foregoing discussion, we can readily appreciate the impossi-
bility of producing a universal preservative, although we can summarize
the essential requirements for selecting a material to preserve a specific
topical formulation. This additive must be compatible with the ingredients
of the formulation; it should be stable to heat, prolonged storage, and
product use conditions; and it must be nonirritant, nontoxic, and nonsensitizing to human tissue.

Information on the use of antimicrobial agents in dermatological and
cosmetic formulations is in various manufacturers' brochures and reviews
(Bean, 1967; Rosen and Berk, 1973; Jacobs, 1975; Boem and Maddox,
1972; Speiser, 1968; Gucklhorn, 1969, 1970, 1971; Wedderburn, 1963,
1964; De Navarre, 1962; Wilkinson, 1973; Block, 1977; Bloomfield, 1978).

TABLE 6.4 Examples of Preservatives used in Topical Preparations

Type	Examples	Usual concentration (%)
Alcohols	Ethyl, isopropyl, chlorbutol, benzyl p-chlorphenyl propanediol, β-phenoxy ethyl, bromonitropropanediol (Bronopol)	70
Acids	Benzoic, dehydroacetic, propionic, sorbic, cinnamic	0.1-0.2
Essential oils	Anethol, citronellol, eugenol, vanillates, etc.	0.001-0.002
Mercurials	Phenylmercuric acetate, borate, nitrate, Thimerosal (Thiomersol)	
Phenols	Phenol, cresol, thymol, halogenated derivatives (e.g., p-chloro-m-cresol)	0.1-0.2
p-Hydroxybenzoates	Methyl, ethyl, propyl, butyl (Parabens)	0.01-0.5[a]
Quaternary ammonium compounds	Benzalkonium chloride, cetylpyridinium chloride, cetrimide	0.002-0.01
Formaldehyde/ formaldehyde donors	Formaldehyde, dimethylol dimethylhydantoin, Dowicil 200	
Others	Trichlorodihydroxydiphenyl ether, chlorhexidine gluconate (Hibitane), chloroform, imidazolidinyl urea (Germall 115), sugars, sulfites	

[a] In Aureomycin Ointment, 3%.
Source: From Katz (1973).

Mathematical models for calculating the concentration of preservatives available within the aqueous phase of an emulsion have been constructed by Bean et al. (1965), Bean et al. (1969), Mitchell and Kazmi (1975), Garrett (1966), Garrett and Woods (1953), and Schwarz (1971).

Table 6.4 illustrates examples of the various classes of preservatives used in topical products; in particular, the Parabens (p-hydroxybenzoates) are versatile and widely employed, as are the quaternaries and formaldehyde donors.

VII. RANCIDITY AND ANTIOXIDANTS

Many prototype pharmaceutical preparations could deteriorate on storage because the therapeutic ingredients or the adjuvants oxidize in the presence of even small amounts of atmospheric oxygen. This decomposition can be particularly troublesome in emulsions because the emulsification process may introduce air into the product and because there is a high interfacial area of contact between the water and the oil.

Many of the harmful processes to which pharmaceutical preparations are prone are "autoxidation" reactions. These are chain reactions which are often initiated by UV radiation in the presence of a trace of oxygen and which heavy metal ions may catalyze. Highly reactive free radicals form, but the addition of very small amounts of antioxidants inhibit the chain reaction. Thus, antioxidants prevent the formation of aldehydes and ketones in fats and oils, thereby suppressing the development of unpleasant odors and the appearance of rancidity.

We can classify antioxidants into three main groups:

The first group, comprising the true antioxidants (or antioxygens), probably inhibit oxidation by reacting with free radicals and blocking the chain reaction. Examples are the tocopherols, alkyl gallates, butylated hydroxyanisole (BHA), butylated hydroxytoluene (BHT), and nordihydroguiaretic acid (NDGA).

The second group of antioxidants, comprising the reducing agents, have a lower redox potential than the chemical which they protect and are therefore more readily oxidized. They often also react with free radicals. Examples are ascorbic and isoascorbic acid and the potassium and sodium salts of sulfurous acid.

The third group comprises the antioxidant synergists. They are sequestering or chelating agents which possess little antioxidant effect themselves but probably enhance the action of a true antioxidant by reacting with those heavy metal ions that catalyze oxidation. The synergist class includes citric acid, tartaric acid, disodium edetate, lecithin, and thiodipropionic acid. Mixtures of true antioxidants may also show synergism.

TABLE 6.5 Some Examples of Antioxidants

Phenolic type:
  Butylated hydroxyanisole (BHA)
  Butylated hydroxytoluene (BHT)
  Nordihydroguiaretic acid (NDGA)
  Propyl gallate, pyrogallol
	Organic acids, alcohols, esters:
	  Ascorbic, citric, malic acids,
	  sorbitol, glycerol, propylene
	  glycol, ascorbyl palmitate

Quinone type:
  Hydroquinone
  Hydroxycoumarins
  Tocopherols
	Amine type:
	  Ethanolamine
	  Lecithin, cephalin
	  Plant and animal phosphatides

Sulfur compounds:
  Thiodipropionic acid (dilauryl,
    distearyl esters)
  Sulfites, bisulfites
  Dithiocarbamates
	Inorganic acids/salts:
	  Phosphoric acid and salts
	  Phosphorous acid and salts

Source: From Katz (1973).

TABLE 6.6 Some Commonly Used Antioxidants and Their Synergists

Antioxidants	Concentration (%)	Synergists
Butylated hydroxyanisole (BHA)	0.005–0.01	Citric and phosphoric acids, lecithin, BHT, NDGA
Butylated hydroxytoluene (BHT)	0.01	Citric and phosphoric acids up to double the weight of BHT and BHA
Propyl gallate α-Tocopherols	0.005–0.15 0.01–0.1	Citric and phosphoric acid
Nordihydroguaiaretic acid (NDGA)	0.001–0.01	Ascorbic, phosphoric, citric acids (25.5% NDGA content) and BHA
Hydroquinone	0.05–0.1	Lecithin, citric acid and phosphoric acid, BHA, BHT

The ideal antioxidant should possess the following properties:

1. Effective at low concentrations
2. Nontoxic, nonirritant, and nonsensitizing
3. Decomposition products should be nontoxic, nonirritant, and nonsensitizing
4. Odorless and should not color the product
5. Stable and effective over a wide pH range
6. Neutral—should not react chemically with other ingredients
7. Nonvolatile

Table 6.5 lists examples of antioxidants, and Table 6.6 details some commonly used antioxidant/synergist combinations.

Data on the types of antioxidants available for purchase, and their recommended uses, may be found in various manufacturers' brochures. Relevant review articles include those of Ostendorf (1965), Scott (1965), Lachman (1968), Chalmers (1971), and WHO (1972, 1974).

REFERENCES

Adams, I., and Davis, S. S. (1973). J. Pharm. Pharmacol. 25:640.
Alexander, A. E., and Johnson, P. (1949). Colloid Science. Oxford Univ. Press, New York.
Anon (1975). Drug Cosmetic Ind. 116(2):36.
Ansel, H. C. (1969). Introduction to Pharmaceutical Dosage Forms. Lea & Febiger, Philadelphia, Chaps. 3, 11, and 14.
Ashley, J. (1955). Australasian J. Pharm. 36:989.
Baer, R. L. (1955). Arch. Dermatol. 71:19.
Bagley, E. B., and Taylor, N. W. (1974). J. Polymer Sci. (Symp.) 45:185.
Baker, H. (1968). Chemist Druggist 190:534.
Barnett, G. (1957). Drug Cosmetic Ind. 80:610, 744.
Barnett, G. (1958). Drug Cosmetic Ind. 83:292.
Barr, M. (1962). J. Pharm. Sci. 51:395.
Barrett, C. W. (1969). J. Soc. Cosmetic Chemists 20:487.
Barrett, C. W., Hadgraft, J. W., and Sarkany, I. (1964a). J. Pharm. Pharmacol. Suppl. 16:104T.
Barrett, C. W., Hadgraft, J. W., and Sarkany, I. (1964b). Br. J. Dermatol. 76:479.
Barrett, C. W., Hadgraft, J. W., Caron, G. A., and Sarkany, I. (1965). Br. J. Dermatol. 77:576.
Barry, B. W. (1968). J. Colloid Interface Sci. 28:82.
Barry, B. W. (1969). J. Pharm. Pharmacol. 21:533.
Barry, B. W. (1970). J. Colloid Interface Sci. 32:551.
Barry, B. W. (1973). J. Pharm. Pharmacol. 25:131.
Barry, B. W. (1975). Adv. Colloid Interface Sci. 5:37.

Barry, B. W. (1976). Dermatologica 152(Suppl. 1):47.
Barry, B. W., and Eccleston, G. M. (1973). J. Texture Studies 4:53.
Barry, B. W., and Grace, A. J. (1970). J. Pharm. Pharmacol. 22(Suppl): 147S.
Barry, B. W., and Grace, A. J. (1971a). J. Texture Studies 2:259.
Barry, B. W., and Grace, A. J. (1971b). Rheol. Acta 10:113.
Barry, B. W., and Grace, A. J. (1971c). J. Pharm. Sci. 60:1198.
Barry, B. W., and Grace, A. J. (1971d). J. Pharm. Sci. 60:814.
Barry, B. W., and Grace, A. J. (1972). J. Pharm. Sci. 61:335.
Barry, B. W., and Meyer, M. C. (1973). J. Pharm. Sci. 62:1349.
Barry, B. W., and Meyer, M. C. (1975). J. Texture Studies 6:433.
Barry, B. W., and Meyer, M. C. (1979a). Int. J. Pharmaceutics 2:1.
Barry, B. W., and Meyer, M. C. (1979b). Int. J. Pharmaceutics 2:27.
Barry, B. W., and Saunders, G. M. (1970a). J. Colloid Interface Sci. 34: 300.
Barry, B. W., and Saunders, G. M. (1970b). J. Pharm. Pharmacol. 22: 139S.
Barry, B. W., and Saunders, G. M. (1971a). J. Colloid Interface Sci. 35: 689.
Barry, B. W., and Saunders, G. M. (1971b). J. Colloid Interface Sci. 36: 130.
Barry, B. W., and Saunders, G. M. (1972a). J. Colloid Interface Sci. 38: 616.
Barry, B. W., and Saunders, G. M. (1972b). J. Colloid Interface Sci. 38: 626.
Barry, B. W., and Saunders, G. M. (1972c). J. Colloid Interface Sci. 41: 331.
Barry, B. W., and Shotton, E. (1967). J. Pharm. Pharmacol. 19(Suppl): 110S.
Barry, B. W., and Shotton, E. (1968). J. Pharm. Pharmacol. 20:242.
Barry, B. W., and Woodford, R. (1974). Br. J. Dermatol. 91:323.
Barry, B. W., and Woodford, R. (1975). Br. J. Dermatol. 93:563.
Barry, B. W., and Woodford, R. (1976). Br. J. Dermatol. 95:423.
Barry, B. W., and Woodford, R. (1977). Br. J. Dermatol. 97:555.
Barry, B. W., and Woodford, R. (1978). J. Clin. Pharm. 3:43.
Bean, H. S. (1967). Pharm. J. ii:289.
Bean, H. S., Heman-Ackah, S. M., and Thomas, J. (1965). J. Soc. Cosmetic Chemists 16:15.
Bean, H. S., Konning, G. H., and Malcolm, S. A. (1969). J. Pharm. Pharmacol. 21:173S.
Beckett, A. H., and Robinson, A. E. (1958). Soap Perfumery Cosmetics 31:454.
Bennett, H., Bishop, J. L., and Wulfinghoff, M. F. (1968). Practical Emulsions. Chemical Publ., New York.
Berneis, K. H., and Münzel, K. (1964). Pharm. Acta Helv. 39:88.

Berneis, K. H., Münzel, K., and Waaler, T. (1964). Pharm. Acta Helv. 39:604.

Birdwell, B. F., and Jesson, F. W. (1966). Nature 209:366.

Blaug, S. (1975). In Remington's Pharmaceutical Sciences, 15th ed. Mack, Easton, Pa., p. 1523.

Block, S. S. (1977). Disinfection, Sterilization, and Preservation, 2nd ed. Lea & Febiger, Philadelphia.

Bloomfield, S. F. (1978). J. Appl. Bacteriol. 45:1.

Boem, E. E., and Maddox, D. N. (1971). Mfg. Chemist Aerosol News 42 (Apr.):41.

Boem, E. E., and Maddox, D. N. (1972). Mfg. Chemist Aerosol News 43 (Aug.):21.

Boylan, J. C. (1966). J. Pharm. Sci. 55:710.

Boylan, J. C. (1967). J. Pharm. Sci. 56:1164.

Breit, R., and Bandmann, H. J. (1973). Br. J. Dermatol. 88:414.

Brode, E. (1968). Arzneim. Forsch. 18:580.

Bruch, C. W. (1971a). Am. Perfumer Cosmet. 86:45.

Bruch, C. W. (1971b). Drug Cosmetic Ind. 108:26.

Burdick, K. H. (1972). Acta Derm. Venereol. (Stockh.) 52(Suppl. 67):19, 24.

Bushnell, L. F. (1965). Pacific Med. Surg. 73:353.

Busse, M. J., Hunt, P., Lees, K. A., Maggs, P. N. D., and McCarthy, T. M. (1969). Br. J. Dermatol. 81(Suppl. 4):103.

Caldwell, I. W., Hall-Smith, S. P., Main, R. A., Ashurst, P. J., Kurton, V., Simpson, W. T., and Williams, G. W. (1968). Br. J. Dermatol. 80:11.

Calnan, C. D. (1962). Proc. R. Soc. Med. 55:39.

Carter, S. J. (1975). Cooper and Gunn's Dispensing for Pharmaceutical Students, 12th ed. Pitman Med. Publ., London.

Casparis, P., and Meyer, E. W. (1935). Pharm. Acta Helv. 10:163.

Castillo, A., and Sune, J. M. (1968). Ars Pharm. 9:367.

Caver, P. M., Gregorio, J., and Nobles, W. L. (1957). Am. J. Pharm. 129:118.

Cerezo, A., and Sune, J. (1970). Trav. Soc. Pharm. Montpellier 30:5.

Chalmers, L. (1971). Soap Perfumery Cosmetics 44:29.

Charm, S. E. (1964). J. Food Sci. 29:483.

Chester, J. F. L. (1967). Soap Perfumery Cosmetics 40:393.

Christie, G. A., and Moore-Robinson, M. (1970). Br. J. Dermatol. 82(Suppl. 6):93.

Christov, K. (1967). Pharmazie 22:251.

Christov, K., Marinov, M., and Todorova, P. (1970). Pharmazie 25:539.

Clark, R. (1963). In Handbook of Cosmetic Science, H. W. Hibbot (Ed.). Pergamon Press, Elmsford, N.Y., pp. 175, 257.

Clark, E. W. (1968). Drug Cosmetic Ind. 103(Sept.):46; (Oct.):74.

Clark, E. W. (1975). J. Soc. Cosmetic Chemists 26:323.

Clark, E. W. (1977). Contact Dermatitis 3:69.

Coates, D. (1973). Mfg. Chemist 44(Aug.):41; (Dec.):19.

Cohen, L. (1956). Soap Chem. Specialities 29:42.

Coldman, M. F., Poulsen, B. J., and Higuchi, T. (1969). J. Pharm. Sci. 58:1098.

Conrad, L. I. (1958). Drug Cosmetic Ind. 83:160.

Conrad, L. I. (1966). J. Soc. Cosmetic Chemists 17:149.

Cooper, J., and Lazarus, J. (1970). In The Theory and Practice of Industrial Pharmacy, L. Lachman, H. A. Lieberman, and J. L. Kanig (eds.). Lea & Febiger, Philadelphia, p. 491.

Courtney, D. L. (1972). Am. Perfumer Cosmet. 87:31.

Criddle, D. W. (1965). Trans. Soc. Rheol. 9:287.

Cronin, E. (1966). Br. J. Dermatol. 78:167.

Davis, S. S. (1969). J. Pharm. Sci. 58:412.

Delonca, H., Dolique, R., and Bardet, L. (1967). Ann. Pharm. Franc. 25:225.

Dempski, R. E., Portnoff, J. B., and Wase, A. W. (1969). J. Pharm. Sci. 58:579.

De Navarre, M. G. (1962). The Chemistry and Manufacture of Cosmetics, 2nd ed., Vols. 1 and 2. Van Nostrand Reinhold, New York.

Dittmar, C. A. (1957). Drug Cosmetic Ind. 81:447.

Dodge, D. W., and Metzner, A. B. (1959). A.I.Ch.E. (Am. Inst. Chem. Engrs.) J. 5:189.

Dolan, M. M., Steelman, R. L., and Tumilowicz, R. R. (1960). Toxicol. Appl. Pharmacol. 2:331.

Dunnigan, A. P. (1968). Proc. Joint Conf. Cosmet. Sci., Toilet Goods Assoc., Washington, D.C., p. 179.

Eccleston, G. M. (1975). J. Pharm. Pharmacol. 27:12P.

Eccleston, G. M. (1976). J. Colloid Interface Sci. 57:66.

Eccleston, G. M. (1977a). J. Pharm. Pharmacol. 29:157.

Eccleston, G. M. (1977b). Cosmetics Toiletries 92(Feb.):21.

Eccleston, G. M. (1980). Br. Pharm. Conf. Commun., 65P.

Epstein, M. B., Wilson, A., Gershman, J., and Ross, J. (1956). J. Phys. Chem. 58:860.

Erdi, N. Z., Cruz, M. M., and Battista, O. A. (1968). J. Colloid Interface Sci. 28:36.

Erös, I., and Kedvessy, Gy. (1969). Acta Pharm. Hung. 39:164.

Evans, S. (1970). Br. J. Dermatol. 82:625.

Everall, J., and Truiter, E. V. (1954). J. Invest. Dermatol. 22:493.

Fabian, Gy., Mozes, Gy., and Vamos, E. (1965). Rheol. Acta 4:6.

Feldmann, R. J., and Maibach, H. I. (1969). J. Invest. Dermatol. 52:89.

Fischer, W. H., Bauer, W. H., and Wiberley, S. E. (1961). Trans. Soc. Rheol. 5:221.

Flynn, G. D. (1979). In Modern Pharmaceutics (Drugs and the Pharmaceutical Sciences, Vol. 7), G. S. Banker and C. T. Rhodes (Eds.). Dekker, New York, p. 263.

Foster, S., Wurster, D. E., Higuchi, T., and Busse, L. W. (1951). J. Am. Pharm. Assoc., Sci. Ed. 40:123.

Franks, A. J. (1964). Soap Perfumery Cosmetics 37:221, 319.

Füller, W., and Münzel, K. (1962). Pharm. Acta Helv. 37:38.

Garnier, J. P. (1971a). Clin. Trials J. (London) 8:55.

Garnier, J. P. (1971b). Pharm. J. 207:475.

Garrett, E. R. (1966). J. Pharm. Pharmacol. 18:589.

Garrett, E. R., and Woods, O. R. (1953). J. Am. Pharm. Assoc., Sci. Ed. 42:736.

Giroux, J., and Schrenzel, M. (1964). Pharm. Acta Helv. 39:615.

Goddard, E. D., and Kung, H. C. (1965). Proc. Ann. Meeting Chem. Spec. Mfr. Assoc., p. 124.

Goodrich, B. F., Manufacturer (n.d.) Carbopol Water Soluble Resins (Service Bulletin). Goodrich, Cleveland, Ohio.

Grace, A. J. (1971). Ph.D. thesis, Council for National Academic Awards, Portsmouth Polytechnic, England.

Gray, C. B. (1943). J. Inst. Petrol. 29:226.

Gretsky, V. M., and Blagovidova, Yu A. (1969). Farmatsiya (Moscow) 18: 16.

Groves, G. A. (1964). Pharm. J. New Zealand 26:247.

Gruntova, Z., Mandak, M., and Duckova, K. (1967a). Ceskoslov. Pharm. 16:263.

Gruntova, Z., Mandak, M., and Duckova, K. (1967b). Farm. Obzor 36: 499.

Gstirner, F. (1970). Indian J. Pharm. 32:73.

Gstirner, F., Kottenberg, D., and Maas, A. (1969). Arch. Pharm. 302: 340.

Gstirner, F., and Meisenberg, R. (1970). Arch. Pharm. 303:872.

Gucklhorn, I. R. (1969). Mfg. Chemist Aerosol News 40(June):23; (July): 38; (Aug.):71; (Sept.):33; (Oct):33; (Nov.):35; (Dec.):43.

Gucklhorn, I. R. (1970). Mfg. Chemist Aerosol News 41(Jan.):42; (Feb.): 30; (Mar.):26; (Apr.):34; (June):44; (July):51; (Aug.):28; (Sept.):82; (Oct.):49; (Nov.):48; (Dec.):50.

Gucklhorn, I. R. (1971). Mfg. Chemist Aerosol News 42(Jan.):34; (Feb.): 35.

Hadgraft, J. W. (1972). Br. J. Dermatol. 87:386.

Heisel, E. B. (1967). In Dermatologic Allergy: Immunology, Diagnosis and Management, L. H. Criep (Ed.). Saunders, Philadelphia, p. 540.

Heyd, A. (1971). J. Pharm. Sci. 60:1343.

Hibbott, H. W. (1963). Handbook of Cosmetic Science. Pergamon Press, Elmsford, N.Y.

Hollis, G. L. (1980). Directory of Surface Active Chemicals: Surfactants U.K., 2nd ed. Tergo-Data, Darlington, England.

Hynniman, C. E., and Lamy, P. (1969). Drug Cosmetic Ind. 105:40.

Idson, B. (1971). In Topics in Medicinal Chemistry, Vol. 4: Absorption Phenomena, J. L. Rabinowitz and R. L. Myerson (Eds.). Wiley (Interscience), New York, p. 181.

Idson, B. (1975). J. Pharm. Sci. 64:901.

Ive, A., and Comaish, S. (1980). Recent Adv. Dermatol. 5:285.

Jacobs, G. (1975). J. Soc. Cosmetic Chemists 26:105.

Jellinek, J. S. (1970). Formulation and Function of Cosmetics. Wiley (Interscience), New York.

Jenkins, G. L., Francke, D. E., Brecht, E. A., and Sperandio, G. J. (1957). The Art of Compounding. McGraw-Hill (Blakiston), New York.

Kato, Y., and Saito, T. (1967). Arch. Pract. Pharm. 27:127.

Katz, M. (1973). In Drug Design (Medicinal Chemistry, Vol. 4), E. J. Ariens (Ed.). Academic Press, New York, p. 93.

Katz, M., and Poulsen, B. (1971). In Handbook of Experimental Pharmacology, B. B. Brodie and J. Gillette (Eds.), Vol. 27, Pt. 1. Springer-Verlag, New York, p. 103.

Katz, M., and Poulsen, B. J. (1972). J. Soc. Cosmetic Chemists 23:565.

Katz, M., and Shaikh, Z. I. (1965). J. Pharm. Sci. 54:591.

Killings, L. O., Ringertz, O., and Silverstolpe, L. (1966). Acta Pharm. Suec. 3:219.

Kinsel, A., and Schindler, H. (1948). Petrol. Refiner 27:124.

Kolvoort, E. C. H. (1938). J. Inst. Petrol. 24:338.

Kostenbauder, H. B. (1959). Am. Perfumer Aromat. 75:28, 32.

Kostenbauder, H. B., and Martin, A. N. (1954). J. Am. Pharm. Assoc., Sci. Ed. 43:401.

Kung, H. C., and Goddard, E. D. (1963). J. Phys. Chem. 67:1965.

Kung, H. C., and Goddard, E. D. (1964). J. Phys. Chem. 68:3465.

Kung, H. C., and Goddard, E. D. (1965). J. Colloid Sci. 20:766.

Lachman, L. (1968). Drug Cosmetic Ind. 102(Jan.):36.

Lachman, L., and Deluca, P. (1970). In The Theory and Practice of Industrial Pharmacy, L. Lachman, H. A. Lieberman, and J. L. Kanig (Eds.). Lea & Febiger, Philadelphia, p. 669.

Lang, W. (1972). Drug Cosmetic Ind. 110:52, 127.

Lang, W. (1974). Am. Perfumer Cosmet. 89:67.

Lawrence, A. S. C. (1958). Discussions Faraday Soc. 25:51, 58.

Lawrence, A. S. C. (1959). Nature p. 1491.

Lawrence, A. S. C. (1961a). Chem. Ind. (London) p. 1764.

Lawrence, A. S. C. (1961b). In Surface Activity and Detergency, K. Durham (Ed.). Macmillan, New York, p. 158.

Lee, J. A., and Nobles, W. L. (1959). J. Am. Pharm. Assoc. 48:92.

Lee, J. A., Caver, P. M., and Nobles, W. L. (1957). Am. J. Pharm. 129:190.

Lemlich, R. (1972). J. Soc. Cosmetic Chemists 23:299.

Lerner, M. R., and Lerner, A. B. (1960). Dermatologic Medications. Year Book Med. Publs., Chicago.

Levy, G., and Schwartz, T. W. (1957). Drug Cosmetic Ind. 81:606.

Lintner, C. J. (1975). In Remington's Pharmaceutical Sciences, 15th ed. Mack, Easton, Pa., p. 1419.

Longworth, A. R., and French, J. D. (1969). J. Pharm. Pharmacol. 21 (Suppl.):1S.

Lorincz, A. L. (1964). In The Evaluation of Therapeutic Agents and Cosmetics, T. H. Sternberg and V. D. Newcomer (Eds.). McGraw-Hill, New York, p. 86.

Lowek, E. S., and Cressey, S. (1957). Drug Cosmetic Ind. 81:450.

McCarthy, T. J. (1972). Am. Perfumer Cosmet. 87:37.

McEwan, P. (1968). Lancet i:45.

Malkinson, F. D. (1964). In The Epidermis, W. Montagna and W. C. Lobitz (Eds.). Academic Press, New York, Chap. 21.

Malkinson, F. D., and Rothman, S. (1963). In Handbuch der Haut und Geschlechtskrankheiten, J. Jadasohn (Ed.), Springer-Verlag, New York.

Mandak, M., Kucera, J., and Verber, V. (1969a). Pharm. Tijdschr. Belg. 46:114.

Mandak, M., Kucera, J., and Verber, V. (1969b). Farmatsiya (Moscow) 18:73.

Mapstone, G. E. (1974). Cosm. Perf. 89:31.

Marriot, R. H. (1961). J. Soc. Cosmetic Chemists 12:89.

Martin, A. N., Swarbrick, J., and Cammarata, A. (1969). Physical Pharmacy. Lea & Febiger, Philadelphia, p. 354.

Mears, E. (1962). J. Reprod. Fertility 4:337.

Meyer, E. (1968). White Mineral Oil and Petrolatum, and Their Related Products, Petroleum Sulphonates and Microcrystalline Waxes. Chemical Publ., New York.

Meyer, M. C. (1978). Ph.D. thesis, Council for National Academic Awards, Portsmouth Polytechnic, England.

Meyer, R. J., and Cohen, L. (1959). J. Soc. Cosmetic Chemists 10:143.

Misek, B., Powers, J., Ruggiero, J., and Skaun, D. (1956). J. Am. Pharm. Assoc. 45:56.

Mitchell, A. G., and Kazmi, S. J. A. (1975). Can. J. Pharm. Sci. 10:67.

Mnyukh, Yu. V. (1963). J. Phys. Chem. Solids 24:631.

Morimoto, K., and Suzuki, S. (1972). J. Appl. Polymer Sci. 16:2947.

Mottram, F. J. (1961). Lab. Pract. 10:767.

Müller, A. (1930). Proc. R. Soc. Lond. A127:417.

Müller, A. (1932). Proc. R. Soc. Lond. A138:514.

Münzel, K. (1968). J. Soc. Cosmetic Chemists 19:289.

Mulley, B. A., and Marland, J. S. (1970). J. Pharm. Pharmacol. 22:243.

Munro, D. D. (1969). Br. J. Dermatol. 81(Suppl. 4):92.

Munro, D. D., and Stoughton, R. B. (1965). Arch. Dermatol. 92:585.

Murray, J. B., and Smith, G. (1968). Pharm. J. i:87.

Mutimer, M. N., Riffkin, C., Hill, J. A., and Cyr, G. N. (1956). J. Am. Pharm. Assoc., Sci. Ed. 45:101, 212.

Myers, G. E. (1969). Can. J. Pharm. Sci. 4:75.

Myers, G. E., and Leslie, G. A. (1969). Can. J. Pharm. Sci. 4:64.

Nelson, W. L., and Stewart, L. D. (1949). Ind. Eng. Chem. 41:2231.

Neuwald, F., and Adam, K. (1954). Deut. Apotheker-Z. 94:1258.

Newcomb, E. A. (1966). J. Soc. Cosmetic Chemists 17:149.

Newton, D. W., Becker, C. H., and Torosian, G. (1973). J. Pharm. Sci. 62:1538.

Nielsen, J. R., and Hathaway, C. E. (1963). J. Mol. Spectr. 10:366.

Nobles, W. L. (1955). Drug Cosmetic Ind. 77:178.

Olszewski, Z., and Kubis, A. (1969). Acta Polon. Pharm. 26:441.

Ory, A. M. (1962). Ph.D. thesis, University of Zurich.

Ostendorf, J. P. (1965). J. Soc. Cosmetic Chemists 16:203.

Ostrenga, J., Haleblian, J., Poulsen, B., Ferrell, B., Mueller, N., and Shastri, S. (1971a). J. Invest. Dermatol. 56:392.

Ostrenga, J., Steinmetz, C., and Poulsen, B. (1971b). J. Pharm. Sci. 60:1175.

Pajor, Zs., Pandula, E., and Peres, T. (1967). Fette Seifen Anstrichmittel 69:855.

Parker, M. S., and Barnes, M. (1967). Soap Perfumery Cosmet. 40:163.

Patel, N. K., and Foss, N. E. (1964). J. Pharm. Sci. 53:94.

Pickthall, J. (1954). Soap Perfumery Cosmet. 27:1270.

Piper, S. H., Chibnall, A. C., Hopkins, S. J., Pollard, A., Smith, J. A. B., and Williams, E. F. (1931). Biochem. J. 25:2072.

Portnoy, B. (1965). Br. J. Dermatol. 77:579.

Poulsen, B. (1970). Br. J. Dermatol. 82(Suppl. 6):49.

Poulsen, B. (1973). In Drug Design (Medicinal Chemistry, Vol. 4), E. J. Ariens (Ed.). Academic Press, New York, p. 149.

Poulsen, B. J., Young, E., Coquilla, V., and Katz, M. (1968). J. Pharm. Sci. 57:928.

Presting, W., and Keil, G. (1956). Chem. Tech. (Berlin) 8:36.

Rawlins, E. A. (Ed.) (1977a). Bentley's Textbook of Pharmaceutics, 8th ed. Balliere Tindall, London, pp. 256, 351.

Rawlins, E. A. (Ed.) (1977b). Bentley's Textbook of Pharmaceutics, 8th ed. Balliere Tindall, London, p. 140.

Regdon, G., and Kovacs, I. (1969). Deut. Apotheker-Z. 109:1893.

Rhodes, E. L. (1971). Clin. Trials J. (London) 8:61.

Richman, M. D., and Shangraw, R. F. (1966). Aerosol Age 11(5):36.

Roberts, G. W. (1960). Lancet i:283.

Rosen, H. S., and Berk, P. A. (1973). J. Soc. Cosmetic Chemists 24:663.

Rothman, S. (1954). Physiology and Biochemistry of the Skin. Univ. Chicago Press, Chicago.

Sagarin, E. (1957). Cosmetics: Science and Technology. Wiley (Interscience), New York.

Saito, S., and Taniguchi, T. (1973). J. Am. Oil Chemists Soc. 50:276.

Salisbury, R., Leuallen, E. E., and Charkin, L. T. (1954). J. Am. Pharm. Assoc., Sci. Ed. 43:117

Sanders, P. (1966). Am. Perfumer Cosmet. 81:62.

Sanders, P. (1970). Principles of Aerosol Technology. Van Nostrand Rheinhold, New York, p. 302.

Sarkany, I., and Hadgraft, J. W. (1969). Br. J. Dermatol. 81(Suppl. 4): 98.

Sarkany, I., Hadgraft, J. W., Caron, C. A., and Barrett, C. W. (1965). Br. J. Dermatol. 77:569.

Saski, W. (1960). Drug Standards 28:79.

Scherl, N. D., and Scherl, B. A. (1973). Dis. Colon Rectum 16:149.

Schindler, M. (1961). Drug Cosmetic Ind. 89:36.

Schrenzel, M. (1964). Pharm. Acta Helv. 39:546.

Schulman, J. H., and Cockbain, E. G. (1940). Trans. Faraday Soc. 36: 651.

Schulte, K. E., and Kassem, M. A. (1963). Pharm. Acta Helv. 38:358.

Schutz, E. (1957). Arch. Exp. Pathol. Pharmakol. 232:237.

Schwarz, T. W. (1971). Am. Perfumer Cosmet. 86:39.

Schwarz, T. W., and Levy, G. (1958). J. Am. Pharm. Assoc. 47:442.

Sciarra, J. J. (1974). J. Pharm. Sci. 63:1815.

Sciarra, J. J. (1975a). Drug Cosmetic Ind. 116(6):58.

Sciarra, J. J. (1975b). In Remington's Pharmaceutical Sciences, 15th ed. Mack, Easton, Pa., p. 1644.

Scott, G. (1965). Atmospheric Oxidation and Antioxidants. Elsevier, New York.

Secard, D. L. (1962). Drug Cosmetic Ind. 90:1.

Seyer, W. F., Patterson, R. F., and Keays, J. L. (1944). J. Am. Chem. Soc. 66:179.

Sherman, P. (1970). Industrial Rheology. Academic Press, New York, p. 377.

Sherman, P. (1971). Rheol. Acta 10:121.

Singiser, R. E., and Beal, H. M. (1958). J. Am. Pharm. Assoc., Sci. Ed. 47:6.

Smith, A. E. (1953). J. Chem. Phys. 21:2229.

Sobrero, A. J. (1960). Fertility Sterility 11:518.

Speiser, P. (1968). Pharm. Acta Helv. 43:193.

Sprowls, J. B. Jr. (1963). Prescription Pharmacy. Lippincott, Philadelphia.

Stein, R. S., and Sutherland, G. B. B. M. (1954). J. Chem. Phys. 22: 1993.

Sternberg, T. H., and Newcomer, V. D. (1964). The Evaluation of Therapeutic Agents and Cosmetics. McGraw-Hill, New York.

Stoughton, R. B., and Frisch, W. (1964). Arch. Dermatol. 90:512.

Streeter, R. E., Caver, P. M., and Nobles, W. L. (1955). J. Am. Pharm. Assoc. 16:671.

Sugai, T., and Higaski, J. (1975). Contact Dermatitis 1:146.

Swafford, W. B., and Nobles, W. L. (1955). J. Amer. Pharm. Assoc. 16: 171.

Swinyard, E. A. (1975). In Remington's Pharmaceutical Sciences, 15th
    ed. Mack, Easton, Pa., p. 1221.
Taylor, N. W., and Bagley, E. B. (1974). J. Appl. Polymer Sci. 18:2747.
Taylor, N. W., and Bagley, E. B. (1975). J. Polymer Sci. 13:1133.
Testa, B., and Etter, J. C. (1973). Pharm Acta Helv. 48:378.
Testa, B., and Etter, J. C. (1975a). Can. J. Pharm. Sci. 10:16.
Testa, B., and Etter, J. C. (1975b). Can. J. Pharm. Sci. 10:20.
Tissot, J., and Osmundsen, P. E. (1966). Acta Derm. Venereol. (Stockh.)
    46:447.
Tsagareishvili, G. V., Bashura, G. S., Lekhan, A. S., and Kovalev, I. P.
    (1969). Soobshch. Akad. Nauk Gruz. S.S.R. 56:345.
Van der Have, J. H., and Verver, C. G. (1957). Petroleum and Its Prod-
    ucts. Pitman Med. Publ., London.
Van Ooteghem, M. (1965). Pharm. Acta Helv. 40:543.
Van Ooteghem, M. (1968). Pharm. Acta Helv. 43:264.
Van Oudtshoorn, M. C. B., and Potgieter, E. J. (1971). Pharm. Weekblad
    106:909.
Vickers, C. F. (1966). In Modern Trends in Dermatology, R. B. McKenna
    (Ed.), Vol. 3. Butterworths, London, Chap. 4.
Vincent, J. M., and Skoulios, A. (1966). Acta Cryst. 20:447.
Warburton, B., and Davis, S. S. (1969). Rheol. Acta 8:205.
Ward, R. B. (1974). Drug Cosmetic Ind. 115(2):50.
Warth, A. H. (1956). The Chemistry and Technology of Waxes. Van Nos-
    trand Rheinhold, New York.
Wedderburn, D. L. (1963). In Handbook of Cosmetic Science, H. W.
    Hibbott (Ed.). Pergamon Press, Elmsford, N.Y., pp. 205, 445.
Wedderburn, D. L. (1964). Adv. Pharm. Sci. 1:195.
Weiner, N. D., Shah, A. K., Kanig, J. L., and Felmeister, A. (1969).
    J. Soc. Cosmetic Chemists 20:215.
Wells, F. V., and Lubowe, I. I. (1964). Cosmetics and the Skin. Van
    Nostrand Reinhold, New York.
WHO (1972). Food Additives Ser. WHO No. 3. (World Health Org., Geneva.)
WHO (1974). Food Additives Ser. WHO No. 5. (World Health Org., Geneva.)
Wilkinson, D. S. (1972). In Mechanisms in Drug Allergy, C. H. Dash and
    H. E. H. Jones (Eds.). Churchill Livingstone, Edinburgh and London,
    p. 85.
Wilkinson, J. B., Ed. (1973). Harry's Cosmeticology, 6th ed. Hill,
    London, England.
Wilkinson, D. S. (1979a). In Texbook of Dermatology, 3rd ed., Vol. 2.
    A. Rook, D. S. Wilkinson, and F. J. G. Ebling (Eds.). Blackwell Sci.
    Publ., Oxford, England, p. 2353.
Wilkinson, D. S. (1979b). In Textbook of Dermatology, 3rd ed., Vol. 2.
    A. Rook, D. S. Wilkinson, and F. J. G. Ebling (Eds.). Blackwell Sci.
    Publ., Oxford, England, p. 2293.
Wolff, J. S., and Meyer, R. J. (1961). Soap Chem. Specialities 77:131.

Wood, J. H., Giles, W. H., and Catacalos, G. (1964). J. Soc. Cosmetic
    Chemists 15:564.
Woodford, R., and Barry, B. W. (1973). Br. J. Dermatol. 89:53.
Woodford, R., and Barry, B. W. (1974a). Curr. Ther. Res. 16:338.
Woodford, R., and Barry, B. W. (1974b). Br. J. Dermatol. 90:233.
Woodford, R., and Barry, B. W. (1977a). Curr. Ther. Res. 21:877.
Woodford, R., and Barry, B. W. (1977b). J. Pharm. Sci. 66:99.
Woodford, R., and Barry, B. W. (1979). Curr. Ther. Res. 26:601.
Zografi, G. (1970). In The Theory and Practice of Industrial Pharmacy,
    L. Lachman, H. A. Lieberman, and J. L. Kanig (Eds.). Lea & Febiger,
    Philadelphia, p. 463.

— 7 —

RHEOLOGY OF DERMATOLOGICAL VEHICLES

I. INTRODUCTION

A wide spectrum of formulations is available for use in topical therapy, ranging from simple solutions, fluid emulsions and suspensions, sprays and aerosols, paints, gels, creams and ointments, to pastes and powders. Such materials range in consistency from fluid to solid. An important category comprises the semisolids, or quasi-solids. Semisolids possess the particular property that they readily deform when we apply them to the skin yet they cling to the body, generally until washed or wiped off. Because of their nature, they are valuable therapeutic aids and drug delivery systems in dermatology, but semisolids are also the most difficult of materials to characterize rheologically because they combine solid behavior and liquid properties within the same material.

Why should we trouble to determine the rheological properties of semisolids? There are many reasons, the most important of which are the following:

1. To aid our fundamental understanding of the physicochemical nature of the vehicle
2. The quality control of ingredients, test formulations, and final products, together with manufacturing processes such as mixing, milling, pumping, stirring, extrusion, filling, and sterilization
3. To study the effects which alterations in the formulation, the temperature, and the storage time have on a product
4. To investigate the capacity of the vehicle to suspend solids or immiscible liquids
5. To assess a topical formulation with respect to patient usage, e.g., the

ease of removal of the preparation from a jar or tube without spillage, or spreadability and adherence to the skin, possibly with correlation with a panel response in texture profiling (Sherman, 1970; Barry and Grace, 1972; Barry and Meyer, 1973)

6. To monitor the effect of the vehicle's consistency on the release of a drug from the preparation and its subsequent percutaneous absorption (bioavailability of the medicament)

In the past, all too often formulators adjusted the consistencies of topical semisolids so as to satisfy cosmetic, compatibility, and stability criteria and they paid little regard to bioavailability considerations. Partly, this was because patients critically evaluate the sensory and cosmetic properties of ointments, creams, pastes, and gels—indeed, more so than they do for any other pharmaceutical product (Martin et al., 1964; Worthington, 1973). The extreme view is that the final purpose of rheological investigations is to establish simple correlations between physical quantities and the sensory response of the average consumer (Langenbucher and Lange, 1969). However, the modern view should emphasize that, although pharmaceutical elegance in a formulation is important, medicated topical products may deliver potent therapeutic agents and their clinical effectiveness (which includes drug bioavailability) is of primary concern.

Much of the published work on the flow properties of pharmaceutical semisolids is confusing or incorrect because the authors have discounted the essential viscoelastic nature of their materials. In general, they have tested their preparations with the implicit assumption that the systems were simply anomalous liquids, or non-Newtonian fluids. Further confusion arises when investigators used single-point or empirical instruments in attempts to establish the flow properties of semisolids. There is no sound justification for this procedure, and this category of instrument will not be considered in this chapter. For details of such apparatus the reader may consult, e.g., Martin et al. (1964) or Sherman (1970).

Nearly all the investigations which are relevant to our discussion of the rheology of topical vehicles use deformation in simple shear. For simplicity, therefore, this chapter will not use a tensor treatment for analysis but will employ only elementary mathematical procedures to treat the geometry of simple shear. The resultant simplification should compensate for the inevitable lack of analytical rigor and loss in generality.

Readers who wish to refresh their knowledge of general pharmaceutical rheology may consult, for example, Dinsdale and Moore (1962), Martin et al. (1964, 1969), Rankell and Lieberman (1970), or Schott (1975). Revevant reviews include those of Barry (1970a) and Barry and Grace (1971a). Sherman (1970) has surveyed industrial rheology, including pharmaceuticals and cosmetics, and Barry (1974) has discussed the continuous shear and viscoelastic properties of topical semisolids.

II. DETERMINATION OF THE RHEOLOGICAL BEHAVIOR OF TOPICAL VEHICLES

Probably the easiest way for us to deal with the flow characteristics of dermatological vehicles is to discuss the features in terms of a limited number of idealized flow classes. Such types of deformation and flow include Newtonian flow, Hookean deformation, plastic and pseudoplastic flow, dilatancy, rheopexy, thixotropy, and irreversible shear breakdown. In a particular rheological test under standardized conditions, a dermatological vehicle may behave quite similarly to one of these ideal flow types. However, the actual type of flow which a vehicle exhibits depends on such factors as the test temperature, the concentration, the dispersed phase volume, the particle size and the particle size distribution, the shear rate and shear stress regime, the past history of the sample, and the type of viscometer we use. It can be misleading to state, for example, that a certain ointment base shows plastic flow, without specifying all the relevant experimental details.

A. Continuous Shear Rheometry

1. Newtonian flow

Ideal viscous liquids obey Newton's law of viscous flow, according to which the flow rate depends on the applied stress. In simple laminar flow (in which streamlines are parallel), if σ represents the shear stress (in units of force per unit area) and $\dot{\gamma}$ (or $d\gamma/dt$) is the shear rate (with units of reciprocal time), then

$$\sigma = \eta \dot{\gamma} \tag{7.1}$$

The proportionality constant, η, is the coefficient of viscosity, which we sometimes abbreviate to "viscosity." The kinematic viscosity, ν, which we derive directly in capillary tube viscometry, equals the viscosity divided by the density, ρ. Some rheological discussions refer to the reciprocal of the viscosity, called the fluidity, ψ. These quantities are therefore related by

$$\eta = \nu\rho = \frac{1}{\psi} \tag{7.2}$$

A representative flow curve, or rheogram, illustrates the linear relationship between shear stress and shear rate (Fig. 7.1). The straight line passes through the origin of the graph. Newtonian fluids include simple liquids such as water, glycerol and propylene glycol, true solutions, and very dilute colloidal systems.

Einstein (1905, 1906, 1911) derived an equation which relates the viscosity, η, of a dilute dispersion or suspension to the viscosity of the

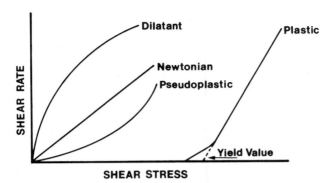

FIG. 7.1 Typical rheograms illustrating Newtonian, dilatant, pseudo-plastic, and plastic flow.

dispersion medium or solvent, η_0, and the volume fraction, ϕ, the volume of the particles per unit volume of the suspension:

$$\eta = \eta_0 (1 + 2.5\phi) \qquad (7.3)$$

This equation only applies to spherical, nondeformable particles under certain limiting conditions: the volume concentration of the particles must be so low that they do not interact; the distances between the particles should be much greater than their diameters; the fluid of the continuous phase must not slip at the particle surface; and η should arise only from the dissipation of energy (viscous drag) as fluid motion changes near the particle surfaces.

At higher concentrations of dispersed phase, the particles begin to interact with each other as their flow patterns in the continuous phase draw closer together and their streamlines eventually overlap. The overall viscosity is then no longer the sum of the effects which arise from individual particles. Guth and Simha (1936) allowed for this hydrodynamic interaction by modifying Eq. (7.3) to yield

$$\eta = \eta_0 (1 + 2.5\phi + 14.1\phi^2) \qquad (7.4)$$

Several workers have amended Eq. (7.4) to forms which we can represent by a polynomial in ϕ:

$$\eta = \eta_0 (1 + a\phi + b\phi^2 + c\phi^3 + d\phi^4 + \cdots) \qquad (7.5)$$

Sherman (1970) provides details of such amendments and also deals with other developments of the Einstein equation, which we will not consider further here.

We also meet with other viscosity coefficients in the literature. We define the relative viscosity, η_r, as the ratio of the viscosity of the dispersion to that of the solvent. From the Einstein equation,

$$\eta_r = \frac{\eta}{\eta_0} = (1 + 2.5\phi) \tag{7.6}$$

The specific viscosity, η_{sp}, is the relative increase in the viscosity of the dispersion over that of the solvent alone:

$$\eta_{sp} = \frac{\eta - \eta_0}{\eta_0} = \frac{\eta}{\eta_0} - 1 \tag{7.7}$$

Thus, the Einstein equation becomes

$$\eta_{sp} = \frac{\eta}{\eta_0} - 1 = 2.5\phi \tag{7.8}$$

Since ϕ, the volume fraction, is directly proportional to the concentration, c, of the dispersed phase, Eq. (7.8) may be expressed as

$$\eta_{sp} = kc \tag{7.9}$$

where k is a constant. As we have already seen in Eq. (7.5), for real systems at finite concentrations of the dispersed phase the equation is usually written as a power series

$$\eta_{sp} = \alpha c + \beta c^2 + \cdots \tag{7.10}$$

We can define a reduced viscosity by dividing the specific viscosity by c:

$$\frac{\eta_{sp}}{c} = \alpha + \beta c + \cdots \tag{7.11}$$

If we plot the reduced viscosity as a function of concentration and extrapolate to c = 0, the intercept yields the intrinsic viscosity, $[\eta]$. We can use the intrinsic viscosity to obtain the average molecular weight of polymers, $\bar{M}$, from

$$[\eta] = K\bar{M}^a \tag{7.12}$$

where K and a are constants for a series of polymers.

2. Non-Newtonian flow

The majority of the vehicles which we use in dermatology do not obey the simple Newtonian relationship when we test them in a continuous shear viscometer. Complex liquid and solid dispersions such as ointments, creams, pastes, and gels fall into this category, which we may subdivide as follows.

a. Plastic flow   Certain materials flow readily, provided that the shear stress is sufficiently high, but they will not flow if the applied shear stress is below a critical value—the yield stress or yield value. Below this stress, the material behaves essentially as an elastic solid. We call this rheological

behavior plastic flow, and materials which exhibit it we name Bingham
bodies after the scientist who first studied their properties (see Reiner,
1943). The rheogram is linear over most of its length, but the extrapolation
of the linear portion intersects the shear stress axis at the yield value instead of passing through the origin as a Newtonian liquid would (see Fig. 7.1).

The equation which describes plastic flow is

$$\sigma - \sigma_y = \eta_{pl}\dot{\gamma} \tag{7.13}$$

where σ_y is the yield value and η_{pl} is the apparent plastic viscosity, which
is analogous to the coefficient of viscosity in Newtonian flow.

In its simplest terms, we can consider plastic flow to arise from the
contact of flocculated particles in a concentrated suspension (Martin et al.,
1964). The particles link together throughout the body of the material, and
before it can flow the material requires a force to overcome both the
van der Waals forces of attraction between the particles and general frictional forces. The yield stress is that required to break down the solid
structure and to initiate flow.

A high yield value may help to maintain an ointment or a cream on the
skin so that it does not run off after application. When we spread the preparation over the diseased area, the imposed shearing forces exceed the
yield value and the application flows.

b. Pseudoplastic flow (shear thinning)   The flow curve for a pseudoplastic material starts at the origin (or it at least approaches the origin at
low shear rates), and there is no yield value. However, the plot is nonlinear
and the consistency decreases with increasing rate of shear (see Fig. 7.1).
We may derive an apparent viscosity at any defined rate of shear from the
reciprocal of the slope of the tangent to the curve at the specified point.
Alternatively, some workers define the apparent viscosity as the reciprocal
of the slope of a line which joins a specified point along the pseudoplastic
curve to the origin of the graph.

Typical pseudoplastic preparations include liquid dispersions of
natural and synthetic gums such as tragacanth, alginates, gelatin, methyl-
cellulose, and sodium carboxymethylcellulose. At rest, these systems
contain entwined long-chain molecules or other aggregated structures. As
the shearing stress increases, the aggregates progressively disrupt and
polymer molecules begin to align their long axes in the direction of flow,
i.e., along the laminar streamlines in a viscometer. The shearing forces
may also release some of the solvent previously associated with the molecules or aggregates. The effective concentration and the size of the dispersed aggregates fall. Both phenomena reduce the internal resistance to
flow and therefore the apparent viscosity reduces, in proportion to the
magnitude of the shear rate. The system appears to thin; hence the alternative designation for this type of flow behavior—shear rate thinning.

Various mathematical formulas define pseudoplastic curves. However, for our purposes the simplest and probably the best approach is to present the complete rheogram for inspection.

c. Dilatant flow and shear thickening Dilatant materials and shear thickening systems increase their resistance to flow as the shear rate rises (see Fig. 7.1). When the agitation ceases, the material becomes fluid again. Suspensions which contain a high concentration of finely divided, deflocculated particles (of the order of 50% v/v) may exhibit dilatant flow. At rest, the particles settle and pack into a mass with a minimum volume. The relatively small quantity of liquid present is sufficient to fill the void volume and to lubricate the particles so that the suspension flows like a liquid at low shear rates. However, if we agitate the mass more vigorously, the bulk increases (or dilates) as the particles attempt to form an open packing and to move past each other. The void volume increases, and the liquid is now insufficient to fill the voids and drains away. The resistance to flow increases because the fluid can no longer completely lubricate the particles. Eventually, the suspension sets to form a firm paste. When shearing ceases, the grains reform the close-packed, minimum void bed. The liquid can now fill the voids and lubricate the particles, and so the consistency again becomes relatively low.

Examples of dilatant formulations include 50% suspensions of potassium silicate or fine starch powder in cold water and various materials at certain stages in the manufacture of paint, printing inks, and pharmaceutical suspensions.

The comments which relate to the definition of an apparent viscosity, the mathematical analysis of the curve, and the value of the full rheogram, as considered for pseudoplastic flow, apply equally to dilatant flow and shear thickening.

d. Pseudoplastic or dilatant flow with yield value Some materials provide evidence of a yield value, but—unlike the rheogram of a Bingham body—their rheograms are nonlinear at greater shear stresses. By analogy with pseudoplastic and dilatant materials, if the flow curve is concave to the shear stress axis, we designate the formulation as a pseudoplastic material with yield value. If the rheogram is convex to the axis, the material is dilatant with yield value.

e. Time effects in continuous shear: thixotropy, antithixotropy, and rheopexy If we stir many concentrated non-Newtonian dispersions, the systems become more mobile with time of stirring. Then, if left undisturbed, they reset to a semisolid consistency with a characteristic time lag for recovery. Freundlich (1935) coined the term "thixotropy" for this phenomenon, which may be defined as "an isothermal and comparatively slow recovery, on standing of a material, of a consistency lost through shearing" (Reiner and Scott Blair, 1967). It is important that the tempera-

ture does not change during the rheological determination, or we may obtain
a false positive result in our test for thixotropy.

Thixotropy proceeds from structural breakdown and reaggregation in
complex materials in which a loose network connects together the sample.
At rest or at very low shear rates, the three-dimensional structure provides the system with some rigidity and the material behaves as a gel. As
a viscometer stresses the sample, the structure begins to disrupt as the
points of contact break and the particles start to align. The material com-
mences flowing, and its consistency decreases progressively with time as
the shear stress and shear rate increase. The substance thus transforms
from a gel to a sol. When we decrease or remove the applied stress, the
internal structure starts to reform but with a time lag, as the particles
which build the network need a period in which to contact each other. The
shapes of rheograms which we obtain for thixotropic materials therefore
depend very much on the rate at which we alter the shear conditions and
the time during which we subject the sample to each shear rate. In addition, the flow curve depends on the previous shear history of the sample,
including the way in which we load it into our viscometer.

Probably the most convenient way in which we can assess thixotropy
is to produce a hysteresis loop in the rheogram of a sample (Green, 1949).
Using a rotational viscometer, preferably in conjunction with an X-Y
plotter, we increase steadily the shear rate or shear stress to obtain readings for the "up curve." At some preset maximum value of the controlled
variable (usually at a designated shear rate achieved after a set sweep
time), we decrease the shear rate steadily to obtain the "down curve."
The up curve coincides with the down curve for a material without thixotropy. For a thixotropic material the two curves form a hysteresis loop,
the area of which measures the extent of thixotropy in the body under the
conditions of the test. This simple assessment of thixotropy is usually
adequate as a means of monitoring structural breakdown in topical vehicles
under shear, although we may also use analytical expressions (Green and
Weltmann, 1943, 1944, 1946a,b; Weltmann, 1943; Green, 1949; Zettlemoyer et al., 1953; Martin et al. 1964).

Thixotropy may be superimposed on a plastic (Bingham) body such as
a bentonite suspension or soft petrolatum, or on a pseudoplastic material
such as a dispersion of a synthetic suspending agent.

We may define antithixotropy as "a comparatively slow fall, on standing
of the sample, of a consistency that was gained as a result of shearing"
(Reiner and Scott Blair, 1967). Antithixotropy arises, therefore, from a
combination of dilatancy with thixotropy; it is a property of some quick-
sands. Figure 7.2 provides diagrams which illustrate such complex flow
properties.

Occasionally, we can accelerate the resolidification of a thixotropic
sol by gentle, regular movements which bring the particles into contact

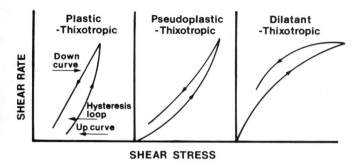

FIG. 7.2 Rheograms depicting various types of thixotropic behavior. The "up curve" denotes the shear stress/shear rate relationship we obtain with increasing shear; the "down curve" represents values we derive by subsequently decreasing the shear.

once more though the energy imparted to the system is insufficient to cause shear thinning. This phenomenon is known as rheopexy (Reiner and Scott Blair, 1967).

f. Further complexities in continuous shear: spurs, turning points and irreversible shear breakdown So far, we have dealt with somewhat idealized types of flow. However, various complications may arise when we attempt to determine the properties of dermatological formulations under continuous shear conditions. An exhaustive treatment of such intricacies is outside the scope of this chapter. However, we can deal with some of the main features if we consider the continuous shear rheometry of two types of formulations that we use widely in dermatology—oil-in-water creams (and the ternary systems which stabilize them and control their consistencies), and soft paraffins and their ointment formulations (Barry, 1974).

Barry and Shotton (1967a) investigated the structure and rheology of a ternary system composed of the mixed emulsifier sodium dodecyl sulfate/cetyl alcohol dispersed in water. They used a Ferranti-Shirley cone and plate viscometer with automatic control and an X-Y plotter (McKennell, 1954, 1956, 1960; Van Wazer et al., 1963). Such a preparation, and the emulsions and creams which we form by adding an "oil" phase such as liquid paraffin, may range in consistency from fluid to gel-like as the mixed emulsifier concentration increases. If we subject the material to a constant shear rate, the shear stress decreases with the time of shearing and we may not reach an equilibrium state even after 30-min treatment. The formulations thus exhibit shear-dependent and time-dependent behavior. If we employ the viscometer in automatic mode, we can display the rheogram in the form of a hysteresis loop (Fig. 7.3).

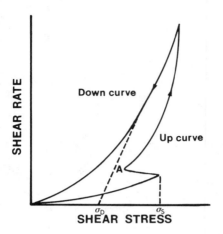

FIG. 7.3 Typical hysteresis rheogram for a semisolid dermatological formulation obtained using an automatic viscometer: σ_D is the dynamic yield value; σ_S is the static yield value; and A is a turning point on the up curve. (From Barry, 1974.)

In general terms, as discussed previously, the hysteresis loop indicates the extent of structural breakdown which takes place during the shearing cycle; a planimeter can measure the loop area. However, an additional, characteristic feature of the rheograms of many topical semisolids is that they form spur points on the up curve. Many investigators have reported spurs and bulges for such diverse systems as colloidal dispersions of graphite (McKennell, 1954), sodium carboxymethylcellulose solutions (De Butts et al., 1957), oil-in-water emulsions (Axon, 1954; Talman et al., 1967, 1968; Talman and Rowan, 1970; Barry and Saunders, 1970a, 1971a, 1972a; Barry and Eccleston, 1973a), procaine penicillin G depot injections (Ober et al., 1958), ointments (Boylan, 1966, 1967), soft paraffins (Davis, 1969a; Barry and Grace, 1970, 1971a,b), fatty alcohol/propylene glycol (FAPG) base (Barry, 1973), and Plastibases (Davis and Khanderia, 1980a). When such bulges and spurs are not experimental artifacts, they form from the same mechanisms which provide yield values for plastic materials, i.e., they indicate the presence of network gel structures. By analogy with traditional yield values, we can accept the spur point as a measure of the strength of a system in which some of the three-dimensional structure must break down before the material can flow significantly. The shear stress at the spur point provides the static yield value, σ_S. This value is an approximation as a strict definition implies that we should determine static yield values only at zero shear rate. Additionally, although investigators often define σ_S as the minimum shear stress required to initiate flow, for topical vehicles this concept is also an approximation, as the value obtained is not independent of the time taken to determine it. Apart from the general axiom of rheology that probably all substances flow under finite stresses provided that the time scale of observation is long enough, viscoelastic measurements indicate that topical vehicles flow however small the applied stress, although the shear rate may be almost zero (Sec. II.B).

After the spur point on the up curve, the rheogram often displays a turning point (A in Fig. 7.3). Some investigators consider that this turning point is an instrumental artifact rather than a property of the material (Enneking, 1958; Levy, 1962). Although this concept may be valid when plug flow occurs in concentric cylinder viscometers, it is not relevant to the cone/plate geometry. Provided that the sample does not fracture within the gap to form slippage planes, at small gap angles the shear rate is essentially uniform throughout the gap and plug flow does not occur (Davis et al., 1968b). In addition, both the spur point and its associated turning point often disappear when we recycle the same sample in the viscometer (Fig. 7.4). This behavior illustrates that both these aspects of the rheogram involve material characteristics.

If we extrapolate the linear portion of the down curve to meet the shear stress axis, the intercept provides a dynamic yield value, σ_D. This yield value is a measure of the energy required to maintain a constant ratio of shear stress to shear rate after some structure has broken down during the up curve cycle. We can increase the time of shear or the shear rate until this dynamic yield value reaches a maximum. According to Martin

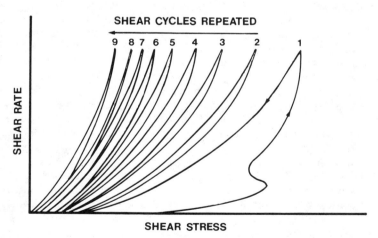

FIG. 7.4 A series of nine rheograms derived on a single sample by using an automatic viscometer to distinguish between thixotropy and irreversible shear breakdown. (From Barry and Shotton, 1967a.)

et al. (1964), this maximum represents the energy needed to disrupt all
the weak, secondary bonds which hold particles together; the dispersed
units then exist solely as primary particles. We may use the magnitude of
the dynamic yield value to predict if a dermatological vehicle will maintain
sufficient semisolid behavior when used under shear, for example, as a
levigating agent (Barry, 1973). For a vehicle which does not recover its
structure after shearing ceases, we should use the dynamic yield stress,
not the static yield value, to assess the consistency of the layer of material
which remains on the skin after application. For systems which do not
produce a hysteresis loop, the ascending and descending curves coincide
so that the static and dynamic yield values are identical.

Figure 7.3 suggests that the material is thixotropic. However, one
should always distinguish between thixotropy and irreversible shear breakdown (or irreversible work softening). In the latter process, any structure
which disrupts under shear, such as during the up curve of the rheogram
cycle, does not reform on standing. In general, few investigators have
specifically studied the phenomenon of irreversible shear breakdown.
Probably this neglect stems from the fact that investigators have not recog-
nized this rheological behavior, or they have confused it with thixotropy,
or workers have simply ignored the property on the basis that it poses an
intractable experimental problem (Scott Blair, 1949; Van Wazer et al.,
1963). To discriminate between thixotropy and irreversible shear breakdown, we test to confirm if the disrupted structure reforms at rest. For
example, Fig. 7.4 illustrates the results of an experiment which produces
a flow curve and then repeats the cycle with the same sample in the viscometer (Barry and Shotton, 1967a). The study generates a series of nine
hysteresis loops after various periods of resting. The characteristic spur
develops only during the initial run. Subsequent rheograms shift towards
the shear rate axis, with the displacement increasing in the order in which
rheograms develop. Loop areas decrease in sequence; the most dramatic
reduction is between the first and the second sweeps. This observation
implies that the majority of the labile structure disrupts during the first
shear cycle. We may therefore conclude that the network structure rebuilds
to a negligible extent under zero flow conditions and that because breakdown
is irreversible the formulation does not display true thixotropy within the
time scale of the experiment.

However, this apparently simple test to confirm thixotropy is not
always conclusive. For materials such as creams and gels which contain
volatile solvents like water and ethanol and for which disconnected structure
may rebuild only slowly, the original flow curve may never reform. This
may be because evaporation at the free surface of the cone-plate gap alters
the consistency of the product during the extended period required for
testing.

We conclude that for most multiphase topical semisolids, pure thixotropy is relatively rare. The usual rheological behavior is a combination
of thixotropy and irreversible shear breakdown.

When workers investigate a rheological problem using a continuous shear method of analysis, they should derive the complete rheogram. To examine the effect of a change in a variable such as temperature or the concentration of an ingredient, it is convenient for us also to plot some parameter derived from the hysteresis loop as a function of the variable. The three parameters we most commonly derive are the loop area, the yield stress (dynamic, static, or both), and the apparent viscosity calculated at some specific point on the rheogram, often at the loop apex. Barry (1974) provides some examples of this procedure using the hysteresis loop method of analysis for topical semisolids.

3. Instrumentation for continuous shear rheometry

a. General instruments The literature describes a wide variety of instruments to measure the consistency of materials. Many of these devices are empirical in that they cannot provide rheological data in the form of stress, strain, and time because we cannot mathematically analyze the geometry of flow which the viscometers impose on the sample. Typical instruments in this category are rotational viscometers with bobs and cups of unusual design, instruments which draw a plate across the material under test, and devices which drop an object onto the sample or squeeze it from a tube. Such contraptions provide empirical data only, and we will not consider them here.

We may classify viscometers either as single-point or multipoint instruments. A single-point apparatus such as a simple capillary viscometer provides only one point on the flow curve, and we therefore use it only for known Newtonian fluids such as simple liquids and solutions. Multipoint instruments provide a range of shear stress/shear rate data for us to plot the full rheogram.

This chapter is not the place for us to consider the various designs, test procedures, and calculations relevant to continuous shear viscometers. Besides the brochures of the various instrument makers, the reader may find information in the texts of Ferry (1970), Van Wazer et al. (1963), Martin et al. (1964), and Sherman (1970). However, it is valuable to consider briefly in a general way the applications and the limitations of the four principal categories of commercially available viscometers: capillary; rolling or falling sphere; coaxial cyclinder; and cone and plate.

Of the various glass capillary viscometers, the Oswald and the Ubbelohde U-tube instruments are suitable for Newtonian viscosity measurements, whereas the Cannon-Fenske, when fitted with an external pressure source, will determine non-Newtonian viscosities. In the variable pressure class, the Instron Rheometer can apply a wide range of shear rates and shear stresses and can measure Newtonian and non-Newtonian viscosities. The Techne Printing Viscometer is suitable for Newtonian liquids, while the Bingham Viscometer is particularly appropriate for high shear studies. By their very nature, however, capillary instruments as a class are not suited to the examination of the many semisolid preparations used in dermatology.

The Hoeppler Viscometer measures the time taken for a steel ball to roll through the sample contained in a glass tube. However, with this method it is difficult to define the shear rate and the shear stress, and therefore the instrument is suitable only for Newtonian liquids. Other rising and falling sphere viscometers suffer from similar disadvantages.

In rotating viscometers, two members enclose the material under test and one member rotates relative to the other about a common axis of symmetry. We use the relationship between the relative angular velocity of the elements and the torque to characterize the flow behavior of the test sample. Typical concentric cylinder instruments include the Stormer, the Haake Rotovisko, the Epprecht Rheomat, and the Portable Ferranti. A relatively new instrument, the Deer Variable Stress Rheometer, can handle both continuous shear and viscoelastic (creep) experiments. As a class, concentric cylinder viscometers can suffer from end effects and from variable shear stresses across the gap between the two cylinders. For plastic materials, the shear stress may be lower than the yield value for a certain distance across the gap but may exceed the yield point for the material in the remainder of the gap. Some of the sample then flows, but the remainder remains stationary. This phenomenon of plug flow, as it is known, can provide quite misleading results when we examine the rheology of a plastic semisolid in a coaxial cylinder viscometer.

Cone-plate viscometers, such as the Ferranti-Shirley, the Weissenberg Rheogoniometer, the Haake Rotovisko, and the Deer Variable Stress Rheometer, shear the test sample between a small-angled cone and a flat plate. These instruments possess the major advantage that, provided the cone angle is small (less than 4°), the shear rate is essentially uniform throughout the sample and plug flow should not present a problem. Both the Weissenberg and the Deer can measure viscoelastic parameters.

Of the various geometries, cone and plate instruments provide the most suitable arrangement for examining the continuous shear rheology of dermatological semisolids. The Ferranti-Shirley is one of the best instruments on the market, and basic research programs have used it to examine topical vehicles. It is therefore worthwhile for us to consider in a little more detail both the advantages and disadvantages of this particular instrument, as such an examination highlights some more of the problems which face an investigator in this field (Barry, 1974).

b. Advantages of the Ferranti-Shirley cone and plate viscometer This viscometer imposes a uniform rate of shear throughout the cone-plate gap, as the angles for the various cones are all less than 4°. For other commercial viscometers, this uniformity may not hold and plug flow may be a serious problem. The instrument comes with a selection of cones of different angles and radii, torque springs, and gear settings. Thus, wide ranges of shear stress and shear rate are available, and we can calculate explicitly those rheological parameters from the geometry of the flow region. The apparatus is convenient and simple to clean, to fill, and to operate. It requires only small sample sizes, of approximately 1 ml, which is an advantage when we deal with expensive substances or for those in short supply, e.g., biological materials, experimental samples, or small tubes of dermatologicals. Because the cone-plate gap holds only a thin layer of material, the sample temperature equilibrates rapidly with excellent temperature control. There are no end effects, and edge effects at the free surface of the sample are negligible. To examine materials which may show time effects such as thixotropy and irreversible shear breakdown, facilities are available which automate the shear cycle.

c. Limitations of the Ferranti-Shirley cone and plate viscometer All continuous shear viscometers possess limitations, and the Ferranti-Shirley is no exception. One of the most important restrictions of any continuous shear method when we apply it to a semisolid is that it does not yield fundamental rheological parameters. Thus, apparent viscosities, yield values, hysteresis loop areas, etc., depend in part on operating variables, and instrumental effects contribute to their magnitudes.

Cone and plate viscometers have a narrow clearance between the rotating members, and the Ferranti-Shirley will not readily measure suspensions of particles greater than about 30 μm. With coarser dispersions, cone-plate viscometers may function like a colloid mill rather than a rheometer! There is no clutch arrangement to allow rapid start and stop at a set shear rate.

The very versatility of the instrument can lead to problems. In automatic mode, different combinations of sweep times and maximum shear rates alter the rheogram shape and interlaboratory comparisons may be difficult (Davis et al., 1968b). Material may not adhere to the viscometer elements but may slip at the cone or plate surfaces, causing artifacts in the rheogram (Jefferies, 1965; Boylan, 1967). To minimize these errors, we can use long sweep times, particularly with the larger cones.

During shear, the test material may fracture within the gap, decreasing the recorded torque. The fracture may then heal, and we may wrongly interpret the rheological behavior as thixotropic (Hutton, 1963). Cavitation or tensile failure may intervene, particularly with samples which possess a high elastic component (Hutton, 1963; Lammiman and Roberts, 1961). Stiggles (1965) has observed this behavior optically, and Lenk (1965) has determined the minimum shear rate at which the substance fractures and then avoids the region of spurious effects.

A common source of trouble in cone-plate viscometry is that the instrument may eject material from the gap. For example, some batches of soft paraffin (petrolatum) provide very irregular rheograms when tested in automatic mode. The viscometer almost completely expels the sample from the gap after the spur point so that the measured torque falls to almost zero (Barry and Grace, 1970). As a general rule, whenever continuous shear rheograms become markedly irregular, we should treat the data with suspicion because of the likelihood of instrumental artifacts. Sometimes one can see material exuding from the gap, but at other times we may be unaware of slippage, shear fracture, and sample expulsion, which can even occur in a reproducible fashion. Thus, congruent repeat rheograms do not provide absolute proof for a "correct" rheogram.

The sample temperature may increase at extreme shear rates because of viscous heating (McKennell, 1956), although in general the Ferranti-Shirley provides excellent thermal control. If the sample does warm up with shearing, hysteresis loops may form under cyclic conditions, even with time-independent materials. Cheng (1965) recommends that to minimize the heating effect we should reduce the time of shearing as much as possible. However, with the larger cones, diminished sweep times may generate a flywheel inertial effect, even for Newtonian liquids (Cheng, 1967). The hysteresis loop develops clockwise, with the down curve lying closer to the stress axis than does the up curve. It is therefore advisable to use sweep times as long as possible when we have to employ large cones to generate sufficient torque. However, we may have to compromise for experiments with volatile samples at raised temperatures. Evaporation at the free surface of the material may produce serious artifacts in the rheogram, even when we use an antievaporation unit (Davis et al., 1968).

During the up and down sweeps of the cone, the acceleration may vary (Barry and Shotton, 1968). For viscoelastic materials with suspended particles, the consistency may fall as particles migrate to the periphery of the cone (Highgate, 1966; Highgate and Whorlow, 1968). Cheng (1968) considered the problem of secondary flow in the cone-plate geometry.

Cones may not be machined truly conical (Cheng and Davis, 1968), although in practice minor deviations are insignificant in the examination of semisolids.

Finally, the process of loading the viscometer inevitably disturbs to some degree the sample structure, and any damaged structure may not have time to reform before a test begins.

d. The role of continuous shear viscometers for examining semisolids When we consider the types of difficulties involved in using a continuous shear viscometer, even one as good as the Ferranti-Shirley, a significant conclusion is forced on us. This is that the interpretation of the data may be seriously in error even though continuous shear experiments are easy to perform and deceptively simple to analyze. We may make a wrong inference, partly because of the instrumental limitations considered previously. However, more fundamentally, the difficulty is that continuous shear methods, when applied to semisolids, monitor the complex phenomenon of structure breakdown and reformation. The rate and magnitude of such dynamic processes depend on the protocol of testing, which does not directly determine true material constants, such as viscosity and elasticity.

Therefore, the benefits of continuous shear methods for examining semisolids are somewhat limited. However, they can be valuable in several situations. Such determinations may predict the performance of the semisolid under the high shear rate conditions met with in manufacture and in use, including application to the skin. We can use the technique to screen rapidly many materials in formulation work. We can partly assess rheological properties and thus impose some quality control specifications on dermatological ingredients such as soft paraffin and the preparations made from them, e.g., creams, ointments and pastes. We may also control unit processes such as mixing, milling, pumping, and filling of semisolids into containers. We can investigate rheological variations within a closely related series of preparations and can evaluate semiquantitative measurements of rheological structure. Finally, we may be able to correlate our results with more fundamental methods of analysis.

Indeed, it is these fundamental methods of analysis which promise a deeper insight into the nature and the behavior of a semisolid. The basic approach may also confirm if instrumental artifacts so dominate a continuous shear method that they obscure the analysis. Fundamental methods should aim to examine the semisolid in its rheological ground state. In such a condition, tests begin with a relaxed specimen which possesses no internal stresses or strains arising from its past history. The rheometer flexes any organized structure, such as gel networks or floccules and aggregates in emulsions and suspensions, without disrupting the infrastructure. The tests are rheologically nondestructive in the sense that, at completion, the sample is unchanged and is identical in all respects to the original material. The method of analysis conforms with linear viscoelastic theory (Alfrey and Gurnee, 1956; Ferry, 1958, 1970; Leaderman, 1958).

B. Viscoelastic Analysis of Semisolids

1. The nature of viscoelastic deformation

If we wished to investigate the mechanical properties of an elastic solid, we could apply the classical theory of elasticity even though we realize that real solids deviate from Hooke's law. Similarly, for a viscous liquid we could use hydrodynamic theory with the knowledge that any real liquid, if measured sufficiently precisely, would deviate slightly from absolute Newtonian behavior. Such deviations are of two types. In the first category, stress deviations occur when the strain rate in a liquid or the strain in a solid is not directly proportional to the stress magnitude but depends on the stress in a more complicated fashion. Secondly, time anomalies are those for which the stress is a function of both the strain and the strain rate. Then the rheological properties have both liquid and solid aspects and the substance is a viscoelastic material. All dermatological semisolids show this degree of rheological complexity. Stress and time anomalies may coexist in a material, and the rheological analysis may be very complicated and even intractable. However, if only time anomalies are present, the material is linearly viscoelastic. Often a semisolid behaves as a linear viscoelastic material provided that the strain remains small; we therefore design viscoelastic rheometers with this criterion in mind. Under such experimental conditions, for a linear viscoelastic material the ratio of stress to strain is independent of the stress magnitude and is a function of time alone. In linear viscoelastic materials, therefore, elastic effects obey Hooke's law and viscous effects are Newtonian, at least at small strains.

We may classify topical vehicles either as viscoelastic liquids or as viscoelastic solids. When we examine such materials with the fundamental viscoelastic technique, the creep test, viscoelastic liquids eventually flow steadily (their deformation increases linearly with time). In contrast, viscoelastic solids approach an equilibrium deformation or zero strain rate. Topical semisolids in general belong to the subsection of viscoelastic liquids.

2. Linear viscoelastic behavior as represented by mechanical models

For a linear viscoelastic material, we can deduce a "rheological equation of state" or a "constitutive equation" which defines the relationship between stress, strain, and time. However, for the nonmathematician it is helpful in comprehending viscoelastic behavior if we duplicate the flow properties of the experimental material by imagining, or even constructing, a model made from a combination of Hookean springs and Newtonian dashpots (Kuhn, 1947; Alfrey, 1948).

If we combine a Newtonian dashpot in series or in parallel with an elastic spring, the composites formed are the simplest mechanical models which are analogs of viscoelastic materials. Figure 7.5 illustrates the two types which we use to represent viscoelastic behavior. In these, a force applied to the model terminals represents a shear stress, the relative displacement of the terminals is analogous to the shear strain, and the rate of displacement represents the rate of shear. Throughout model deformation, the system must not distort so that all parallel lines remain so. Each dashpot possesses a frictional resistance, defined as the ratio of force to velocity, which is analogous to a coefficient of viscosity, and we assign to each spring a stiffness (force/displacement) which is analogous to a shear modulus.

a. The Maxwell model This mechanical model combines a dashpot containing a purely viscous liquid of viscosity, η, in series with a purely elastic spring of shear modulus, G (Fig. 7.5). The material which it represents, when stressed, will respond elastically to give an approximately instantaneous response because of the deformation of the spring,

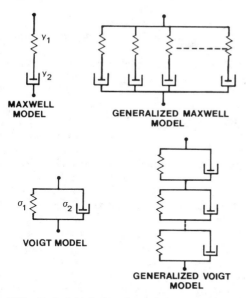

FIG. 7.5 Mechanical models consisting of springs and dashpots which we may use to represent viscoelastic behavior.

yet the substance also exhibits viscous flow as the dashpot moves. As the model elements link together as in a chain, under any external force the stresses in the spring and in the dashpot are equal. However, the total strain or deformation is the addition of the strains experienced by the dashpot and the spring. Thus,

$$\gamma = \gamma_1 + \gamma_2 \tag{7.14}$$

where γ_1 is the elastic strain; γ_2 is the viscous strain; and γ is the total strain.

When we apply a shear stress, σ, to the model, the spring extends instantaneously and, according to Hooke's law,

$$\gamma_1 = \frac{\sigma}{G} = J\sigma \tag{7.15}$$

where J, the elastic compliance, is defined as the reciprocal of G. Note that G is not a relaxation modulus as defined only in the particular time pattern used in stress relaxation experiments (Ferry, 1970). Applying Newton's law—Eq. (7.1)—to Eq. (7.14) and emphasizing that stresses and strains are functions of time, we obtain

$$\dot{\gamma}(t) = \dot{\gamma}_1(t) + \dot{\gamma}_2(t) = \frac{\dot{\sigma}(t)}{G} + \frac{\sigma(t)}{\eta} \tag{7.16}$$

If we apply a constant shear stress to the Maxwell model, then $\sigma(t) = 0$, Eq. (7.16) reduces to Newton's law, and the model simplifies to a Newtonian dashpot.

The ratio of shear viscosity to shear modulus, which has the dimensions of time, is known as the relaxation time

$$\tau = \frac{\eta}{G} = \eta J \tag{7.17}$$

In a stress relaxation test, we constrain the specimen at a fixed deformation and measure the stress required to maintain this deformation as it decreases or relaxes with time. The Maxwell model is particularly useful for representing this behavior, if we imagine that we suddenly pull out the terminals of the model to a fixed extension. The force required to hold this deformation decreases with time as the motion of the dashpot allows the spring to relax. The relaxation time is the time taken for the stress to relax to $1/e$ of its initial value when we hold the strain constant (e is the natural number).

Mechanical models mimic the properties of real materials. It is unlikely that we could represent such complex preparations as topical semi-solids by a single relaxation time involving a lone coefficient of viscosity and one elastic compliance. However, we can combine in parallel as many Maxwell elements as we require, each with its own relaxation time, to form the generalized Maxwell model. For most purposes a combination of a relatively few parallel elements, providing a discrete spectrum of relaxation times, will simulate a real material. Alternatively, we can extend the analogy to an infinite number of elements and so arrive at a continuous spectrum of relaxation times.

b. The Voigt or Kelvin model If we combine a spring and a dashpot in parallel (see Fig. 7.5) we can represent a material in which the response to an external force does not occur instantaneously but a viscous resistance retards the movement. Under such an external force, the strains in the spring and in the dashpot are equal (γ) but the total stress, σ, is the sum of that in the spring, σ_1, and that in the dashpot, σ_2:

$$\sigma = \sigma_1 + \sigma_2 \tag{7.18}$$

As for the Maxwell model, by Newton's and Hooke's laws, the differential equation which relates stress, strain, and time is

$$\sigma(t) = G\gamma(t) + \eta\dot{\gamma}(t) \tag{7.19}$$

For a constant strain, the strain rate $\dot{\gamma}(t) = 0$ and the Voigt model reduces to an uncoupled spring.

The parameter $\tau = \eta/G$ is the retardation time; it represents the time required for the strain to relax to $1/e$ of its starting value when we suddenly reduce the stress to zero. The retardation time will be long, that is, the strain recovers slowly, if η (which characterizes the "internal friction" of the material) is large compared to the rigidity modulus, G. If the internal friction is negligible measured against the rigidity, then the strain recovers rapidly and the retardation time is short. The viscosity associated with a Voigt body is sometimes called the internal viscosity because it relates to the internal friction which delays, although it does not prevent, the complete recovery of a strained material which is essentially a solid (Alfrey and Gurnee, 1956).

To generalize the Voigt model so that it can represent real, complex semisolids, we construct a model by combining a set of Voigt elements in series, each with a different retardation time. If we apply a constant shear stress to this model, then to obtain the total strain, which is time dependent, we add together the strains for each constituent element.

The generalized Voigt model represents a viscoelastic solid because it does not sustain unlimited, nonrecoverable viscous flow. However, if in one of the Voigt elements we omit a spring (or allocate a zero modulus), the element degenerates to a simple dashpot which does provide unlimited flow under constant stress. A Voigt model which contains such a degenerate element (an uncoupled dashpot) corresponds to a viscoelastic liquid. The companion degenerate Voigt element is an unretarded spring, i.e., an element with a zero viscosity dashpot. If we include such an element in our model, we have allowed for a certain amount of instantaneous elastic behavior within the material. If we combine both degenerate elements with a generalized Voigt model, it is equivalent to our adding a Maxwell element to the model.

One of the simplest, most important, and most widely used experiments for studying the viscoelastic behavior of topical semisolids is the creep test. In creep analysis, we impose a stress on a sample at zero time and maintain its constant. The response of the sample in terms of its development of strain with time provides the data for a viscoelastic analysis. We can derive the shear behavior which follows the application of such a constant stress to a generalized model containing a finite number of Voigt elements and a Maxwell element as follows (Warburton and Barry, 1968). For the Voigt elements, let each retardation time, τ_i, be associated with a shear modulus, G_i, and a shear or Newtonian viscosity, η_i. Let σ be the constant shear stress. At a time, t, after the onset of the stress, the stress in the ith element σ_i equals σ and the strain in this element is γ_i. By substituting the parameters for this element into Eq. (7.19) we have

$$\sigma_i = \gamma_i G_i + \frac{d\gamma_i}{dt} \eta_i \qquad (7.20)$$

Rearranging Eq. (7.20)

$$\frac{d\gamma_i}{\sigma_i - \gamma_i G_i} = \frac{1}{\eta_i} dt \qquad (7.21)$$

Defining the retardation time for the ith element as $\tau_i = \eta_i/G_i = \eta_i J_i$, Eq. (7.21) becomes

$$\frac{d\gamma_i}{(\sigma_i/G_i) - \gamma_i} = \frac{dt}{\tau_i} \tag{7.22}$$

On integration without limits

$$-\ln\left(\frac{\sigma_i}{G_i} - \gamma_i\right) = \frac{t}{\tau_i} + k_1 \tag{7.23}$$

At the beginning of the test, $t = 0$, $\gamma_i = 0$; therefore $k_1 = -\ln(\sigma_i J_i)$ and

$$\ln\left(\frac{\sigma_i J_i - \gamma_i}{\sigma_i J_i}\right) = -\frac{t}{\tau_i} \tag{7.24}$$

Thus, the strain in the ith element is

$$\gamma_i = \sigma_i J_i \left[1 - \exp\left(-\frac{t}{\tau_i}\right)\right] \tag{7.25}$$

and the compliance is

$$J_i(t) = J_i \left[1 - \exp\left(-\frac{t}{\tau_i}\right)\right] \tag{7.26}$$

The total strain in the generalized Voigt model is the sum of the strains in the individual elements. Thus, compliances in series are also additive, and for n Voigt elements in series we can write

$$J(t) = \sum_{i=1}^{n} J_i \left[1 - \exp\left(-\frac{t}{\tau_i}\right)\right] \tag{7.27}$$

The model represented by Eq. (7.27) simulates a viscoelastic solid. To represent real, viscoelastic liquids we may extend the equation to include the limiting conditions, τ_i equals zero and infinity. For zero retardation time one of the Voigt elements simplifies to an elastic spring with its modulus represented by G_0 and its compliance defined as J_0. This element corresponds to the instantaneous elastic response of the substance. To allow for unlimited Newtonian flow, a second Voigt element reduces to a viscous dashpot of compliance $J_N(t)$. Applying Newton's law to this element

$$\sigma = \eta_0 \frac{d\gamma_N}{dt} \tag{7.28}$$

where $d\gamma_N/dt$ is the rate of viscous strain of the uncoupled dashpot. Integrating

$$\gamma_N = \frac{\sigma t}{\eta_0} + k_2; \quad \text{when } t = 0, \ \gamma_N = 0, \ k_2 = 0$$

Then

$$J_N(t) = \frac{t}{\eta_0} \tag{7.29}$$

Finally, for a real viscoelastic liquid, which most dermatological semi-solids are, we reach

$$J(t) = J_0 + \sum_{i=1}^{n} J_i \left[1 - \exp\left(-\frac{t}{\tau_i}\right) \right] + \frac{t}{\eta_0} \tag{7.30}$$

where $J(t)$ represents the overall creep compliance in the test; J_0 is the instantaneous elastic compliance; the middle term on the right-hand side of the equation provides the contribution from the Voigt elements; and the last term represents unretarded viscous flow.

3. The Boltzmann superposition principle

The Voigt and Maxwell models illustrate one of the necessary characteristics of a linear viscoelastic material, which is that the rheological behavior must satisfy the Boltzmann superposition principle (see Leaderman, 1943; Ferry, 1970). In essence, the principle is that, if we subject our material to a series of known stresses, the net effect on the strain must be the aggregate of the effects of each of the individual stresses. We can express this in a more formal way: "The value of a characteristic function of a system is equal to the sum of all changes induced in the system by the driving functions which have been applied to it throughout its past history" (Van Wazer et al., 1963). In a particular experiment, for a material which disobeys the Boltzmann principle, we may not analyze the test on the basis of linear viscoelastic theory.

4. Experimental methods for viscoelastic analysis

In recent years, investigators have employed two main techniques to determine the viscoelastic properties of dermatological formulations — creep testing and oscillatory testing. These procedures will be discussed in this section, together with mathematical methods that are useful for transforming creep data into oscillatory parameters, and vice versa.

a. The creep test We can use two main geometries in creep to examine the properties of pharmaceutical semisolids: the cone and plate arrangement or the concentric cylinder arrangement. With the cone-plate geometry, because of the relatively low consistency of many pharmaceutical products, it can be difficult experimentally to remain in the linear region of strain throughout the time scale of the experiment. As the shear stress is inversely proportional to the cube of the radius, we might decrease the value of the shear stress for a set applied torque by increasing the radii of the cone and the plate. However, the edge gap might then become so wide that more mobile material would flow out. We could decrease the cone angle to compensate for this effect, but then we would reduce the angular movement allowed for any particular strain, as the strain is inversely proportional to the cone angle. This restriction on angular movement can lead to difficulties in measurement. The evaporation of volatile solvents, such as water, from hydrophilic preparations like creams and gels compounds the experimental difficulties. We can overcome these obstacles if we use the concentric cylinder geometry to solve the problems of the evaporation of water and the requirements of a low applied shear stress. There is a limited surface available from which water can evaporate, yet a large area ensures that the applied torque produces a low shear stress.

Because of the low stresses which we must use with typical dermatological formulations designed to spread easily, it is important that the rheometer should be as frictionless as possible. Static or moving friction forces, of a magnitude which may be negligible in a continuous shear viscometer, could easily be similar to the applied torque in a creep viscometer. Thus, for topical semisolids, simple adaptations of commercial coaxial cylinder viscometers so as to form creep viscometers are not satisfactory (Sherman, 1968, 1970). Purpose-designed instruments use air bearings to provide near frictionless supports, either compressed air or an induction motor to apply the torque, and noncontact transducers to measure the strain. Warburton and Barry (1968) designed a simple, inexpensive creep viscometer which has been further improved (Davis et al., 1968a; Davis, 1969b; Barry and Saunders, 1969; Barry and Grace, 1970; Barry, 1971, 1974). A commercially available instrument developed from this is the Deer Variable Stress Rheometer, which provides cone and plate, parallel plate, and concentric cylinder geometries; we may also use it as a continuous shear viscometer.

To obtain accurate results from creep tests with dermatological formulations, it is advisable to adopt a standardized procedure (Barry, 1974). In essence, however, the technique is simple: we apply a constant stress, record the strain as a function of time, and obtain the recovery curve when we remove the stress. We normally analyze the data in the form of a compliance curve, i.e., the strain divided by the stress, so that we produce the same curve regardless of the magnitude of the applied stress, provided that linear viscoelastic conditions prevail.

We may interpret creep curves in their raw form, we may derive continuous or discrete spectra of retardation times, or we may transform the curves mathematically to provide dynamic data. This last procedure allows us to predict how the material would behave in an oscillatory test, without actually vibrating the sample.

b. Creep analysis

Discrete Spectral Analysis. We can analyze creep curves graphically (Inokuchi, 1955; Warburton and Barry, 1968; Sherman, 1968, 1970; Barry, 1974) or by using a computer (Davis and Warburton, 1968).

Figure 7.6 illustrates a creep and recovery curve typical of that which many topical semisolids yield. The inset mechanical model mimics the viscoelastic behavior. For many dermatological materials the model consists of a Maxwell unit in series with a few (often three) Voigt units. If we separate the Maxwell unit so that the spring and dashpot attach to each end of the model, the arrangement is convenient for discussion. For a fit requiring three Voigt units, we make n = 3 in Eq. (7.30).

Recall that $J(t)$ represents the total creep compliance at any time t. It is a monotonically nondecreasing function of time, and the shape and the magnitude of the creep compliance curve is fundamentally important in viscoelastic theory; we may relate other rheological parameters to this curve.

We obtain J_0, the residual or initial shear compliance, by dividing the instantaneous shear strain by the constant shear stress. In the mechanical model, the initial compliance is that of the residual spring which represents primary chemical bonds in our test material stretching elastically. Operationally, J_0 is often ill-defined but we take as an approximation the value of $J(t)$ at as short a time as the rheometer and its associated recorder

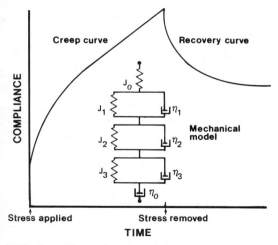

FIG. 7.6 Typical creep and recovery curves for a viscoelastic dermatological formulation. The mechanical model which simulates the rheological behavior consists of three Voigt units in series with a Maxwell unit.

will respond. The value thus depends in part on the swiftness with which we impose the constant stress and the inertia of the viscometer elements and the recording apparatus. To resolve in further detail molecular mechanisms which operate on a short time scale, dynamic methods are more suitable (see Sec. II.B.4.c).

In Fig. 7.6, J_1, J_2, and J_3, the shear compliances of Voigt units 1 to 3, represent the contributions of the retarded elastic region to the total compliance. The Voigt units symbolize those parts of the molecular and colloidal structure of the dermatological in which secondary bonds break and reform during the test. The retardation times are those which such processes require; and as bonds form and disrupt at different rates, a material exhibits a spectrum of retardation times. For the majority of dermatological semisolids, the method of discrete spectral analysis yields a finite line spectrum of between two and five Voigt elements. Of course, in a complex, multiphase system such as an oil-in-water cream, very many secondary bonds operate with different retardation times. A discrete spectral method groups these bonds into a few categories, by averaging similar retardation times. It is difficult to resolve individual retardation times if there are more than 10 and if the smallest spacing between any two adjacent times is less than five times greater than the smaller retardation time (Warburton and Barry, 1968).

The dashpot of the Maxwell element represents the residual or uncoupled viscosity, η_0. We obtain its value from the reciprocal of the slope of the creep curve after an extended period of testing, when the compliance is linear with time. From the start of this linear region, we have already applied the stress for a time sufficient to ensure that all the Voigt units have essentially fully extended, after which period further deformation is viscous and is nonrecoverable. Mathematically, a Voigt unit extends exponentially and therefore requires infinite time; see Eq. (7.30). However, for practical purposes we take the onset of the linear region to be the point at which further curvature becomes negligible. For dermatologicals, a useful rule of thumb is to run the creep experiment until one-third to one-half of the total curve is linear. A typical creep curve would require a total stress time of the order of 90 min.

A residual viscosity appears in nearly all pharmaceutical semisolids so far tested, implying that they are viscoelastic liquids. This unretarded viscosity means that the material cannot have a static yield value as strictly defined (see Sec. II.A.2). Any stress, however small, produces flow provided that the period of observation is long enough. This phenomenon emphasizes the approximate nature of much of the continuous shear rheology of semisolids: η_0 is usually very large, often reaching 10^{10} poise, and it is many orders of magnitude greater than the usual apparent viscosities which we determine in continuous shear.

The recovery curve, which is that part of the compliance curve developed after the removal of the shear stress, allows us to ensure that the

creep curve remained within the domain of linear viscoelasticity. Barry
(1974) has provided further details of this analysis.

After we have developed a creep curve for a topical semisolid, we
may use the data in several ways. We can simply consider the entire creep
curve, or segments or points taken from it at particular experimental times.
Alternatively, we can analyze the data in the form of line spectra and their
associated models. Some examples of these approaches will now be considered.

Figure 7.7 illustrates the creep curves that we obtain for three oil-in-
water creams stabilized by different mixed emulsifiers of a general class
used to formulate topical creams (Barry, 1970b). For all three preparations, the mechanical model consists of three Voigt units and one Maxwell
unit; thus the creep curves are similar in shape but differ in magnitude.

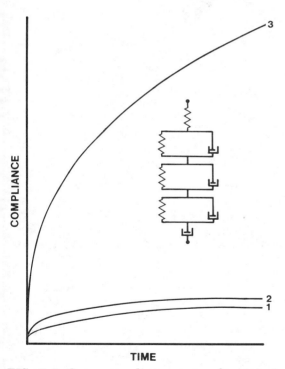

FIG. 7.7 Creep compliance curves for topical oil-in-water creams stabilized by different mixed emulsifier blends based on sodium dodecyl sulfate
and (1) cetyl alcohol, (2) cetostearyl alcohol, and (3) stearyl alcohol. The
mechanical model represents the rheological behavior of the formulations.
(From Barry, 1970b.)

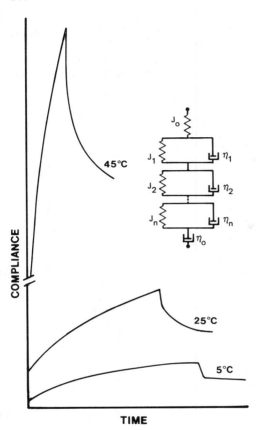

FIG. 7.8 Variation with temperature of creep compliance curves for white soft paraffin (petrolatum). The mechanical model represents the visco-elastic properties of the material. (From Barry and Grace, 1971b.)

The first curve is from an emulsion stabilized with the mixed emulsifier sodium dodecyl sulfate/cetyl alcohol. It is very similar in magnitude to curve 2 for which the stabilizer is sodium dodecyl sulfate/cetostearyl alcohol. However, curve 3 (sodium dodecyl sulfate/stearyl alcohol) differs markedly, as it has a much higher creep compliance. Such a rheological analysis assists us to deduce the nature of the viscoelastic networks which hold globules together in these self-bodied creams. For the cream with stearyl alcohol (curve 3) the network is weaker and more diffuse than the colloidal structures in the cetyl or cetostearyl alcohol creams.

Soft paraffin (petrolatum) is a common ingredient in ointments and creams, and pharmaceutical investigators have studied its rheological properties in some detail. Figure 7.8, taken from the work of Barry and Grace (1971b), illustrates how the creep behavior of a sample varies with temperature. At low-to-moderate temperatures (up to 25°C), the high-consistency material shows complex viscoelastic properties which require five Voigt units together with a Maxwell unit to simulate the creep compliance curve. If we warm the sample, some crystal-crystal and crystal-amorphous hydrocarbon bonds break and the material starts to melt. The compliance increases dramatically, and the model representation simplifies to three Voigt units and a Maxwell element.

Barry and Saunders (1970b, 1971b, 1972b) provide examples of the way in which increasing temperature modifies the viscoelastic behavior of creams containing mixed emulsifiers. Barry and Meyer (1979a) studied the effect of temperature and other variables on the creep behavior of Carbopol gels. To a first approximation, such gels behave as elastic solids.

Figure 7.8 illustrates the viscoelastic properties of one sample of soft paraffin. These materials are variable substances, however, and common quality control procedures do little to define their rheological properties (Barry and Grace, 1971b). Creep tests demonstrate how rheologically variable an official material can be. Figure 7.9 displays curves for five samples of white soft paraffin, all of which comply with pharmacopoeial standards, yet there is an almost eightfold variation between the curves (Barry and Grace, 1970). Figure 7.9 also demonstrates the accuracy with which we may analyze creep curves into mechanical models using Eq. (7.30). The data points were derived from a theoretical reconstitution of the creep curve using the model analysis, and they all lie on the original plots.

The creep technique, like viscoelastic methods in general, does not irreversibly disrupt colloidal network structures. We can therefore use creep experiments to investigate the kinetics of structure buildup in a semisolid without breaking the structure as it forms. A continuous shear

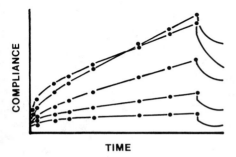

TIME

FIG. 7.9 Creep compliance curves for five samples of white soft paraffin (petrolatum) of pharmacopoeial grade. The points are data reconstituted from the creep test; see Eq. (7.30). (From Barry and Grace, 1970.)

method of analysis does not have this advantage. As an example of the use
of the creep method in kinetics, we can consider the effects of work softening and recovery on the rheological properties of soft paraffin (Barry and
Grace, 1971d). Typically, material may work soften during mixing, milling,
and pumping operations in the manufacturing process of an ointment or
during high shear viscometry. A patient may also work soften a topical
dermatological when rubbing it into the skin. Figure 7.10 illustrates that
soft paraffin possesses a high consistency in the unworked state but also
that the network structure readily fractures on working. Thus, the creep
compliance curve derived 0.5 hr after we apply a standardized working
procedure indicates the presence of a weaker structure. However, if soft
paraffins remain essentially undisturbed, they recover to some extent the
three-dimensional matrix responsible for their consistency. The way in
which the creep curves shift towards the unworked state as the material
ages reveals this structural recovery. The time scale for this process can
be quite long: the diagram makes clear that recovery is still not complete
even 10 days after the work softening process.

To provide an example of the use of discrete viscoelastic parameters,
we can turn to work performed on the self-bodying action of mixed emulsifiers in oil-in-water emulsions. A blend of sodium dodecyl sulfate with a
long-chain alcohol such as cetyl alcohol can both stabilize an emulsion and
also control its consistency between wide limits. The mixed emulsifier
forms a viscoelastic network in the continuous phase, and we can see the

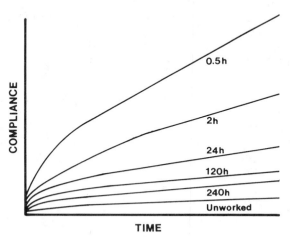

TIME

FIG. 7.10 Creep compliance curves which indicate structural rebuilding
in a sample of soft paraffin, worked and then allowed to recover. Numbers
on the curves refer to the time, in hours, since the work-softening process.
(From Barry and Grace, 1971c.)

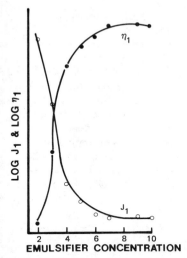

FIG. 7.11 Compliance (J_1) and viscosity (η_1) of the first Voigt unit as functions of mixed emulsifier concentration for liquid paraffin in water emulsions. (From Barry, 1968.)

way in which the network strengthens with increased concentration of the blend if we plot individual model parameters as functions of concentration. For example, Figure 7.11 provides such plots for the compliance and viscosity of the first Voigt unit, the element with the longest retardation time (Barry, 1968). The viscosity increases sharply as the concentration of mixed emulsifier increases, but the graph then levels off at 10% concentration. The compliance plot descends steeply at first and then forms a plateau. The initial dramatic changes in the compliance and viscosity plots reflect the extent of structure buildup in the aqueous phase of the emulsions. Semisolid creams form once networks are extensive enough to link globules together. Any further additions to this network have a less obvious effect on rheological properties, and the graphs flatten.

Continuous Spectral Analysis. We can manipulate a creep curve to produce a continuous retardation spectrum. Such a spectrum represents viscoelastic behavior in a more general way than the creep compliance, but the spectrum can be tedious to produce. In essence, we increase the number of Voigt units to infinity and we define the retardation spectrum, L, by the continuous analog of Eq. (7.30) to yield

$$J(t) = J_0 + \int_{-\infty}^{\infty} L(\tau)\left[1 - \exp\left(-\frac{t}{\tau}\right)\right] d \ln \tau + \frac{t}{\eta_0} \tag{7.31}$$

where L is a distribution function with the dimensions of compliance (Ferry, 1970). This treatment acknowledges that in a complex topical semisolid the many difference molecular and particle interactions provide a wide range of retardation times, with adjacent times in the spectrum differing infinitesimally. We need a logarithmic treatment because the complete spectrum may extend over many orders of magnitude on the time scale. The maxima in such a spectrum represent concentrations of retardation processes as determined by their contributions to the compliance. The processes are elastic strain mechanisms which are time dependent and which ultimately operate at the molecular level. Several approximation techniques can determine retardation spectra (Williams and Ferry, 1953; Haar, 1950; Leaderman, 1958). Pharmaceutical scientists have used the method of Alfrey (1948), as developed by Schwarzl (1951) and Schwarzl and Staverman (1952, 1953), to investigate topical semisolids, in the following manner.

We may calculate the distribution function using a first-order approximation method with the aid of Eq. (7.32):

$$L(\tau) \approx \frac{d}{d \ln t} \left[J(t) - \frac{t}{\eta_0} \right] \tag{7.32}$$

The method has the disadvantage that we must develop the creep curve until the material reaches a steady state of flow, so as to derive η_0. For some dermatological vehicles, this process could take hours. In investigations in which the materials rapidly change their rheological properties, the time scale of the creep experiment may equal or exceed the characteristic time of the process under investigation. Examples of such studies include recovery after work softening or the rate of development of lattice structure in self-bodied emulsions.

We avoid this difficulty if we use a second-order approximation method according to Eq. (7.33):

$$L(\tau) \approx \frac{d}{d \ln t} \left[J(t) \frac{dJ(t)}{d \ln t} \right] \bigg|_{t=2\tau} \tag{7.33}$$

To use Eq. (7.33), we develop a creep curve (for only a few minutes in a kinetic experiment) and plot it as a function of ln t. We measure the gradient at selected times, subtract the values from the appropriate values of compliance, and again plot the results with respect to ln t. We generate Eq. (7.33) by taking the gradients of this curve (Barry, 1974).

Equations (7.32) and (7.33) have been used in studies on water-in-oil emulsions and food products (Sherman, 1967; Whitehead and Sherman, 1967; Shama and Sherman, 1970), oil-in-water emulsions (Barry and Saunders, 1972c; Barry and Eccleston, 1973a), and paraffin-containing materials (Barry and Grace, 1971c,d).

Figure 7.12 provides us with an example of the use of continuous spectrum analysis; here we can compare the $L(\tau)$ plots for a sample of soft

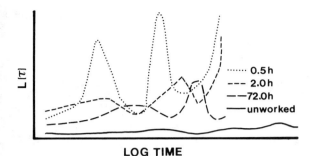

FIG. 7.12 Continuous spectral analysis of soft paraffin, unworked and then worked and allowed to recover for the stated period (hours). (From Barry and Grace, 1971d.)

paraffin when unworked and then when work softened and allowed to recover. Figure 7.10 illustrates the creep curves which provide the data for Fig. 7.12 via Eq. (7.33). The changes in rheological behavior arising from the work-softening process are obvious, and the way in which the curves gradually approach the plot for the unworked material shows the manner in which structure recovers on resting.

Figures 7.13 and 7.14 illustrate spectra which demonstrate the kinetics of structure buildup in self-bodied emulsions. When we use an ionic mixed emulsifier, such as cetrimide/cetostearyl alcohol, to stabilize an oil-in-water cream, the formulation achieves a satisfactory consistency within a short time. Thus, Fig. 7.13 shows that the emulsion increases in consistency within 2.5 hr because the height of the spectrum decreases. Each individual peak diminishes in height as the number of secondary bonds located around the peak time increases. With additional storage time, the maxima in the spectra move toward longer times. This lateral shift suggests that the additional structure which forms during storage may be slightly different at the molecular level to that present initially. With a nonionic emulsifier such as cetomacrogol/cetostearyl alcohol, the spectra are different (Fig. 7.14). Molecular interactions continue during storage to provide additional structure, and so the cream takes many hours to reach its final semisolid consistency. Therefore, spectral heights reduce markedly during the first day of storage. The trend whereby as the creams age the peaks move toward longer times is more obvious with nonionic emulsions than with ionic creams.

Figures 7.13 and 7.14 emphasize the sensitivity of the creep method for examining dermatological formulations at the fundamental level. The technique does not significantly disrupt the structure under investigation, and we may use the measurements to monitor structure at rest or in a rheologically excited state, provided that the state does not relax significantly during the period we require to produce the creep curve.

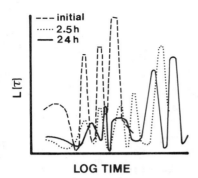

FIG. 7.13 Continuous retardation spectra for an oil-in-water cream stabilized by the ionic mixed emulsifier cetrimide/cetostearyl alcohol and aged for the stated times (hours). (From Barry and Saunders, 1972c.)

c. Dynamic (sinusoidal) analysis If we perform experiments in which the stress and strain vary sinusoidally at a frequency f Hz or ω rad sec^{-1}, where $\omega = 2\pi f$, we can supplement a transient experiment such as creep and we can obtain rheological information corresponding to very short times. A periodic experiment at frequency ω is qualitatively equivalent to a transient experiment at time $t = 1/\omega$. For a dermatological semisolid which we test in the linear viscoelastic region, the amplitudes of stress

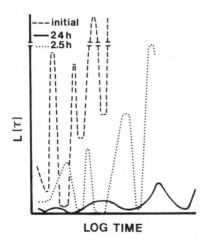

FIG. 7.14 Continuous retardation spectra for an oil-in-water cream stabilized by the nonionic mixed emulsifier cetomacrogol/cetostearyl alcohol and aged for the stated times (hours). (From Barry and Saunders, 1972c.)

and strain are proportional and the stress and strain waves alternate sinusoidally at the same frequency but are out of phase. This phase angle varies
between 0° for a Hookean solid and 90° for a Newtonian liquid. Barry (1974)
has provided an elementary treatment of these concepts with further details.

In a dynamic experiment the stress and the strain are sine or cosine
functions, and we may treat them as rotating vectors. The vector magnitudes are equivalent to the amplitudes of the peak strain and the peak stress
(γ_0 and σ_0, respectively). One revolution of the vector equals one cycle of
oscillation.

The stress and strain are complex variables, σ^* and γ^*, respectively,
defined as

$$\gamma^* = \gamma_0 \exp(i\omega t) \tag{7.34}$$

$$\sigma^* = \sigma_0 \exp[i(\omega t + \phi)] \tag{7.35}$$

where ϕ is the phase angle between stress and strain and $i^2 = -1$.

The complex shear modulus G^* is defined as

$$G^* = \frac{\sigma^*}{\gamma^*} \tag{7.36}$$

We can separate the complex shear modulus into an in-phase or real component G', which is the ratio of the stress in phase with the strain to the
strain, and an out-of-phase or imaginary component G'', the stress 90° out
of phase with the strain divided by the strain

$$G^* = G' + iG'' \tag{7.37}$$

The absolute modulus, $|G^*|$, is the ratio of peak stress to peak strain

$$|G^*| = \frac{\sigma_0}{\gamma_0} = (G'^2 + G''^2)^{1/2} \tag{7.38}$$

and the tangent of the phase angle, $\tan \phi$, is the loss tangent ($\tan \phi = G''/G'$).

Each dynamic measurement at a given frequency simultaneously yields
two independent parameters to characterize the visoelastic behavior, either
G' and G'', or $|G^*|$ and ϕ.

Another method expresses dynamic data in the form of a complex compliance, J^*, which we define as the reciprocal of the complex modulus:

$$J^* = \frac{1}{G^*} = \frac{\gamma^*}{\sigma^*} \tag{7.39}$$

and

$$J^* = J' - iJ'' \tag{7.40}$$

Thus we resolve the complex compliance into J', an in-phase real component (strain in phase with stress, divided by stress) and an out-of-phase
imaginary component J'' (strain 90° out of phase with stress, divided by
stress).

The in-phase modulus and compliance, G' and J', represent solid-like behavior as they are associated with the storage of energy during a periodic deformation: springs conserve energy during stretching. Therefore, we also call these parameters the storage modulus and the loss modulus, respectively. Parameters G'' and J'' relate to the dissipation of energy as heat (which occurs in a flowing liquid), and therefore we style them as the loss modulus and the loss compliance. The absolute compliance $|J^*|$ is the ratio of peak strain amplitude to peak stress amplitude, i.e., it is the reciprocal of the absolute modulus $|G^*|$, which we defined previously.

An alternative method for expressing dynamic data is in terms of a complex dynamic viscosity η^*. The complex viscosity is the complex stress divided by the complex rate of strain:

$$\eta^* = \frac{\sigma^*}{\gamma^*} \tag{7.41}$$

We can resolve the complex viscosity into a real part η' (the component of stress in phase with the rate of strain, divided by the rate of strain) and an imaginary part η'' (the component of stress $90°$ out of phase with the rate of strain, divided by the rate of strain).

A valuable relationship is

$$\eta^* = \eta' - \frac{iG'}{\omega} \tag{7.42}$$

For a purely viscous liquid, η' does not alter with change in frequency and G' is zero. The loss modulus relates to η' by

$$G'' = \eta'\omega \tag{7.43}$$

We can appreciate how a viscoelastic material behaves when it oscillates if we consider the generalized Maxwell model (see Fig. 7.5). Imagine that we grip the terminals of the model and pull it in and out. At very low frequencies of oscillation, there is sufficient time in each cycle for the dashpots to move to extensions which far exceed the deformations of the springs; energy dissipates and the sample behaves as a viscous liquid. At the other extreme, at very high frequencies, the dashpots have little time to move but the springs can elongate and contract, as we assume that their responses are instantaneous. Each cycle of deformation stores energy, and the material behaves as an elastic solid. At intermediate frequencies, springs and dashpots move to a comparable extent, both liquid and solid behavior become apparent, and we are taking measurements in the viscoelastic domain. We may relate this frequency response to the retardation or relaxation time, $\tau = \eta/G$. If $1/\omega$ is much less than τ, elastic deformation dominates the behavior; if $1/\omega$ is much greater than τ, viscous flow predominates. The system demonstrates viscoelastic behavior when $1/\omega$ lies between these two extremes.

Depending on conditions, we can undertake periodic experiments over an extreme frequency range (10^{-5} to 10^{8} Hz). However, any one technique will usually span only a few decades of frequency. To cover a greater range, we can combine data from more than one method.

In an oscillatory experiment we can either apply to the material a small sinusoidal shear stress and measure the resulting shear strain or we can impose a sinusoidal shear strain and record the shear stress. In steady state sinusoidal tests, these methods are equivalent. For the inspection of dermatological vehicles, workers have used the Weissenberg Rheogoniometer, which imposes a sinusoidal strain. Examples of such work include the studies of Barry and Shotton (1967b), Warburton and Davis (1969), Barry and Grace (1971a, c), Davis (1971a, b, 1973), Barry and Eccleston (1973a, b, c), and Barry and Meyer (1979b).

As an example of the forced oscillatory technique, Figs. 7.15 and 7.16 illustrate the variations with frequency of the storage modulus and the dynamic viscosity for oil-in-water emulsions stabilized by the mixed emulsifier cetomacrogol/cetostearyl alcohol (Barry and Eccleston, 1973a, b). As the frequency of oscillation increases, at first, G' increases and η' decreases. This behavior conforms with the mechanical model analogy described above. The frequency at which G' suddenly falls and η' abruptly rises in the resonance frequency of the Rheogoniometer; Barry (1974) discusses the cause of such discontinuities. As the mixed emulsifier increases in concentration, the phase angles for the creams approach zero and the

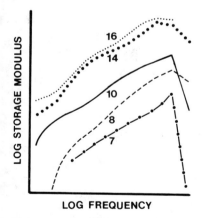

FIG. 7.15 Variation of storage modulus with frequency of oscillation for oil-in-water emulsions stabilized by the mixed emulsifier cetomacrogol/cetostearyl alcohol. Numerals on curves provide the approximate percentage of mixed emulsifier. (From Barry and Eccleston, 1973b.)

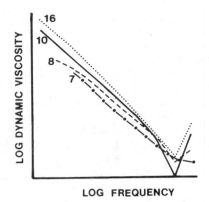

LOG FREQUENCY

FIG. 7.16 Variation of dynamic viscosity with frequency of oscillation for oil-in-water emulsions stabilized by the mixed emulsifier cetomacrogol/cetostearyl alcohol. Numerals on curves provide the approximate percentage of mixed emulsifier. (From Barry and Eccleston, 1973b.)

formulations become more solid-like. The self-bodying phenomenon becomes apparent in the way in which the storage moduli and the dynamic viscosities increase throughout the measured frequency range as the mixed emulsifier concentration rises. Thus emulsion plots lie in ascending order of concentration with respect to the G' or η' axes.

Figure 7.17 provides plots of the dynamic viscosity, the storage modulus, the loss modulus, and the loss tangent (tan ϕ) for three topical creams, aqueous cream, cetrimide cream, and chlorhexidine cream (Davis, 1971a). For each cream, G' is greater than G'', indicating that elastic properties dominate viscous behavior. The loss tangent (the tangent of the phase angle) is a measure of the ratio of energy lost to energy stored in a cyclic deformation. Because we can determine them so readily, spectra of log tan ϕ versus log frequency (consistency spectra) may be useful in quality control, in storage tests, or in formulation experiments (Davis, 1971a; Barry, 1974).

The general aim in dynamic testing is to cover as wide a range of frequency as feasible so as to define the properties of our test material as fully as possible. However, if we wish to examine the effects of changes in a variable such as concentration or temperature, it is difficult to assimilate easily the many curves which we obtain. Then a useful procedure is for us to select representative low, intermediate, and high test frequencies and to plot the viscoelastic functions against the variable of interest at these selected frequencies. Barry and Eccleston (1973b, c) have provided examples of this method of approach.

Oscillatory instruments are expensive. However, as a periodic experiment at a frequency ω is qualitatively equivalent to a creep test at time $t = 1/\omega$, we can deduce oscillatory data from a creep curve without actually

vibrating the material. Thus we can use a creep viscometer to provide
oscillatory data by employing a mathematical transformation procedure.

d. Transformation of creep measurements to dynamic parameters In
the previous subsection we saw how we could express the rheological properties of a dermatological semisolid in the form of complex elasticities,
compliances, or viscosities. Taking as an example the complex compliance
J*, we can resolve this into a storage compliance J' and a loss compliance
J". We can transform creep measurements into dynamic data to provide
values for these as a function of frequency.

Provided that the material is linear viscoelastic, the transformation
is feasible but the procedure is difficult, as it uses linear integral transformations (Leaderman, 1958; Ferry, 1970). Thus, Fourier sine and
cosine transformations calculate J' and J" from creep compliance, but
tedious calculations and basic difficulties may arise (Schwarzl and Struik,
1967/68). However, we can avoid integration by using simple numerical
formulas for these interconversions. Many approximation methods exist
(Leaderman, 1954, 1958; Ferry, 1970); Schwarzl (1969) devised one suitable for our purpose.

Numerical Calculation of Storage Compliance from Creep Compliance.
Various numerical formulas calculate $J'(\omega)$ given $J(t)$. The calculation

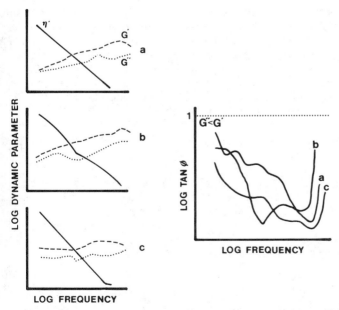

FIG. 7.17 Dynamic viscosity data for: (a) chlorhexidine cream; (b) aqueous
cream; and (c) cetrimide cream. (From Davis, 1971a.)

employs readings of the creep compliance at times which differ by a factor of 2. We may derive the values of $J(t)$ from an experimental creep curve, or we may record them digitally with a logarithmic clock and printer. The formulas, which increase in complexity but decrease in relative error, are of the form

$$J'(\omega) \approx A'(t) \tag{7.44}$$

where $t = 1/\omega$.

The simplest formula is

$$J'(\omega) \approx 1.86J(t) - 0.86J(2t) \tag{7.45}$$

Although Eq. (7.45) is simple, it is quite accurate for small phase angles. Thus, when $\tan \phi$ is less than 0.1, the equation produces a relative error smaller than 1.5%.

We must use more complicated formulas for larger values of $\tan \phi$. The most complex of these takes the form

$$J'(\omega) \approx J(t) - 0.0007[J(32t) - J(16t)] - 0.0185[J(16t) - J(8t)]$$

$$+ 0.197[J(8t) - J(4t)] - 0.778[J(4t) - J(2t)]$$

$$- 0.181[J(t) - J(t/2)] - 0.049[J(t/4) - J(t/8)] \tag{7.46}$$

Equation (7.46) is accurate whatever the value of $\tan \phi$. The relative error always lies between -0.8 and $+0.8\%$. In most practical situations, the formula will be more accurate than the error bounds imply and will easily be within the limits required for a dermatological investigation.

If we have already analyzed the creep curve according to the discrete spectral method, we can use the exact interrelationships of Ferry (1970) to derive our parameters. For a real viscoelastic liquid, which we represent by a generalized Voigt model together with a residual spring and a residual dashpot according to Eq. (7.30), we obtain

$$J'(\omega) = J_0 + \sum_{i=1}^{n} \frac{J_i}{1 + \omega^2 \tau_i^2} \tag{7.47}$$

Numerical Calculation of Loss Compliance from Creep Compliance. There are several numerical formulas for the calculation of the loss compliance from the creep compliance, of the general form

$$J''(\omega) \approx A''(t) \tag{7.48}$$

The simplest of these is a crude approximation

$$J''(\omega) \approx 2.12[J(t) - J(t/2)] \tag{7.49}$$

For $\tan \phi$ equal to 1 the error bounds are $+16$ and -16%, and the error may be even greater for smaller values of $\tan \phi$. Thus, Eq. (7.49) is restricted to materials with phase angles approaching $90°$.

A much better approximation is

$$J''(\omega) \approx -0.470[J(4t) - J(2t)] + 1.674[J(2t) - J(t)]$$

$$+ 0.198[J(t) - J(t/2)] + 0.620[J(t/2) - J(t/4)]$$

$$+ 0.012[J(t/4) - J(t/8)] + 0.172[J(t/8) - J(t/16)]$$

$$+ 0.043[J(t/32) - J(t/64)] + 0.012[J(t/128) - J(t/256)] \qquad (7.50)$$

The upper bound of the relative error for Eq. (7.50) will always be less than 2.7%. The lower bound depends on tan ϕ in a complicated fashion. The relative error will be better than -4% when tan ϕ is in the region $0.05 <$ tan $\phi < \infty$. For tan ϕ smaller than 0.05, the lower bound falls rapidly to -75% at tan $\phi = 0.001$. Thus, Eq. (7.50) never yields values for $J''(\omega)$ which are essentially too high, but it could provide results which are too low when tan ϕ is small. We can formulate an expression which copes with all values of the loss tangent, but this uses an infinite series. However, for most practical circumstances, Eq. (7.50) is more accurate than the error bounds imply.

When we have made a discrete spectral analysis, we can use an exact equation (Ferry, 1970):

$$J''(\omega) = \sum_{i=1}^{n} \frac{J_i \omega \tau_i}{1 + \omega^2 \tau_i^2} + \frac{t}{\eta_0} \qquad (7.51)$$

We can similarly deduce values for G', G'', η', and η'' (Barry, 1974). We can also perform the reverse procedure and convert dynamic data into transient results (Schwarzl and Struik, 1967/68; Struik and Schwarzl, 1969).

In an extensive study of the viscoelastic properties of a semisolid topical formulation, we may need to determine its properties over a frequency scale of 10 or more decades. No single experimental technique will encompass this range. We can investigate the high-frequency (or short-time) region with a dynamic method such as oscillation while reaching the long-time (or low-frequency) range by a transient technique such as creep. We can then unify the data, as discussed previously, to illustrate the rheological behavior over the entire frequency (or time) range, but using only one type of response function. For example, we can complete the transient response at short times, when a creep experiment is inaccurate because of the inertia of the viscometer, if we use data calculated from the harmonic response derived in oscillation.

Figure 7.18 illustrates such a procedure, which exploits creep and oscillatory experiments. The experimental material is an oil-in-water cream stabilized by a cationic mixed emulsifier (Eccleston et al., 1973). Values of G' and η' appear as functions of frequency. At high frequencies we obtain the parameters directly from a Weissenberg Rheogoniometer, and at low frequencies we convert creep measurements into dynamic parameters. The agreement between the two sets of data is excellent.

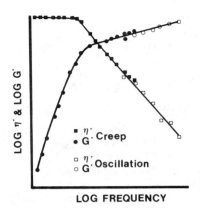

LOG FREQUENCY

FIG. 7.18 Dynamic data for an oil-in-water cream stabilized by cetrimide/ cetostearyl alcohol. Low-frequency data were derived by the mathematical transformation of a creep compliance curve; high-frequency data were obtained with a Weissenberg Rheogoniometer employed in oscillatory mode. (From Eccleston et al., 1973.)

Barry and Meyer (1979b), working with Carbopol gels, have provided an example of how to combine data using the exact interrelationships of Eqs. (7.47) and (7.51).

C. Scheme for the Rheological Analysis of Semisolids

In light of the discussion so far, we may consider devising a general proto- col for determining the rheological properties of a dermatological semi- solid. The depth and extent of such a program will naturally depend on the nature of the problem and the facilities and time available for its solution. The present author has used the protocol outlined below to examine various dermatological formulations. The investigator may expand or contract the methodology according to the particular problem and his interests (see Barry, 1974). The program considers, in sequence, the behavior of the material when handled, its continuous shear properties, and finally its viscoelastic properties.

1. Preliminary examination of the dermatological material

We can gain a considerable amount of valuable qualitative information about a material by simply observing how a sample behaves when handled. This knowledge may also be useful when we assess the validity of subsequent rheological tests, particularly when instrumental artifacts may affect the results. If we invert an open container of the material, does the sample

flow out readily or does it remain in the vessel? If it remains, this suggests
that the formulation possesses a significant elastic component (or yield
stress, in terms of continuous shear rheometry), although a very high viscosity liquid would also do this. The material may pour from the container
but also recoil elastically; again, a prominent elastic element exists in the
substance. If we stir a test sample with a mechanical propeller and a portion climbs up the shaft (the Weissenberg effect), then a normal force is
evident and viscoelastic behavior is dominant. For an emulsion, does it
crack when we rub it into the skin? If so, the formulation may also crack
when we test it in a high shear rate viscometer, and this instability could
provide erroneous rheological data. When we spread the application on the
skin, does the sample fracture, roll up, or recoil elastically? Such behavior
may have its counterpart in anomalous continuous shear rheograms, particularly in the cone-plate geometry, because part of the sample may fracture and eject from the gap. Does the semisolid decrease in consistency as
we rub it (indicating thixotropy or irreversible shear breakdown), or does
it increase (suggesting rheopexy or antithixotropy)?

Ductility is an important property of some ointment bases; it is the
ability of a material to form filaments on extension—as, for example, when
we remove a sample from its container. Thus, highly ductile soft paraffins
of long fiber length produce elongated, thin strands. Low ductile materials
break sharply in a way similar to a brittle fracture in a solid. These paraffin grades behave differently in manufacturing processes such as extrusion
filling, and also when a patient removes a sample from a container. Barry
and Grace (1971a) correlated ductility with total creep compliance at long
time intervals.

Some manufacturers incorporate polymers, such as polyisobutylenes
of relatively low molecular weight, into soft paraffins, causing the flow
characteristics to alter. We may often detect these additives if we place
a sample on the palm of the hand and clap. The polymer falls out in the
form of fine, fibrous particles.

2. Continuous shear analysis

For the continuous shear analysis of a dermatological semisolid, the
most satisfactory general purpose instrument is a cone and plate apparatus
with automatic programming and an X-Y plotter, e.g., the Ferranti-Shirley
viscometer. We should avoid empirical, single-point instruments and those
multipoint instruments for which we cannot derive the rheological variables
of shear stress and shear rate because we cannot analyze the geometry of
flow, e.g., paddle-type instruments.

A standard procedure when we examine a novel semisolid with a
Ferranti-Shirley is to select the largest cone possible to provide maximum
torque, to select the longest sweep time to minimize instrumental effects,
and then to record automatically the rheograms in the following two regimes:
(a) 0 to 10 to 0 rpm, and (b) 0 to 100 to 0 rpm. In general, we avoid shear

rates greater than that represented by 100 rpm, as they often produce
serious errors because of, for example, turbulence, fracture, or ejection
of material from the gap, or cracking of emulsion bases.

The rheograms which we obtain for dermatological vehicles are often
hysteresis loops. When the loop area is so small that it approaches instrumental error, we can confirm its presence by performing a similar test
with a different apparatus geometry, e.g., a concentric cylinder arrangement. This test may use a manual procedure rather than automatic programming, and it will usually employ lower shear rates. Therefore the
rheological conditions will not relate directly to those of the cone-plate
experiment, but the procedure should allow us to decide if the hysteresis
loop obtained with the standard test is a material property or if the rheogram is only an instrumental artifact.

We can then repeat these experiments to cover the temperature range
of interest, including, for a topical material, skin and body temperature.
The nature of further tests depends on the particular problems which the
investigator faces.

For both dermatological and cosmetic use, it is important that formulations should have maximum acceptability to patients and consumers, besides possessing the correct physicochemical and biopharmaceutical properties. Spreadability plays an important role in the patient's assessment
and acceptance of a topical product. Some authors have assessed spreadability using the theoretical equation for plane laminar flow between parallel
plates (Henderson et al., 1961; Langenbucher and Lange, 1969; Mitsui et al.,
1971), whereas others have made evaluations by a correlation with non-
Newtonian viscosities (Van Ooteghem, 1967; Suzuki and Watanable, 1970;
Suzuki et al., 1970).

Barry and Grace (1972) developed a method for assessing the shear
stress/shear rate relationship which operates when we spread topical lipophilic (oily) preparations on the skin. A panel of volunteers compared a
series of formulations, which varied in consistency from mobile liquids to
stiff semisolids, with a range of Newtonian silicone oils of different viscosities, by spreading the materials on the inner surface of the forearm.
The panel indicated the oil that appeared to possess the same spreading
properties as each test formulation. Flow curves of the materials were
obtained with a Ferranti-Shirley Cone and Plate Viscometer, and the inter-
section of the rheogram of the test preparation and the selected Newtonian
oil provided estimates of the shearing conditions which operate during
spreading of a dermatological formulation on the skin. A double logarithmic
plot of shear stress against shear rate provided a Master Curve. The panel
then rated the same preparation in terms of preferred spreadability; these
data, superimposed on the Master Curve, suggested the optimum and preferred shearing conditions for maximum patient acceptability. Barry and
Meyer (1973) extended the work to hydrophilic preparation by deriving
Master Curves for oil-in-water emulsions and aqueous gels. These Master

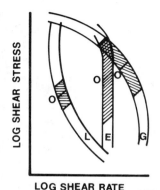

FIG. 7.19 Combination of Master Curves for spreadability for lipophilic (L), hydrophilic gels (G), and oil-in-water emulsions (E), illustrating the acceptable range of viscosities for spreading on the skin (shaded area) and the optimum values (solid line, O). (From Barry and Meyer, 1973.)

Curves differed in shape, area, and position of the preferred region from those obtained for lipophilic products. Figure 7.19 is a composite diagram which illustrates the Master Curves obtained with lipophilic preparations, hydrophilic gels, and oil-in-water emulsions.

Workers have determined the spreadability characteristics of official creams and ointments, and FAPG base, by using the Master Curve concept and the Ferranti-Shirley viscometer (Barry, 1973; Barry and Meyer, 1975).

The general procedure for continuous shear rheometry which we have just discussed provides a sound basis for assessing the rheological behavior of a material under moderate shear rate conditions. However, a final caution is that all the instrumental techniques we have outlined in this chapter employ laminar flow conditions, whereas many industrial processes occur in turbulent flow.

3. Viscoelastic analysis

The final stage in a basic rheological analysis is to submit the material to a small strain procedure. The simplest such technique is the creep test. We determine the limit of viscoelastic linearity and produce the creep curve within this region so as to provide rheological information which we can interpret at the molecular level. We may use the data in the form of the entire experimental creep curve or portions taken from it. We may also express the results as mechanical models and line spectra or as continuous spectra. If we do not have access to an oscillatory instrument but require dynamic parameters, we can mathematically transform the creep curve to provide oscillatory data. If available, we can use an oscillatory viscometer to derive directly the behavior of the material under periodic excitation. If

both creep and oscillatory rheometers are available, we can unify the data
to assess material properties over an extended frequency range.

III. CORRELATION OF RHEOLOGICAL PARAMETERS
WITH DRUG BIOAVAILABILITY

In the introduction to this chapter, we listed some of the many reasons why
investigators determine the rheology of topical semisolids. We concluded
that an important field of research is that which studies the effect of the
consistency of a dermatological formulation on the release of a drug. The
base should not hinder drug release, but it should make the medicament
fully available for percutaneous absorption. A literature search, however,
leads to the depressing conclusion that studies very rarely correlate the
rheological parameters of semisolids with bioavailability data at a fundamental level. Some reports discuss the theme, and they occasionally infer
that the investigators have successfully correlated their rheological measurements with drug-release parameters. However, such papers seldom
treat their data fundamentally, particularly with respect to the rheological
section of the study.

   In the domain of general statements, Erös et al. (1970) wrote that
suitable rheological characteristics are important in determining how an
ointment releases an effective agent. Martin et al. (1969) commented that
the rheology of a particular product can affect biological availability. Similar assertions occur in the works of, e.g., Van Abbe (1959, 1969), Idson
(1971), Skauen et al. (1949), Munzel (1971), Sherman (1970), Larry and
Hymnimen (1969), and Barr (1962). Occasionally the literature reports a
lack of correlation between the "viscosity" of a pharmaceutical preparation
and its therapeutic activity (Nogami and Hanamo, 1958; Giroux and Schrenzel,
1964; Brocades, 1972).

   If we consider specific investigations, we can select three reports from
the literature which represent typical cases in point (Khanderia, 1976):

   Whitworth and Stephenson (1971) plotted the diffusion rate constant
derived from in vitro experiments against the "viscosity" of the vehicles
determined with a Brookfield viscometer. (Nonrheologists occasionally use
the misnomer "viscosity" to describe the consistency of a semisolid.) The
complex vehicles (two emulsions and two ointments) each contained up to
six components, and the analysis of the results did not distinguish between
the types. The authors claimed to have determined the viscosity of each
formulation and that in some instances this parameter correlated with diffusion rates.

   In several investigations with topical bases, Khristov and his associates
reported that drug release was related to rheological characteristics. For
example, they attempted to correlate yield values and plastic viscosities,
determined with a rotational viscometer, with the diffusion of drugs into an

agar gel. The vehicles were complex and contained hydroxypropylmethyl-cellulose, calcium soap, liquid paraffin, cotton seed oil, and water. However, the authors concluded that the rheological parameters were inversely proportional to the release rate of the medicaments (Khristov et al., 1969).

Finally, Erös and Kedvessy (1972) claimed that they had illustrated "a direct relationship between structure-viscosity index, yield stress and diameter of ring indicating diffusion of salicylic acid into agar gel." They measured their rheological parameters with a parallel plate plastometer, which does not provide fundamental data.

Similar types of investigations were reported by Wood et al. (1962), Khristov (1964, 1967, 1969a,b), Khristov and Dragonova (1967), Khristov et al. (1970), Norn (1964), Cid (1968), Erös et al. (1970), Popovicia and Ionescu (1970), and Ritschel et al. (1974).

The problems which arise when we attempt to analyze experiments of the type just considered may be grouped into three categories, with any one paper usually presenting difficulties in more than one class. Some obstacles relate to the drug and vehicle system, others to the nature of the viscometer and the rheological parameter, while the remaining problems involve the drug-release test method (Khanderia, 1976).

Most studies with topical semisolids have used complex, multicomponent vehicles which were usually also multiphase systems. The investigators have neglected possible interactions between components of the formulation and between components and the drug. They have compared quite different colloidal systems without due consideration of their dissimilar structures. For example, some workers have compared simple bases and multicomponent vehicles with oil-in-water or water-in-oil emulsion bases. They appear to have selected their drugs on criteria of familiarity, ready availability, and ease of assay, rather than on physicochemical considerations relevant to a drug-release and rheological study.

We have already seen in this chapter that topical semisolids are rheologically complex and that it is not easy to define and to measure their fundamental flow characteristics. Workers in the topical bioavailability area often select instruments such as penetrometers and the Brookfield viscometer, and so they derive nonfundamental or empirical parameters. The most important observation we can make on the subject of the correlation of topical rheology with bioavailability is that rheological measurements on semisolids do not correspond with the conditions which exist in the environment surrounding the diffusing molecule. Published studies on complex semisolids have not answered the crucial question: What is the true rheological environment which a diffusing drug molecule experiences, and how can we measure it?

Some drug-release studies have employed simple in vitro release methods and have extrapolated the results to derive conclusions with respect to percutaneous absorption. A classic release test, such as diffusion of a drug into an agar plate—or its passage through a porous synthetic membrane into a sink—can only relate to the release of the drug from the vehicle as the test assumes that the rate-limiting step exists within the formulation or the artificial membrane. Occasionally, workers employ in vivo methods to correlate pharmacological effects with vehicle rheology. They may neglect the fact that the rate-limiting step in the overall percutaneous absorption process usually resides in the diffusional step in the stratum corneum. Such experiments may also neglect the effects which different vehicles may have on the permeability of the skin, e.g., increased hydration with occlusive ointments, or the penetration-enhancing potential of low-molecular-weight solvents (see Chap. 4, Sec. III.C). Sometimes, the treatment of drug release data has overlooked fundamental considerations, such as the difference between a single phase and a multiphase vehicle, whether or not the diffusant is in solution or as a suspension, where the rate-limiting step arises, and thermodynamic relationships in general.

Although the literature proposes no satisfactory general mathematical relationship to connect topical drug availability with fundamental rheological parameters of semisolids, the trends which are apparent suggest that under certain circumstances a rheological contribution may control drug release. Academic workers have recently approached the problem anew, by selecting suitable model semisolid vehicles and by carefully defining their rheological examination (Khanderia, 1976; Davis and Khanderia, 1980a,b, 1981a,b). They selected a range of Plastibases, semisolid vehicles containing polyethylene distributed as small crystallites and amorphous filaments in a mineral oil. The series met the requirements that the vehicles should be relatively simple in composition and structure and should provide a range of consistencies and that the gels should be stable over a normal temperature span (from 0° to 50°C). With respect to vehicle-drug interactions, an impor-

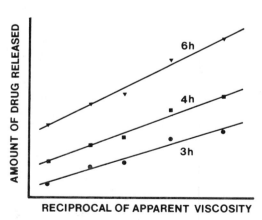

RECIPROCAL OF APPARENT VISCOSITY

FIG. 7.20 Release of salicylic acid from Plastibases correlated with the apparent viscosity derived in continuous shear. (From Khanderia, 1976.)

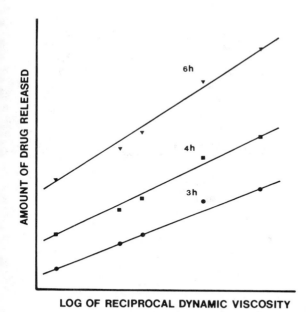

AMOUNT OF DRUG RELEASED

6h

4h

3h

LOG OF RECIPROCAL DYNAMIC VISCOSITY

FIG. 7.21 Release of salicylic acid from Plastibases correlated with
dynamic viscosity derived in oscillation. (From Khanderia, 1976.)

tant consideration was that the chemical potential or thermodynamic activity
of the drug at any set concentration should not vary with the composition of
the base. The concept was that one should be able to vary the rheological
characteristics of the vehicle without at the same time inevitably altering
the thermodynamic activity of the diffusant. Then one could do a truly controlled experiment with only one variable changing in an orderly manner.
The vehicles had to be inert so as to reduce drug-vehicle bonding to a
minimum. For in vivo experiments in human volunteers, the bases should
not inflame, irritate, or sensitize the skin. The Plastibase series fulfilled
all these criteria.

The drugs used were salicylic acid and methyl salicylate; release
studies employed a Silastic membrane and an aqueous sink. In vivo studies
in humans included a skin irritation procedure and a urinary excretion
determination following topical application.

Davis and Khanderia concluded that the in vitro release of salicylic
acid and methyl salicylate from the Plastibases complied with the suspension
and the solution models discussed earlier (Chap. 4, Sec. III.D). The release of salicylic acid into saline related linearly to the reciprocal of the
apparent viscosity of the vehicle as derived with a Ferranti-Shirley Cone
and Plate Viscometer (Fig. 7.20). The amount released was a similar

function of the log of the reciprocal of the dynamic viscosity (as derived from oscillatory testing at low frequency; see Fig. 7.21). In vivo studies confirmed these results. For this series of experiments with salicylic acid the drug was in suspension in the vehicles, and it was concluded that the consistency of the base can be an important factor when drug dissolution in the vehicle is a rate-determining factor.

However, methyl salicylate is soluble in Plastibase and its release into saline was independent of the consistency of the gel. Again, in vivo results supported this finding. It was concluded that for methyl salicylate the rate-determining step for percutaneous absorption resided in the transport step through the skin and not in the vehicle.

An important finding of the aforementioned work is that the authors, using conventional continuous shear viscometry and creep and dynamic testing, still could not identify the rheological environment of a diffusing molecule in a semisolid, even for relatively simple gels. The best that they could do was to derive simple arbitrary relationships between the "microviscosity" which the diffusing molecule experiences, as deduced theoretically from the Stokes-Einstein equation, and the macroviscosity determined experimentally. However, very recently the microviscosities of Carbopol gels have been determined by photon correlation spectroscopy, and the reciprocals have been correlated with the release of salicylates in vitro (Al-Khamis, 1981).

A satisfactory, fundamental correlation of the rheological parameters of topical semisolids in general with the bioavailability of an incorporated drug remains a goal for the future.

SYMBOLS

G	shear modulus
G^*	complex shear modulus
$|G^*|$	absolute shear modulus
G'	storage shear modulus
G''	loss shear modulus
G_0	initial, residual, uncoupled, instantaneous shear modulus (creep)
G_i	shear modulus of the ith Voigt unit
J	creep shear compliance, elastic shear compliance
J^*	complex shear compliance
$|J^*|$	absolute shear compliance
J'	storage shear compliance

J''	loss shear compliance
J_0	initial, residual, uncoupled, instantaneous shear compliance (creep)
J_i	shear compliance of ith Voigt unit
J_N	Newtonian shear compliance (creep)
K	constant
L	retardation spectrum
$\bar{M}$	average molecular weight
a	constant
b	constant
c	constant, concentration
d	constant
e, exp	natural number
f	frequency of oscillation (Hz)
i	square root of minus 1
k, k_1, k_2	constants
t	time

α	constant
β	constant
γ	shear strain
γ^*	complex shear strain
$\dot{\gamma}$	shear rate
$\dot{\gamma}^*$	complex shear rate
γ_0	peak shear strain (oscillation)
γ_N	shear strain of Newtonian region of creep curve
η	coefficient of viscosity
η^*	complex dynamic viscosity
η'	real component of complex dynamic viscosity; dynamic viscosity
η''	imaginary component of dynamic viscosity

η_0 residual or uncoupled shear viscosity (creep); solvent viscosity

η_i shear viscosity of ith Voigt unit

η_{pl} apparent plastic viscosity

η_r relative viscosity

η_{sp} specific viscosity

$[\eta]$ intrinsic viscosity

ν kinematic viscosity

ρ density

σ shear stress

σ^* complex shear stress

σ_0 peak shear stress (oscillation)

σ_D dynamic yield stress or dynamic yield value

σ_s static yield stress or static yield value

σ_y yield stress or yield value

τ relaxation or retardation time

τ_i retardation time of ith Voigt unit

ϕ phase angle between stress and strain (oscillation); volume
fraction of suspension

ψ fluidity

ω frequency of oscillation (rad sec^{-1})

∞ infinity

REFERENCES

Alfrey, T. T. (1948). Mechanical Behavior of High Polymers. Wiley
    (Interscience), New York.
Alfrey, T. T., and Gurnee, E. F. (1956). In Rheology, Theory and Appli-
    cations, F. R. Eirich (Ed.), Vol. 1. Academic Press, New York and
    London, p. 387.
Al-Khamis, K. I. (1981). Ph.D. thesis, University of Nottingham, England.
Axon, A. (1954). J. Pharm. Pharmacol. 6:830.
Barr, M. (1962). J. Pharm. Sci. 51:395.
Barry, B. W. (1968). J. Colloid Interface Sci. 28:82.
Barry, B. W. (1970a). J. Texture Studies 1:405.

Barry, B. W. (1970b). J. Colloid Interface Sci. 32:551.
Barry, B. W. (1971). J. Soc. Cosmet. Chem. 22:487.
Barry, B. W. (1973). J. Pharm. Pharmacol. 25:131.
Barry, B. W. (1974). Adv. Pharm. Sci. 4:1.
Barry, B. W., and Eccleston, G. M. (1973a). J. Texture Studies 4:53.
Barry, B. W., and Eccleston, G. M. (1973b). J. Pharm. Pharmacol. 25:
244.
Barry, B. W., and Eccleston, G. M. (1973c). J. Pharm. Pharmacol. 25:
394.
Barry, B. W., and Grace, A. J. (1970). J. Pharm. Pharmacol. 22(Suppl.):
147S.
Barry, B. W., and Grace, A. J. (1971a). J. Texture Studies 1:259.
Barry, B. W., and Grace, A. J. (1971b). Rheol. Acta 10:113.
Barry, B. W., and Grace, A. J. (1971c). J. Pharm. Sci. 60:814.
Barry, B. W., and Grace, A. J. (1971d). J. Pharm. Sci. 60:1198.
Barry, B. W., and Grace, A. J. (1972). J. Pharm. Sci. 61:335.
Barry, B. W., and Meyer, M. C. (1973). J. Pharm. Sci. 62:1349.
Barry, B. W., and Meyer, M. C. (1975). J. Texture Studies 6:433.
Barry, B. W., and Meyer, M. C. (1979a). Int. J. Pharm. 2:1.
Barry, B. W., and Meyer, M. C. (1979b). Int. J. Pharm. 2:27.
Barry, B. W., and Saunders, G. M. (1969). J. Pharm. Pharmacol. 21:607.
Barry, B. W., and Saunders, G. M. (1970a). J. Colloid Interface Sci. 34:
300.
Barry, B. W., and Saunders, G. M. (1970b). J. Pharm. Pharmacol. 22
(Suppl):139S.
Barry, B. W., and Saunders, G. M. (1971a). J. Colloid Interface Sci. 35:
689.
Barry, B. W., and Saunders, G. M. (1971b). J. Colloid Interface Sci. 36:
130.
Barry, B. W., and Saunders, G. M. (1972a). J. Colloid Interface Sci. 38:
616.
Barry, B. W., and Saunders, G. M. (1972b). J. Colloid Interface Sci. 38:
626.
Barry, B. W., and Saunders, G. M. (1972c). J. Colloid Interface Sci. 41:
331.
Barry, B. W., and Shotton, E. (1967a). J. Pharm. Pharmacol. 19(Suppl):
110S.
Barry, B. W., and Shotton, E. (1967b). J. Pharm. Pharmacol. 19(Suppl):
121S.
Barry, B. W., and Shotton, E. (1968). J. Pharm. Pharmacol. 20:167.
Barry, B. W., and Warburton, B. (1968). J. Soc. Cosmetic Chemists 19:
725.
Boylan, J. C. (1966). J. Pharm. Sci. 55:710.
Boylan, J. C. (1967). J. Pharm. Sci. 56:1164.
Brocades Ltd. (1972). Chemist Druggist p. 762.

404   Dermatological Formulations

Cheng, D. C.-H. (1965). Rheol. Acta 4:257.
Cheng, D. C.-H. (1967). Nature 216:1099.
Cheng, D. C.-H. (1968). Chem. Eng. Sci. 23:895.
Cheng, D. C.-H., and Davis, J. B. (1968). Rheol. Acta 7:85.
Cid, E. (1968). Farmaco [Prat.] 23:474 (cited by Khanderia, 1976).
Davis, S. S. (1969a). J. Pharm. Sci. 58:412.
Davis, S. S. (1969b). J. Sci. Instr. [2] 2:102.
Davis, S. S. (1971a). J. Pharm. Sci. 60:1351.
Davis, S. S. (1971b). J. Pharm Sci. 60:1356.
Davis, S. S. (1973). J. Texture Studies 4:15.
Davis, S. S., and Khanderia, M. S. (1980a). Int. J. Pharm. Tech. Prod. Mfr. 1(2):11.
Davis, S. S., and Khanderia, M. S. (1980b). Int. J. Pharm. Tech. Prod. Mfr. 1(3):15.
Davis, S. S., and Khanderia, M. S. (1981a). Int. J. Pharm. Tech. Prod. Mfr. 2(1):13.
Davis, S. S., and Khanderia, M. S. (1981b). Int. J. Pharm. Tech. Prod. Mfr. 2(2):33.
Davis, S. S., and Warburton, B. (1968). J. Pharm. Pharmacol. 20(Suppl):836.
Davis, S. S., Deer, J. J., and Warburton, B. (1968a). J. Sci. Instr. [2] 1:933.
Davis, S. S., Shotton, E., and Warburton, B. (1968b). J. Pharm. Pharmacol. 20(Suppl):157S.
De Butts, E. H., Hudy, J. A., and Elliott, J. H. (1957). Ind. Eng. Chem. 49:94.
Dinsdale, A., and Moore, F. (1962). Viscosity and Its Measurement. Chapman & Hall, London.
Eccleston, G. M., Barry, B. W., and Davis, S. S. (1973). J. Pharm. Sci. 62:1954.
Einstein, A. (1905). Ann. Phys. 17:549.
Einstein, A. (1906). Ann. Phys. 19:289, 371.
Einstein, A. (1911). Ann. Phys. 24:591.
Enneking, H. (1958). Rheol. Acta 1:234.
Erös, I., Kata, M., and Kedvessy, G. (1970). Acta Pharm. Hung. 40:64 (cited by Khanderia, 1976).
Erös, I., and Kedvessy, G. (1972). Deut. Apotheker-Z. 112:665 (cited by Khanderia, 1976).
Ferry, J. D. (1958). In Rheology: Theory and Applications, F. R. Eirich (Ed.), Vol. 2. Academic Press, New York, p. 433.
Ferry, J. D. (1970). Viscoelastic Properties of Polymers, 2nd ed. Wiley, New York.
Freundlich, H. (1935). Thixotropy (Actualités Scientifiques et Industrielles, No. 267), Hermann, Paris.
Giroux, J., and Schrenzel, M. (1964). Pharm. Acta Helv. 39:615.
Green, H. (1949). Industrial Rheology and Rheological Structures. Wiley, New York.

Green, H., and Weltmann, R. N. (1943). Ind. Eng. Chem. (Anal.) 15:201.
Green, H., and Weltmann, R. N. (1944). J. Appl. Phys. 15:414.
Green, H., and Weltmann, R. N. (1946a). Ind. Eng. Chem. (Anal.) 18:167.
Green, H., and Weltmann, R. N. (1946b). In Colloid Chemistry, J.
    Alexander (Ed.), Vol. 6. Van Nostrand Reinhold, New York, p. 328.
Guth, E., and Simha, R. (1936). Kolloid-Z. 74:266.
Haar, D. Ter (1950). Physica 16:719, 839.
Henderson, N. L., Meer, P. M., and Kostenbauder, H. B. (1961). J.
    Pharm. Sci. 50:788.
Highgate, D. (1966). Nature 211:1390.
Highgate, D., and Whorlow, R. W. (1968). In Polymer Systems: Deforma-
    tion and Flow, R. E. Wetton and R. W. Whorlow (Eds.). Macmillan,
    New York, p. 251.
Hutton, J. F. (1963). Nature 200:646.
Idson, B. (1971). J. Soc. Cosmetic Chemists 22:615.
Inokuchi, K. (1955). Bull. Chem. Soc. Japan 28:453.
Jefferies, H. D. (1965). Rheol. Acta 4:241.
Khanderia, M. S. (1976). Ph.D. thesis, University of Aston in Birminham,
    England.
Khristov, K. (1964). Pharmazie 19:134 (cited by Khanderia, 1976).
Khristov, K. (1967). Pharmazie 22:251 (cited by Khanderia, 1976).
Khristov, K. (1969a). Farmatsiya (Sofia) 17:331 (cited by Khanderia, 1976).
Khristov, K. (1969b). Farmatsiya (Sofia) 19:1 (cited by Khanderia, 1976).
Khristov, K., and Draganova, L. (1967). Pharmazie 22:208 (cited by
    Khanderia, 1976).
Khristov, K., Gluzman, M., and Levitskaya, I. (1969). Farmatsiya (Sofia)
    19:15 (cited by Khanderia, 1976).
Khristov, K., Gluzman, M., Todorova, P., and Daschevskaja, I. (1970).
    Pharmazie 25:344 (cited by Khanderia, 1976).
Kuhn, W. (1947). Helv. Chim. Acta 30:487.
Lammiman, K. A., and Roberts, J. E. (1961). Lab. Pract. 10:816.
Langenbucher, F., and Lange, B. (1969). Pharm. Acta Helv. 45:572.
Larry, P., and Hymnimen, C. E. (1969). Drug. Cosmetic Ind. 105:40,
    153.
Leaderman, H. (1943). Elastic and Creep Properties of Filamentous Mate-
    rials and Other High Polymers. Textile Foundation, Washington, D.C.
Leaderman, H. (1954). In Proc. 2nd Int. Congr. Rheol., V. G. W. Harri-
    son (Ed.). Butterworths, London, p. 203.
Leaderman, H. (1958). In Rheology: Theory and Applications, F. R.
    Eirich (Ed.), Vol. 2. Academic Press, New York, p. 1.
Lenk, R. S. (1965). Rheol. Acta 4:282.
Levy, G. (1962). J. Pharm. Sci. 51:947.
McKennell, R. (1954). In Proc. 2nd Int. Cong. Rheol., V. G. W. Harrison
    (Ed.). Butterworths, London, p. 350.
McKennell, R. (1956). Anal. Chem. 28:1710.

McKennell, R. (1960). The Instrument Manual, 3rd ed. United Trade Press, London, p. 284.

Martin, A. N., Banker, G. S., and Chun, A. H. C. (1964). Adv. Pharm. Sci. 1:1.

Martin, A. N., Swarbrick, J., and Cammarata, A. (1969). Physical Pharmacy, 2nd ed. Lea & Febinger, Philadelphia, p. 497.

Mitsui, T., Morosawa, K., and Otake, C. (1971). J. Texture Studies 2: 339.

Munzel, K. (1971). Pharm. Acta Helv. 46:513.

Nogami, H., and Hanamo, M. (1958). Chem. Pharm. Bull. 6:249.

Norn, M. (1964). Dansk Tidsskr. Farm. 38:95 (cited in Khanderia, 1976).

Ober, S. S., Vincent, H. C., Simon, D. E., and Frederick, K. J. (1958). J. Am. Pharm. Assoc., Sci. Ed. 47:667.

Popovicia, A., and Ionescu, M. (1970). Farmatsiya (Sofia) 18:545 (cited in Khanderia, 1976).

Rankell, A., and Lieberman, H. A. (1970). In The Theory and Practice of Industrial Pharmacy, L. Lackman, H. A. Lieberman, and J. L. Kanig (Eds.). Lea & Febiger, Philadelphia, p. 49.

Reiner, M. (1943). Ten Lectures on Theoretical Rheology. Wiley (Interscience), New York.

Reiner, M., and Scott-Blair, G. W. (1967). In Rheology, F. E. Eirich (Ed.), Vol. 4. Academic Press, New York, Chap. 9.

Ritschel, W. A., Siegel, E. G., and Ring, P. E. (1974). Drug Res. 24:907.

Schott, H. (1975). In Remington's Pharmaceutical Sciences, 15th ed. Mack, Easton, Pa., p. 350.

Schwarzl, F. (1951). Physica 17:830.

Schwarzl, F. R. (1969). Rheol. Acta 8:6.

Schwarzl, F., and Staverman, A. J. (1952). Physica 18:791.

Schwarzl, F., and Staverman, A. J. (1953). Appl. Sci. Res. A4:127.

Schwarzl, F., and Struik, L. C. E. (1967/68). Ad. Mol. Relaxation Processes 1:201.

Scott Blair, G. W. (1949). A Survey of General and Applied Rheology, 2nd ed. Pitman Med. Publ., London, p. 76.

Shama, F., and Sherman, P. (1970). J. Texture Studies 1:196.

Sherman, P. (1967). J. Colloid Interface Sci. 24:107.

Sherman, P. (1968). Emulsion Science. Academic Press, New York.

Sherman, P. (1970). Industrial Rheology. Academic Press, New York.

Skauen, D. M., Cyr, G. N., Christian, J. E., and Lee, C. O. (1949). J. Am. Pharm. Assoc., Sci. Ed. 38:618.

Stiggles, J. S. (1965). J. Sci. Instr. 42:162.

Struik, L. C. E., and Schwarzl, F. R. (1969). Rheol. Acta 8:134.

Suzuki, K., and Watanabe, T. (1970). Am. Perfumery Cosmet. 85:115.

Suzuki, K., and Watanabe, T. (1971). J. Texture Studies 2:431.

Suzuki, K., Matsumoto, S., Watanabe, T., and Ono, S. (1970). Kogyo Kagaku Zasshi 73:774.

Talman, F. A. J., and Rowan, E. M. (1970). J. Pharm. Pharmacol. 22: 338.

Talman, F. A. J., Davies, P. J., and Rowan, E. M. (1967). J. Pharm. Pharmacol. 19:417.

Talman, F. A. J., Davies, P. J., and Rowan, E. M. (1968). J. Pharm. Pharmacol. 20:513.

Van Abbe, N. J. (1959). Pharm. J. 111.

Van Abbe, N. J. (1969). Pharmaceutical and Cosmetic Products for Topical Administration. Heinemann, London, p. 98.

Van Ooteghem, M. (1967). J. Pharm. Belg. 22:147.

Van Wazer, J. R., Lyons, J. W., Kim, K. Y., and Colwell, R. E. (1963). Viscosity and Flow Measurement: A Laboratory Handbook of Rheology. Wiley (Interscience), New York.

Warburton, B., and Barry, B. W. (1968). J. Pharm. Pharmacol. 20:255.

Warburton, B., and Davis, S. S. (1969). Rheol. Acta 8:205.

Weltmann, R. N. (1943). J. Appl. Phys. 14:343.

Whitehead, J., and Sherman, P. (1967). Food Technol. 21:107.

Whitworth, C. W., and Stephenson, R. E. (1975). Can. J. Pharm. Sci. 10:89.

Williams, M. L., and Ferry, J. D. (1953). J. Polymer Sci. 11:169.

Wood, J. H., Giles, W. H., and Catacolos, G. (1964). J. Soc. Cosmetic Chemists 15:565.

Wood, J. A., Wait Rising, L., and Hall, N. A. (1962). J. Pharm. Sci. 51:668.

Worthington, H. E. C. (1973). Acta Derm. Venereol. (Stockh.) 53(Suppl. 70):29.

Zettlemoyer, A. C., Lower, G. W., and Walker, W. C. (1953). J. Colloid Sci. 8:116.

AUTHOR INDEX

Underlined numbers give the page on which the complete reference is listed.

SUBJECT INDEX

A

Abnormalities, skin, 21-24
Absorbents, 37
Absorption
  bases, formulation, 310-311
  percutaneous, biological factors,
    129-145
  blood flow, 137-138
  complexity, 127-129
  methods for studying, 234-280
  physicochemical factors, 145-
    213
  properties influencing, 127-213
  regional skin sites, 133, 135
  skin condition, 130-133
  skin metabolism, 135-137
  species differences, 138-145
  summary, 119
  rate, dimensional analysis, 57
Acantholysis, 5
  after friction, 20
Accelerants (see also Penetration
    enhancers)
  and reservoir formation, 117
Accelerated stability tests, 332
Acceptability
  of formulations, 330-331

[Acceptability]
  and spreadability of semisolids,
    394-395
Acetic acid, dimerization, 81
Acetone
  in aerosols, 323
  effect on skin permeability, 131
  in paints, 300
Acetylcysteine, percutaneous ab-
    sorption, 139-140
Acetylsalicylic acid
  effect of temperature on perme-
    ation, 160
  penetration and hydration, 158
  skin diffusion, 248-249
Acid mantle, of skin, 16
Acids
  acetic, benzoic, boric, as germi-
    cides, 34
  association in polymers, 85
  fatty, composition in o/w creams,
    320
  in mixed emulsifiers, 314-315
  and percutaneous absorption, 130
Acne
  bioassays, 255
  conglobata, 28
  explosive facial, of females, 28